Immunosenescence

Methods and Protocols

Edited by

Albert C. Shaw

Section of Infectious Diseases, Department of Internal Medicine, Yale School of Medicine, New Haven, CT, USA

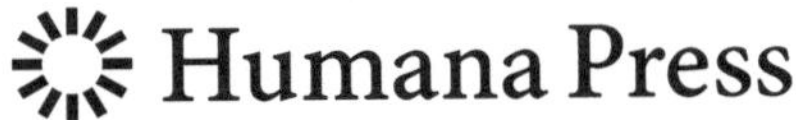 Humana Press

Editor
Albert C. Shaw
Section of Infectious Diseases
Department of Internal Medicine
Yale School of Medicine
New Haven, CT, USA

ISSN 1064-3745 ISSN 1940-6029 (electronic)
Methods in Molecular Biology
ISBN 978-1-4939-4418-7 ISBN 978-1-4939-2963-4 (eBook)
DOI 10.1007/978-1-4939-2963-4

Springer New York Heidelberg Dordrecht London

Humana Press is a brand of Springer
Springer Science+Business Media LLC New York is part of Springer Science+Business Media (www.springer.com)

Preface

The United Nations estimates that, by 2050, the number of adults over age 60 will rise to over two billion worldwide and will exceed the number of individuals under age 15 for the first time in human history. This aging of the worldwide population has profound social implications and will undoubtedly influence the distribution and delivery of healthcare; notably, older adults are at increased risk for organ-specific dysfunction such as cardiovascular and renal disease, as well as increased rates of neurodegeneration and epithelial malignancies, to name a few examples. Older adults are also at risk for increased morbidity and mortality from infectious diseases and poor responses to vaccinations. In some cases, this increased risk is for specific infectious syndromes, such as sepsis, or reactivation of varicella zoster virus infection or tuberculosis. At the same time, aging of adults with chronic viral infections such as HIV disease will result in immunologic changes that reflect the convergence of immune dysregulation of chronic infection and of aging. This burden of acute and chronic disease in older adults in part results from age-associated changes in the immune system, or immunosenescence. This volume contains protocols employed by experts in the field to study the protean effects of immunosenescence on innate and adaptive immune responses and includes cell biology and biochemical methods for analyses of telomere dysfunction, autophagy, and protein oxidation. Genomic approaches for the analysis of antigen receptor repertoire, microRNAs, and DNA methylation are also discussed. While in no way comprehensive, this volume is intended to provide a mixture of basic and advanced protocols that will be useful for immunologists in general and investigators in aging biology in particular.

This edition of *Methods in Molecular Biology* would not have been possible without the efforts of the chapter authors, and I am grateful to them for taking time from their busy schedules to contribute. I would also like to thank Professor John Walker, the Editor-in-Chief of this series, for inviting me to edit this volume and for his constant support, and would also like to thank Patrick Marton, David Casey, and the team at Humana Press. We all hope that this edition will facilitate cross-fertilization and future advances aimed at improving the health of older adults.

New Haven, CT   *Albert C. Shaw*

Contents

Contributors

MARK ASQUITH • *Division of Pathobiology and Immunology, Oregon National Primate Research Center, Beaverton, OR, USA*

ARUNABH BHATTACHARYA • *Cellular and Structural Biology, University of Texas Health Science Center at San Antonio, San Antonio, TX, USA; Barshop Institute for Longevity and Aging Studies, University of Texas Health Science Center at San Antonio, San Antonio, TX, USA*

BONNIE B. BLOMBERG • *Department of Microbiology and Immunology, University of Miami Miller School of Medicine, Miami, FL, USA*

YAIR BOTBOL • *Department of Pathology, Albert Einstein College of Medicine, Bronx, NY, USA*

SCOTT D. BOYD • *Department of Pathology, Stanford University, Stanford, CA, USA*

ALEAH L. BRUBAKER • *Integrative Cell Biology, Loyola University Chicago, Health Sciences Division, Maywood, IL, USA; Burn and Shock Trauma Institute, Loyola University Chicago, Health Sciences Division, Maywood, IL, USA; Immunology and Aging Program, Loyola University Chicago, Health Sciences Division, Maywood, IL, USA; Stritch School of Medicine, Loyola University Chicago, Health Sciences Division, Maywood, IL, USA*

CARMEN CAMPOS • *Department of Immunology, IMIBIC, Reina Sofia University Hospital, University of Cordoba, Cordoba, Spain*

STEWART R. CARTER • *Burn and Shock Trauma Institute, Loyola University Chicago, Health Sciences Division, Maywood, IL, USA; Department of Surgery, Loyola University Chicago, Health Sciences Division, Maywood, IL, USA; Stritch School of Medicine, Loyola University Chicago, Health Sciences Division, Maywood, IL, USA*

SANDY CHANG • *Department of Laboratory Medicine, Yale School of Medicine, New Haven, CT, USA; Department of Pathology, Yale School of Medicine, New Haven, CT, USA*

ASISH R. CHAUDHURI • *UT Southwestern Medical Center, Dallas, TX, USA; Barshop Institute for Longevity and Aging Studies, University of Texas Health Science Center at San Antonio, San Antonio, TX, USA; Departments of Biochemistry, University of Texas Health Science Center at San Antonio, San Antonio, TX, USA; South Texas Veterans Health Care System, San Antonio, TX, USA*

PRADYOT DASH • *Department of Immunology, St. Jude Children's Research Hospital, Memphis, TN, USA*

ERIN M. DEBIASI • *Department of Internal Medicine, Section of Pulmonary, Critical Care and Sleep Medicine, Yale School of Medicine, New Haven, CT, USA*

COLIN DELANEY • *Department of Internal Medicine, University of Michigan Medical School, Ann Arbor, MI, USA*

ALEXANDRE DE LENCASTRE • *Department of Biological Sciences, Quinnipiac University, Hamden, CT, USA*

ALAIN DIAZ • *Department of Microbiology and Immunology, University of Miami Miller School of Medicine, Miami, FL, USA*

DEBORAH DUNN-WALTERS • *Department of Immunobiology, King's College London School of Medicine, London, UK*

CARL FORTIN • *Department of Medicine, Duke University Medical Center, Durham, NC, USA*

DANIELA FRASCA • *Department of Microbiology and Immunology, University of Miami Miller School of Medicine, Miami, FL, USA*

TAMAS FÜLÖP • *Research Center on Aging, Department of Medicine, Immunology Postgraduate Programme, Faculty of Medicine and Health Sciences, Université de Sherbrooke, Sherbrooke, QC, Canada*

SANJAY K. GARG • *Department of Internal Medicine, University of Michigan Medical School, Ann Arbor, MI, USA*

BETH GENTLEMAN • *Advanced Medical Research Institute of Canada, Sudbury, ON, Canada*

KRISTEN HABERTHUR • *Department of Molecular Microbiology and Immunology, Oregon Health and Science University, Portland, OR, USA*

RYAN HAMILTON • *Cellular and Structural Biology, University of Texas Health Science Center at San Antonio, San Antonio, TX, USA; Barshop Institute for Longevity and Aging Studies, University of Texas Health Science Center at San Antonio, San Antonio, TX, USA*

ERICA L. HERZOG • *Department of Internal Medicine, Section of Pulmonary, Critical Care and Sleep Medicine, Yale School of Medicine, New Haven, CT, USA*

XINYUAN HU • *Department of Internal Medicine, Section of Pulmonary, Critical Care and Sleep Medicine, Yale School of Medicine, New Haven, CT, USA*

KATHERINE J.L. JACKSON • *Department of Pathology, Stanford University, Stanford, CA, USA*

SAMIT R. JOSHI • *Section of Infectious Diseases, Department of Internal Medicine, Yale School of Medicine, New Haven, CT, USA; Bristol-Myers Squibb, Inc., Wallingford, CT, USA*

INSOO KANG • *Section of Rheumatology, Department of Internal Medicine, Yale School of Medicine, New Haven, CT, USA*

DAVID KIPLING • *Department of Pathology, Cardiff University, Cardiff, UK*

ELIZABETH J. KOVACS • *Integrative Cell Biology, Loyola University Chicago, Health Sciences Division, Maywood, IL, USA; Burn and Shock Trauma Institute, Loyola University Chicago, Health Sciences Division, Maywood, IL, USA; Immunology and Aging Program, Loyola University Chicago, Health Sciences Division, Maywood, IL, USA; Department of Surgery, Loyola University Chicago, Health Sciences Division, Maywood, IL, USA; Stritch School of Medicine, Loyola University Chicago, Health Sciences Division, Maywood, IL, USA*

MICHAEL D. LEIPOLD • *Institute for Immunity, Transplantation and Infection, Stanford University, Stanford, CA, USA*

YI LIU • *Department of Pathology, Stanford University, Stanford, CA, USA; Biomedical Informatics Training Program, Stanford University, Stanford, CA, USA*

FERNANDO MACIAN • *Department of Pathology, Albert Einstein College of Medicine, Bronx, NY, USA*

HOLDEN T. MAECKER • *Institute for Immunity, Transplantation and Infection, Department of Microbiology and Immunology, Stanford University, Stanford, CA, USA*

JANET E. MCELHANEY • *Advanced Medical Research Institute of Canada, Sudbury, ON, Canada*

ILHEM MESSAOUDI • *Division of Biomedical Sciences, University of California, Riverside School of Medicine, Riverside, CA, USA*

CHRISTINE MEYER • *Division of Pathobiology and Immunology, Oregon National Primate Research Center, Beaverton, OR, USA*

SUBHASIS MOHANTY • *Division of Pathobiology and Immunology, Oregon National Primate Research Center, Beaverton, OR, USA; Molecular Microbiology and Immunology, Oregon Health and Science University, Portland, OR, USA; Division of Biomedical Sciences, School of Medicine, University of California, Riverside, CA, USA*

RUTH R. MONTGOMERY • *Section of Rheumatology, Department of Internal Medicine, Yale School of Medicine, New Haven, CT, USA*

EVAN W. NEWELL • *Singapore Immunology Network, Singapore, Singapore*

ALEJANDRA PERA • *Department of Immunology, IMIBIC, Reina Sofia University Hospital, University of Cordoba, Cordoba, Spain*

FENG QIAN • *Section of Rheumatology, Department of Internal Medicine, Yale University School of Medicine, New Haven, CT, USA; State Key Laboratory of Genetic Engineering and Ministry of Education Key Laboratory of Contemporary Anthropology, School of Life Sciences, Fudan University, Shanghai, China*

REKHA RAI • *Department of Laboratory Medicine, Yale School of Medicine, New Haven, CT, USA*

KRISHNA M. ROSKIN • *Department of Pathology, Stanford University, Stanford, CA, USA*

BEATRIZ SANCHEZ-CORREA • *Immunology Unit, Department of Physiology, University of Extremadura, Caceres, Spain*

ALBERT C. SHAW • *Section of Infectious Diseases, Department of Internal Medicine, Yale School of Medicine, New Haven, CT, USA*

MIN SUN SHIN • *Section of Rheumatology, Department of Internal Medicine, Yale School of Medicine, New Haven, CT, USA*

FRANK SLACK • *Cancer Center at BI-Deaconess Medical Center, Department of Pathology, Harvard Medical School, Boston, MA, USA*

RAFAEL SOLANA • *Department of Immunology, IMIBIC, Reina Sofia University Hospital, University of Cordoba, Cordoba, Spain*

RAQUEL TARAZONA • *Immunology Unit, Department of Physiology, University of Extremadura, Caceres, Spain*

PAUL G. THOMAS • *Department of Immunology, St. Jude Children's Research Hospital, Memphis, TN, USA*

CHEN WANG • *Department of Pathology, Stanford University, Stanford, CA, USA*

GEORGE C. WANG • *Department of Immunology, St. Jude Children's Research Hospital, Memphis, TN, USA; Center of Excellence in Geriatric Medicine, Newton Medical Center, Sparta, NJ, USA*

ROCHELLE WEI • *Barshop Institute for Longevity and Aging Studies, University of Texas Health Science Center at San Antonio, San Antonio, TX, USA*

YU-CHANG WU • *Randall Division of Cell and Molecular Biophysics, King's College London School of Biomedical Science, London, UK*

RAYMOND YUNG • *Department of Internal Medicine, University of Michigan Medical School, Ann Arbor, MI, USA*

Chapter 1

Isolation of Lipid Rafts from Human Neutrophils by Density Gradient Centrifugation

Carl Fortin and Tamas Fülöp

Abstract

Neutrophils are present within minutes to the site of aggression in the body making them one of the first cells of the immune system to be in contact with incoming threats. The cell functions of neutrophils are elicited through the engagement of surface receptors, some of which are located in a specific region of the membrane called lipid rafts, a functionally segregated region of the membrane enriched with cholesterol and distinct species of sphingomyelin and glycerophospholipids. Lipid rafts are relatively resistant to detergent extraction and this can be taken advantage of to isolate them from the rest of the cell membrane. This chapter will describe a reliable method to obtain lipid rafts from detergent-resistant membrane fractions of human neutrophils. Cells are lysed in an HEPES solution containing 0.5 % Triton X-100, supernatants are mixed with a 42 % sucrose solution, which is then overlaid with a 35 % and 5 % sucrose solution. The gradient is centrifuged for 16 h and the resulting fractions can be further analyzed by immunoblotting or subjected to immunoprecipitation.

Key words Human, Neutrophils, Sucrose, Lipid raft, Flotillin, Detergent-resistant membrane

1 Introduction

Neutrophils are present within minutes to the site of aggression in the body making them one of the first cells of the immune system to be in contact with incoming threats. Neutrophils are well known for their phagocytic and antimicrobial capacities. But, their contribution to the immune response goes well beyond clearance of debris at the site of infection [1]. Indeed, neutrophils locally secrete an impressive array of mediators such as regulatory proteases [2] and cytokines/chemokines [3] that have a profound influence on the shaping of the ensuing immune response.

As in any other cells of the immune system, the cellular functions of neutrophils are elicited through the engagement of surface receptors [4]. It was reported that some of these receptors [4–7] are located in a specific region of the membrane called lipid rafts. Lipid rafts are highly fluctuating, both in size and composition,

Albert C. Shaw (ed.), *Immunosenescence: Methods and Protocols*, Methods in Molecular Biology, vol. 1343, DOI 10.1007/978-1-4939-2963-4_1, © Springer Science+Business Media New York 2015

domains of the membrane enriched in sphingolipids, cholesterol, and proteins (including receptor and adapter proteins). The best-known example of the physiological relevance of lipid rafts is T-cell activation. Indeed, the interaction between the antigenic peptide and the TCR occurs in the central part of the immunological synapse, a functionally segregated region of the membrane enriched with cholesterol and distinct species of sphingomyelin and glycerophospholipids [8]. More simply put, lipid rafts can aggregate (a phenomenon called coalescence) upon cell stimulation and this results in an increased physical proximity for all molecules involved in ligand–receptor signaling. Lipid rafts are, however, not only relevant for T-cell activation, but, as reviewed elsewhere [9], have broad biological roles including virus budding and membrane trafficking.

A crucial characteristic of lipid rafts is that they are relatively resistant to detergent extraction. Taking advantage of this characteristic, this chapter will describe a reliable method to obtain lipid rafts from detergent-resistant membrane (DRM) fractions of human neutrophils. To facilitate the detection of lipid raft-associated proteins by immunoblotting, a small volume gradient and 1 mL ultracentrifuge tubes are used.

2   Materials

Prepare all solutions using double-distilled water and molecular biology grade reagents. The solutions are stored at 4 °C and not filtered, unless indicated otherwise.

2.1 Stock Solutions for Inhibitors (See Note 1)

1. Phenylmethanesulfonyl fluoride (PMSF): For a 250 mg bottle, add 14.35 mL of DMSO. This is your 100 mM stock solution. Use at 1 mM final.

2. DL-Dithiothreitol (DTT): To prepare a 1 M stock solution, add 1 mL of water to 154 mg of powder. Discard after use. Use at 1 mM final.

3. Sodium Fluoride (NaF): To prepare a 1 M stock solution, add 1 mL of water to 42 mg of powder. Discard after use. Use at 10 mM final.

4. Sodium pyrophosphate dibasic ($Na_2H_2PO_7$): To prepare a 1 M stock solution, add 1 mL of water to 222 mg of powder. Discard after use. Use at 2 mM final.

5. β-Glycerophosphate disodium salt hydrate: To prepare a 1 M stock solution, add 1 mL of water to 216 mg of powder. Use at 25 mM final.

6. Diisopropylfluorophosphate (DFP): Depending on your provider, DFP will be in powder or liquid form. Use at 1 mM

final. DFP is extremely toxic, open under a fume hood. Discard the product upon the appearance of a yellow color.

7. Sodium orthovanadate (Na_3VO_4): Orthovanadate must be activated (*see* **Note 2**). Use at 1 mM final. Because of its high pH (pH 10), adding too much of the orthovanadate solution will cause unwanted cell lysis.

2.2 Solutions Required for Neutrophil Lysis	1. Solution A: PBS 1× pH 7.4 containing all the inhibitors mentioned in Subheading 2.1 (*see* **Note 3**).
	2. Solution B: 25 mM HEPES, 100 mM NaCl, 2 mM EDTA, pH 6.9. Add about 100 mL water to a glass beaker. Weight 1.49 g HEPES, 1.46 g NaCl, 0.146 g EDTA, and add to the beaker. Mix until the solution is colorless and adjust the pH to 6.9. Put the solution into a 250-mL graduated cylinder and complete to 250 mL with water. Filter the solution through a 250 mL 0.45 μm filter unit. Discard after 3 months.
2.3 Sucrose Gradient	1. 85 % sucrose solution (*see* **Note 4**): Weigh 42.5 g sucrose and add to a glass beaker containing 10 mL of solution B. Mix overnight with a small stir bar and, when the sucrose is dissolved, complete to 50 mL with solution B. Discard after 3 months.
	2. 35 % sucrose solution (*see* **Note 5**): Weigh 17.5 g sucrose and add to a glass beaker containing 25 mL of solution B. Mix with a small stir bar until the sucrose is dissolved and complete to 50 mL with solution B. Discard after 3 months.
	3. 5 % sucrose solution (*see* **Note 5**): Weigh 2.5 g sucrose and add to a glass beaker containing 25 mL of solution B. Mix with a small stir bar until the sucrose is dissolved and complete to 50 mL with solution B. Store the solution at 4 °C and discard after 3 months.
2.4 Centrifugation	Tubes: 1 mL polycarbonate thick wall centrifuge tubes (11 × 34 mm, Beckman) were used with the TLA-120.2 rotor in a Beckman Optima MAX centrifuge.

3 Methods

3.1 Neutrophil Stimulation	When working with primary cells, such as neutrophils, it is essential to follow some guidelines to prevent accidental cell activation and reduce variability between donors. As neutrophils as extremely sensitive to endotoxins, the entire cell isolation procedure must be carried out under endotoxin-free conditions. Therefore, this means using sterile, apyrogenic plasticware, sterilized and baked glassware (LPS survives autoclaving), and low-endotoxin serum/FBS. Equally important is to avoid heat shock, which can activate the cells.

To do so, always isolate cells at room temperature (no refrigeration during centrifugation) and do not put human neutrophils on ice. It is better to leave human neutrophils at room temperature if you need a short break (15–30 min). Before stimulation, let the cells equilibrate at 37 °C in a water bath for about 15 min. If pre-incubating for 30 min or more with inhibitors, then no prior equilibration is necessary. Also, never exceed a final concentration of 0.3 % DMSO or any other vehicle (some vehicles kill primary cells and others activate them); it is best to aim for 0.1 % by preparing your stock solutions at 1000× so as to use 1 μL in 1 mL, which makes 0.1 % final. In addition, a common mistake made when working with neutrophils is to resuspend them at a high cell density. For most of the readouts, this can result in unwanted activation, false positives, and high backgrounds. Freshly isolated cells must be immediately resuspended (avoid making bubbles) in RPMI + 5 % serum (FBS or autologous) at a final concentration of no more than 3—10×10^6 cells/mL. Stimulation should be done at 37 °C in a water bath with occasional (5–10 min) gentle shaking to avoid cell sedimentation, especially when using a higher cell density. Finally, do not ever use a vortexer to resuspend neutrophils. As a starting point, we suggest that 1×10^7 neutrophils in 1 mL be used.

3.2 Stopping the Stimulation

1. If using 15 or 50 mL conicals, centrifuge for 5 min at $200 \times g$ to pellet the cells. If stimulation was done in microcentrifuge tubes, quickspin (4–5 s at max speed) to pellet the cells. Remove supernatant by aspiration.

2. Gently resuspend the cells in 200 μL of ice-cold solution A with a tip and transfer, if needed, in microcentrifuge tubes.

3. Incubate 10 min on ice.

3.3 Cell Lysis

1. Pellet the cells by doing a quickspin (4–5 s at max speed).

2. Remove supernatant by aspiration (*see* **Note 6**).

3. Resuspend the cells in 150 μL solution B containing freshly made inhibitors (Subheading 2.1) and 0.5 % Triton X-100.

4. Incubate 10 min on ice.

5. Centrifuge 5 min at max speed to pellet cell debris.

6. Proceed immediately to gradient preparation (Subheading 3.4).

3.4 Preparing the Sucrose Gradient

1. Add 150 μL of the 85 % sucrose solution in the bottom of 1 mL polycarbonate thick wall centrifuge tubes (*see* **Note 7**).

2. Add the supernatant from cell lysis (Subheading 3.3, **step 5**) and mix well. The goal is to dilute the 85 % sucrose solution to a 42.5 % sucrose solution.

3. Gently overlay with 500 μL of 35 % sucrose solution (*see* **Note 8**).

4. Carefully add 300 μL of 5 % sucrose solution.

5. Load tubes into the rotor (*see* **Note 9**).

3.5 Centrifugation	1. Centrifuge at $78,288 \times g$ overnight at 4 °C. This speed results in an average rcf of $78,000 \times g$ and a max rcf of $96,000 \times g$ in a TLA-120.2 rotor (*see* **Note 10**).

3.6 Harvest

1. Put a 96-well plate on ice.

2. Carefully remove the tubes from the rotor and put on ice avoiding any disturbance of the gradient.

3. Collect nine 100 µL fractions, starting from the top of the gradient, and put each fraction in a different well. Using the rows of a 96-well plate as a means to separate samples and wells to aliquot fractions greatly facilitates the handling of a large number of samples.

4. Boil fractions in an equal volume of pre-heated 2× Laemmli sample buffer and resolve by gel electrophoresis according to standard protocols [10]. Alternatively, an immunoprecipitation can be performed on fractions to enhance the detection of low abundance proteins (*see* **Note 11**).

4   Notes

1. All inhibitor solutions should be made fresh except for PMSF, β-Glycerophosphate, DFP, and Na_3VO_4. In addition, solution A should have a yellow color when DTT is added; otherwise, discard your DTT and make a fresh solution.

2. Orthovanadate should be activated for maximal phosphotyrosyl phosphatase-blocking activity. The procedure outline below actually depolymerizes the vanadate, which is most potent as a monomer [11]. First, prepare a 200 mM solution of orthovanadate (3.68 g in 100 mL water). Then, adjust to pH 10 (the solution will be yellow). Third, boil until the solution becomes colorless (about 10 min) and let it cool to room temperature. Fourth, readjust to pH 10 and repeat the previous step only if there is still some yellow coloration. Most of the time, only one boiling step is required. Aliquot in small volumes and store at −20 °C. Discard aliquot after use.

3. PBS 1× is diluted from a 10× stock solution. PBS 10×: Add about 800 mL water to a glass beaker. Weigh 80 g NaCl, 2 g KCl, 11.5 g Na_2HPO_4, and 2 g KH_2PO_4 and add to the beaker. Mix until the salts are dissolved and adjust the pH to 7.4. Put the solution into a 1-L graduated cylinder and complete to 1 L with water. Filter the solution through a 500 mL 0.45 µm filter unit and store at room temperature. To make the 1× solution, dilute with distilled water.

4. The 85 % sucrose solution takes a long time to prepare and heating does not make all that sucrose dissolve faster. So, plan accordingly.

5. The 35 and 5 % sucrose solution can easily be made in a 50 mL conical: add the powder in 25 mL of solution B and vortex until the sucrose is dissolved. Complete to 50 mL.

6. Freezing the cell pellets to continue the protocol later is not a good idea.

7. Try to keep the ultracentrifuge tubes on ice, whenever possible, during the gradient preparation.

8. All the sucrose solutions must be ice-cold before use.

9. The rotor as well as the centrifuge must be pre-chilled at 4 °C. Do not put the rotor on ice but in a cold room. Always use the rotor's support because if the diodes at the bottom of the rotor get dirty, the centrifuge will not reach its speed.

10. This centrifugation speed only applies to a 0.950 mL gradient centrifuged in 1 mL tubes in a TLA-120.2 rotor. The optimal centrifugation speed will have to be experimentally determined by each user. To do so, set-up a gradient as described in this chapter and subject all nine fractions to immunoblotting against Flotillin-1, a known lipid raft marker [12]. If the centrifugation speed is adequate, Flotillin-1 distribution will be discontinuous, as showed by us in figure 2A of Fortin et al. [13]. In addition, larger tubes can be used but cell numbers and total volume of the gradient must be scaled up accordingly [12, 14].

11. We have presented in this chapter a method to isolate lipid rafts from 1×10^7 human neutrophils. The detection of a large number of proteins by immunoblotting with this amount of cells should be possible. If you are trying to detect a low-abundance protein, you can try at first to increase cell numbers in solution B (with inhibitors and Triton) to 4×10^7. A wiser alternative, however, is to disrupt a large number of neutrophils (1×10^8 cells) by nitrogen cavitation according to a standard protocol. Resulting cavitates are then centrifuged at a maximum speed in a microcentrifuge for 10 min at 4 °C in order to get rid of nuclei and granules. Supernatants, which contain cell membranes, are then centrifuged for 1 h at $100,000 \times g$. After washing, cell membranes are dissolved directly in solution B containing inhibitors and 0.5 % Triton X-100 (as in Subheading 3.3) for 10 min and the gradient is made as described in Subheading 3.4. This enhances the detection of low-abundance proteins and ensures that no neutrophil-derived proteases degrade your target, which is a genuine risk if you simply increase cell numbers in solution B.

Acknowledgments

This work was supported by grants from the Canadian Institutes of Health Research (CIHR) (No. 106634 and No. 106701), the Université de Sherbrooke, and the Research Center on Aging.

References

1. Mantovani A, Cassatella MA, Costantini C, Jaillon S (2011) Neutrophils in the activation and regulation of innate and adaptive immunity. Nat Rev Immunol 11:519–531

2. Borregaard N (2010) Neutrophils, from Marrow to Microbes. Immunity 33:657–670

3. Scapini P, Lapinet-Vera JA, Gasperini S, Calzetti F, Bazzoni F, Cassatella MA (2000) The neutrophil as a cellular source of chemokines. Immunol Rev 177:195–203

4. Fulop T, Larbi A, Douziech N, Fortin C, Guerard KP, Lesur O, Khalil A, Dupuis G (2004) Signal transduction and functional changes in neutrophils with aging. Aging Cell 3:217–226

5. Fortin CF, Lesur O, Fulop T Jr (2007) Effects of TREM-1 activation in human neutrophils: activation of signaling pathways, recruitment into lipid rafts and association with TLR4. Int Immunol 19:41–50

6. David A, Fridlich R, Aviram I (2005) The presence of membrane proteinase 3 in neutrophil lipid rafts and its colocalization with FcγRIIIb and cytochrome b558. Exp Cell Res 308:156–165

7. Bournazos S, Hart SP, Chamberlain LH, Glennie MJ, Dransfield I (2009) Association of FcγRIIa (CD32a) with lipid rafts regulates ligand binding activity. J Immunol 182:8026–8036

8. Zech T, Ejsing CS, Gaus K, de Wet B, Shevchenko A, Simons K, Harder T (2009) Accumulation of raft lipids in T-cell plasma membrane domains engaged in TCR signalling. EMBO J 28:466–476

9. Simons K, Gerl MJ (2010) Revitalizing membrane rafts: new tools and insights. Nat Rev Mol Cell Biol 11:688–699

10. Gallagher SR (2012) One-dimensional SDS gel electrophoresis of proteins. Curr Protoc Protein Sci 10(1):1–44, Chapter 10, Unit 10 1

11. Gordon JA (1991) Use of vanadate as protein-phosphotyrsine phosphatase inhibitor. Methods Enzymol 201:477–482

12. Sitrin RG, Emery SL, Sassanella TM, Blackwood RA, Petty HR (2006) Selective localization of recognition complexes for leukotriene B4 and Formyl-Met-Leu-Phe within lipid raft microdomains of human polymorphonuclear neutrophils. J Immunol 177:8177–8184

13. Fortin CF, Sohail A, Sun Q, McDonald PP, Fridman R, Fulop T (2010) MT6-MMP is present in lipid rafts and faces inward in living human PMNs but translocates to the cell surface during neutrophil apoptosis. Int Immunol 22:637–649

14. Hill WG, An B, Johnson JP (2002) Endogenously expressed epithelial sodium channel is present in lipid rafts in A6 cells. J Biol Chem 277:33541–33544

Chapter 2

Flow Cytometry Analysis of NK Cell Phenotype and Function in Aging

Raquel Tarazona, Carmen Campos, Alejandra Pera, Beatriz Sanchez-Correa, and Rafael Solana

Abstract

Natural killer (NK) cells represent a subpopulation of lymphocytes involved in innate immunity, defined recently as group 1 of innate lymphoid cells (ILCs). NK cells are cytotoxic lymphocytes with a relevant role in the destruction of transformed cells as virus-infected or tumor cells, as well as the regulation of the immune response through cytokine and chemokine production that activates other cellular components of innate and adaptive immunity. In humans, NK cell subsets have been defined according to the level of expression of CD56. Aging differentially affects NK cell subsets and NK cell function. Here, we describe protocols for the delineation of NK cell subsets and the analysis of their functional capacity using multiparametric flow cytometry.

Key words NK cell subsets, Density gradient separation, Flow cytometry, CD107a/b degranulation assay, Cytotoxicity

1 Introduction

In peripheral blood, human natural killer (NK) cells represent between 5 and 20 % of lymphocytes. They are classically defined by the expression of CD56 and/or CD16 and the absence of T- and B-cell receptors [1]. According to the level of expression of CD56 and CD16, NK cells can be divided into four subsets: $CD56^{bright}$ $CD16^{negative}$, $CD56^{bright}$ $CD16^{+}$, $CD56^{dim}$ $CD16^{+}$, and $CD56^{negative}$ $CD16^{+}$ cells. An additional $CD56^{dim}$ $CD16^{negative}$ subset has been also defined [2]. Recently, $CD56^{bright}$ cells have been placed as a more immature stage of NK cells than $CD56^{dim}$ cells; in addition, CD57 is expressed in more mature and highly cytotoxic NK cells and $CD57^{+}$ NK cells are less responsive to cytokine stimulation [3, 4].

Age can affect cell number, cell subset distribution, and NK cell function as demonstrated previously [5–7]. It has been described that per cell NK cell cytotoxicity is usually decreased whereas CD16-mediated antibody-dependent cell cytotoxicity

Albert C. Shaw (ed.), *Immunosenescence: Methods and Protocols*, Methods in Molecular Biology, vol. 1343,
DOI 10.1007/978-1-4939-2963-4_2, © Springer Science+Business Media New York 2015

(ADCC) is preserved in the elderly [6, 7]. Whereas the number of NK cell is maintained or increased in the elderly, a decline in the more immature CD56^{bright} NK cell subset and an increase in CD56^{dim} cells and in CD57 expression have been reported. NK cell differentiation has been proposed as a continuous process supporting a gradual shift from CD56^{bright} to CD56^{dim} CD57^{negative} and finally to CD56^{dim} CD57$^+$ NK cells [6, 8, 9]. Thus, the alterations observed in NK cells in the elderly can be explained by a remodeling of NK cell subsets, with a decrease in the immature CD56^{bright} subset and the accumulation of more differentiated CD56^{dim} CD57$^+$ NK cells that may also explain many of the functional features of NK cells observed in elderly individuals [6, 7]. The inclusion of anti-CD57 antibody in panels designed to determine NK cell subsets in elderly individuals therefore gives us additional relevant information about NK cell differentiation status.

The mean fluorescence intensity of natural cytotoxicity receptors (NCR) NKp30 and NKp46 has been used to classify NCR^{bright} (NKp30^{bright} NKp46^{bright}), NCR^{discordant} (NKp30^{bright}NKp46^{dull} or NKp30^{dull}NKp46^{bright}) or NCR^{dull} (NKp30^{dull} NKp46^{dull}) phenotypes [10]. We have observed that the majority of healthy young individuals have a NCR^{bright} phenotype, whereas elderly individuals as well as young and elderly leukemia patients frequently display a NCR^{dull} or NCR^{discordant} phenotype [11, 12].

DNAM-1 has been recently emerged as an important regulator of NK cell function. DNAM-1 triggers NK cell-mediated cytotoxicity and IFN-γ production upon engagement with its ligands CD155 and CD112. Recent evidence suggests that DNAM-1 ligands can be induced by cellular stress, strengthening the role of this receptor on NK cell function. DNAM-1 expression has been found to be reduced in the elderly [6, 11–13].

The analysis of the effect of aging and CMV seropositivity on the expression of CD94, CD94/NKG2C, and CD94/NKG2A on NK cell subsets has showed that CMV seropositivity is associated with the expression of CD94/NKG2C dimers and CD57 on the major CD56dimCD16+ and the dysfunctional CD56−CD16+ NK cell subsets. A significant decrease on the expression of the CD94/NKG2A inhibitory receptor is found in the CD56−CD16+ NK cell subset from elderly CMV seropositive individuals compared to young individuals (Campos et al. 2014, Experimental Gerontology, in press). No significant changes have been reported so far on the expression or function of NKG2D on elderly individuals [6]. In addition, in recent years, degranulation assays quantifying CD107a surface expression have been applied to NK cells. CD107a expression correlates with NK cell activity [14], enabling the simultaneous analysis of NK cell markers and the functionality of NK cells.

Technical advances in flow cytometry over the last decade have allowed the analysis on a per cell basis of NK cell subsets and their characteristic phenotypes along with the study of NK cell function in the different subsets. Here, we present protocols and provide advice regarding the analysis of age-associated changes in NK cell phenotype and function.

2 Materials

2.1 Cells, Media, and Solutions

1. Whole blood collected in sodium heparin vacutainer tubes (2–3 tubes by donor) (*see* **Note 1**).

2. Sterile Phosphate Buffered Saline (PBS) 1×.

3. NK cell-susceptible target cells (e.g. K562 or 721.221) are required for functional experiments.

4. Density gradient cell separation medium for mononuclear cells as Histopaque-1077 containing Ficoll and sodium diatrizoate (Sigma-Aldrich).

5. Complete culture medium (RPMIc): RPMI-1640 supplemented with 10 % heat-inactivated fetal bovine serum (FBS) and 2 mM L-glutamine or 1 % of Glutamax (GIBCO) and penicillin (50 U/ml)-streptomycin (50 U/ml).

6. Materials for freezing cells: Cold Freezing Media (Heat inactivated and filtered FBS with 20 % of Dimethylsulfoxide (DMSO)). Cryovials, freezing container (e.g. Mr. Frosty, Nalgene) and isopropyl alcohol.

7. Optional, for NK cell isolation: NK cell-negative isolation kit (Miltenyi) or Rosette Sep human NK cell enrichment cocktail (StemCell Technologies, Grenoble, France).

8. Materials for proliferation assays: CellTrace CFSE proliferation kit, from Invitrogen. Prepare CFSE aliquots at a concentration of 5 mM (10 µl). Store at −20 °C.

9. Human recombinant IL-2 [15] in vials containing 50,000 IU/ml. Store at −20 °C.

10. Flow cytometry buffer.

11. Trypan Blue solution (0.4 %), Neubauer chamber and coverslips.

12. Plasticware: 30 ml sterile universal tubes, sterile pipettes, 15 ml sterile polypropylene conical tubes and 96-well plates, U bottom.

2.2 Monoclonal Antibodies

1. Analysis of NK cell subsets: monoclonal antibodies (mAb) against CD56 (B159 from BD Pharmingen), CD16 (3G8 from BD Pharmingen or VEP13 from Miltenyi Biotec) and CD3 (BW264/56 from Miltenyi Biotec or SP34-2 or SK7 from BD Biosciences) labeled with the appropriate combination of fluorochromes.

2. Study of NK cell activating receptors: mAb against Natural Cytotoxicity Receptors (NCRs) NKp30 (p30-15), NKp46 (9E2) and NKp44 (p44-8.1); NKG2D (1D11); DNAM-1 (CD226) (DX11); CD94 (HP-3D9) from BD Pharmingen and NKG2C (134591) from R&D Systems.

3. Study of NK cell inhibitory receptors: mAb against KIR (e.g. pan KIR2D, NKVFS1, Miltenyi Biotec), CD85j (ILT2) (GHI/75, BD Pharmingen), CD94 and NKG2A (131411, R&D Systems).

4. Antibodies against CD107a (H4A3, BD Pharmingen) for degranulation assays.

5. Antibodies against NK cell effector molecules: perforin (δG9), granzymes A (CB9) and B (GB11) from BD Pharmingen, and cytokines as IFN-γ (45–15) and TNF-α (CA2) from Miltenyi Biotec.

Other combinations of mAbs and fluorochromes from different suppliers can also be used.

2.3 Equipment Required

1. Inverted microscope.

2. Thermostated centrifuge.

3. Cell culture incubator at 37 °C and 5 % CO_2.

4. Freezer (−80°) and a liquid nitrogen (N_2) tank.

5. Flow Cytometer.

3   Methods

Carry out all procedures in sterile conditions unless otherwise specified.

3.1 Peripheral Blood Mononuclear Cell (PBMC) Isolation by Gradient Density

1. Dilute whole blood from each vacutainer at least 2× with PBS. Carefully layer the diluted blood suspension over the Histopaque separation medium (7 ml, ~ 3:1 proportion) in a 30 ml universal tube.

2. Centrifuge at $400 \times g$ for 20 min at room temperature (RT) in a swinging bucket rotor without brake.

3. Aspirate the mononuclear cell layer at the interphase and deposit it in a new 30 ml tube. Fill with 1× PBS to the brim and centrifuge at $300 \times g$ for 5 min.

4. Discard supernatant and resuspend cell pellet in 10 ml of PBS. Centrifuge at $300 \times g$ for 5 min and then discard supernatant and resuspend cell pellet again in 10 ml of PBS.

5. Count cells in a Neubauer chamber using Trypan blue for assessment of viability.

3.2 Freeze–Thaw Procedures

Cryopreservation of blood samples is frequently required for lymphocyte storage for further analysis. Performing a high-quality freezing procedure will improve cell viability and cell recovery after thawing.

1. After counting the previously isolated cells, remove supernatant and resuspend cell pellet with FBS at a concentration of 5–6×10^6 cells/0.9 ml per cryovial and place them on ice. Then add drop by drop 0.9 ml of cold freezing media (containing 20 % of DMSO) to each vial to be frozen, for a final concentration of 10 % DMSO in FBS solution. It is important to deposit the freezing media slowly and do not pipette the cell suspension, instead invert the tube once carefully (*see* **Note 2**).

2. Freeze vials overnight in a –80 °C freezer using a freezing container filled with isopropyl alcohol (some freezer containers do not require alcohol) to ensure standardized cooling rate of –1 °C/min required for successful cryopreservation of cells.

3. Transfer vials to liquid N_2 tank for long-term storage (*see* **Note 3**).

4. Thaw procedure: Warm 8 ml of complete culture media. Remove vial from liquid N_2 tank and hold in 37 °C water bath until sides are thawed but centre remains frozen. Add the warm media to the partially frozen cells and gently pour cells into a 30 ml tube. Do not shake the vial. It is important to remove DMSO as soon as possible. Centrifuge at $250 \times g$ for 5 min. Discard supernatant and resuspend pellet in 10 ml of PBS if the cells are going to be marked for cytometry analysis or in 10 ml of RPMIc if the cells are going to be used for functionality assays. Count cells using Trypan blue to calculate cell viability (*see* **Note 4**).

3.3 Flow Cytometry Analysis of NK Cell Phenotype

The protocol and antibody panels presented here are standardized for the analysis on a 7-color MACSQuant flow cytometer (Miltenyi). Antibody incubation was performed for 20 min at 4 °C unless otherwise specified. We recommend performing titration experiments to obtain the optimal concentration for each antibody batch.

1. For the analysis of human NK cell subsets: $CD56^{bright}CD16^{negative}$, $CD56^{bright}CD16^+$, $CD56^{dim}CD16^+$ and $CD56^{negative}$ $CD16^+$ populations, PBMCs (0.3×10^6 to 10^6) obtained as indicated in Subheading 3.1 were labeled with anti-CD3PerCP, anti-CD56 PE-Cy7, and anti-CD16 APC-Cy7.

2. Further characterization of NK cell subsets is done by using mAb against different surface markers such as CD57 (clone TB03, Miltenyi Biotec), a marker of activated/senescent cells that we include in all tubes, and antibodies against activating and inhibitory receptors such as NKG2D, NKp46, NKp30, DNAM-1 and CD94 together with NKG2A or NKG2C. Table 1 is a representative multicolor antibody panel used for seven-color flow cytometry analysis of NK cells.

Table 1
Example of an antibody panel for seven-color flow cytometry analysis of NK cells

	VioBlue	FITC	PE	PerCP	PE-Cy7	APC	APC-Vio770 or APC-Cy7
	Isotope controls						
Phenotype	CD57 Biotin/ antibiotin VB	DNAM-1	NKp30	CD3	CD56	NKp46	CD16
	CD57 Biotin/ antibiotin VB	CD94	NKG2C	CD3	CD56	NKG2D	CD16
	CD57 Biotin/ antibiotin VB	CD85j	Pan-KIR2D	CD3	CD56	NKG2A	CD16
Analysis of effector molecules and degranulation	CD57 Biotin/ antibiotin VB	Granzyme B	TNF-α	CD3	CD56	INF-γ	CD16
	CD57 Biotin/ antibiotin VB	INF-γ	TNF-α	CD3	CD56	CD107a	CD16
	CD57 Biotin/ antibiotin VB	Perforin	Granzyme A	CD3	CD56	CD107a	CD16

3. Once staining of surface molecules is accomplished, cells are fixed and permeabilized using BD Cytofix/Cytoperm fixation/permeabilization kit (BD Biosciences) and then stained with antibodies against the intracellular cytotoxic effector molecules perforin and granzymes A and B.

4. Cell acquisition is performed gating on the lymphocyte region using forward scatter (FSC) vs. side scatter (SSC) and then gating on $CD3^{negative}$ cells and finally a dot plot of CD56 vs. CD16 will show the four NK cell subsets (Fig. 1). Acquire at least 10^5 cells within the lymphocyte gate (*see* **Note 5**).

3.4 NK Cell Cytotoxicity and Cytokine Production in Response to K562 and 721.221 Cell Lines

As CD107a expression has been directly correlated with CD8+ T cell and NK cell cytotoxicity, this marker is used for the degranulation assays.

1. Use either freshly isolated PBMCs or cryopreserved PBMCs (*see* Subheading 3.2).

2. PBMCs are resuspended at 1×10^6 cells/ml in RPMIc and rested overnight at 37 °C in a standard incubator (humidified CO_2 atmosphere).

3. The following day, PBMCs are placed in a 96-well plate at 1.5×10^6 cells/ml (200 μl final volume). First, anti-CD16 APC-Vio770 (Miltenyi Biotec) is added to all wells and the plate is incubated for 15 min at RT. Next, Anti-CD107a-APC (BD Biosciences) antibody is added. The recommended antibody dilution for CD107a conjugate is 1:10 for up to 10^7 cells/100 μl. For each individual a positive control containing

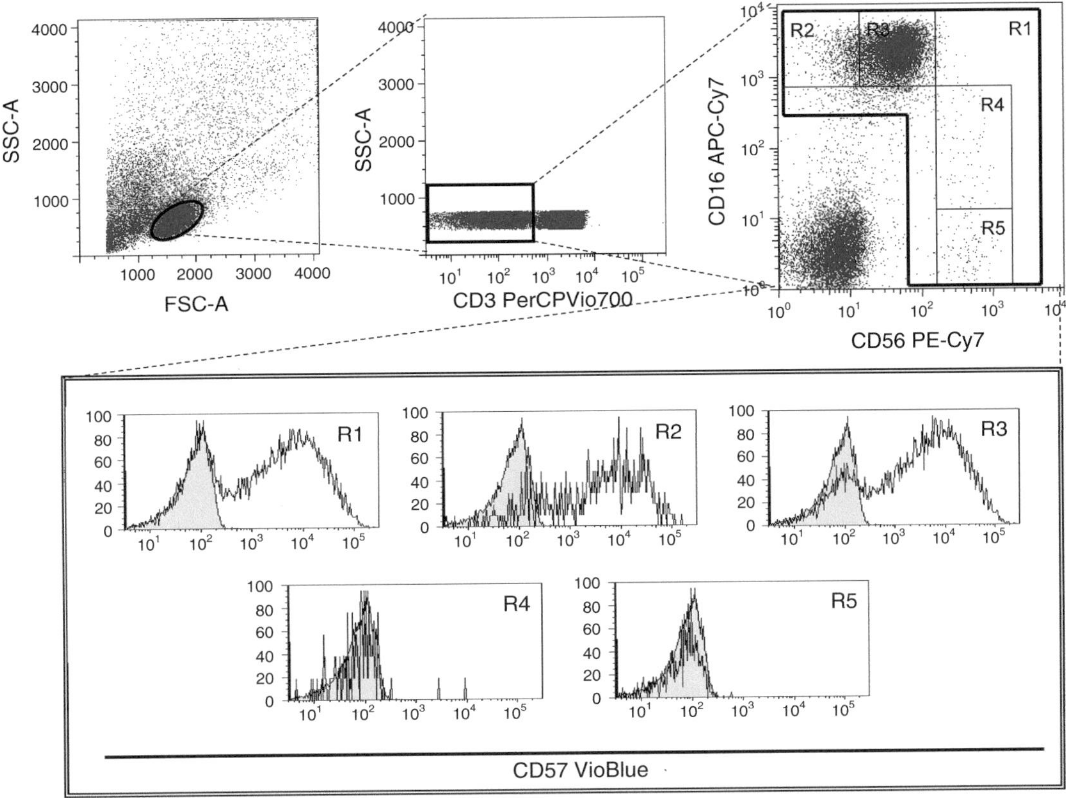

Fig. 1 Representative analysis of NK cell subsets by flow cytometry. Lymphocyte gating is performed according to FSC and SSC parameters, then CD3-negative lymphocytes are selected and the analysis of CD56 and/or CD16 expression is represented in a dot plot in order to select the different NK cell subsets. Regions R1 to R5 represent, total NK cells, CD56[negative] CD16+, CD56[dim] CD16+, CD56[bright] CD16+ and CD56[bright] CD16[negative] NK cells respectively. Histograms represent CD57 expression for each subset

PMA and ionomycin at a final concentration of 50 ng/ml and 1 µg/ml (respectively) was included, as well as a negative control without stimuli, to measure spontaneous stimulation. For stimulation with K562 and 721.221 cell lines the cell target:NK cell ratio recommended is 1:1. This ratio is determined by estimating the NK cell proportion in PBMCs by flow cytometry or by using purified NK cells.

4. The plate is then placed in a standard incubator (37 °C, humidified CO_2 atmosphere) and, after 1 h, each well receives the addition of monensin (Golgistop, 0.67 µl/ml; BD Biosciences) and brefeldin A (Golgi Plug 1 µg/ml; BD Biosciences) (*see* **Note 6**). Cells are then incubated for an additional 4 h. Following incubation, cells are washed twice with PBS (4 °C) and stained with surface antibodies (anti-CD56, anti-CD3). Cells are then fixed and permeabilized and subsequently stained intracellularly with antibodies against IFN-gamma and TNF-alpha for 30 min. For isotype controls

follow the same protocol as samples. All antibodies used must be titred before use. Stained cells can be analyzed by flow cytometry the following day.

3.5 Analysis of Cell Proliferation by CFSE Staining

1. Separate and isolate PBMCs from blood samples as described in Subheading 3.1 (*see* **Note 7**).

2. Count the cells with a Neubauer chamber and calculate viability with Trypan blue solution.

3. Take a few cells (~200,000 cells) to perform a pre-purification analysis (using surface markers CD3 and CD56 and their corresponding isotype controls).

4. Purify cells using a purification kit and count purified cells obtained (*see* Subheading 2.1.7).

5. Take a few cells to make a post-purification cytometry (~100,000 cells) using anti-CD3 and anti-CD56 mAb and quantify its efficiency (*see* **Note 8**).

6. Centrifuge the remaining volume at $300 \times g$, 5 min (to remove any residual separation solution after purification). Decant and resuspend the pellet.

7. Add to the pellet 1 ml of PBS + CFSE (1 μM final concentration) and incubate for 3 min at RT in the dark and shake the sample (manually mixing).

8. Stop reaction by adding 10 ml of cold medium and centrifuge at $200 \times g$ for 10 min at 20 °C. Decant and resuspend in 10 ml of RPMIc, wash twice.

9. Resuspend the pellet in RPMIc to a final concentration of 250,000 cell/200 μl per well (just over 10^6/ml). Usually we use four wells per donor: two for isotype control (stimulated and unstimulated) and two for sample (stimulated and unstimulated).

10. Add 2 μl of rhIL-2 (so that the final concentration of rhIL-2 is 500 IU/ml) to the corresponding wells and incubate at 37 °C and 5 % CO_2 during 24 h.

11. The next day, take 50 μl from one of the unstimulated wells (best use cells from the isotype control well), acquire the cells in the cytometer and set the setting (value) for FL1 (CFSE fluoresces on this channel). Thus, we establish the beginning of proliferation. To do this, we set the voltage for FL1 between 10^3 and 10^4. If we have sufficient cells also set the voltages for the rest of the channels (since unlabeled cells may also emit auto-fluorescence).

12. Incubate for 5 days.

13. At the end of 5 days, centrifuge the plate at $300 \times g$ for 5 min at 20 °C. Decant the supernatant and wash twice with 200 μl of cold sterile 1× PBS. Label the cells with mAb against CD56,

CD3 and CD16 (in any color except FITC, which corresponds to CFSE) and other surface markers of interest, like CD57.

14. Wash with 200 µl of cold sterile 1× PBS. Centrifuge at $300 \times g$ for 5 min at 10 °C, decant and resuspend with 200 µl of 1× PBS or cytometry buffer. Acquire the cells the same day.

15. Analyze the data using the FlowJo software (Tree Star Inc V.7.2.1, Ashland, OR. USA). With this program you can calculate the "proliferation index" which represents the number of cell divisions, not counting the cells that have not entered into division.

4 Notes

1. It has been observed that for flow cytometry analysis, sodium heparin performs better than citrated-based anticoagulants maintaining cell viability.

2. Do not freeze more than five vials at the same time to ensure that cell processing is performed quickly.

3. Using this technique we have increased cell viability after thawing (>90 %) compared with the use of 10 % DMSO freezing media directly deposited on cell pellet.

4. For analysis of NK cell function viability of cell suspension should be greater than 90 %.

5. APC and PE labeled antibodies against NKG2A and NKG2C respectively cannot be used simultaneously due to fluorescence quenching.

6. Monensin is required for the CD107a assay and brefeldin A or monensin for intracellular cytokine detection. Check which transport inhibitor is recommended for the detection of a given cytokine.

7. For proliferation assays freshly isolated PBMCs perform better than cryopreserved PBMCs.

8. Perform the cytometry purification control on the same day of purification.

Acknowledgement

This work was supported by grants PS09/00723 and PI13/02691 (to R.S.) from the Spanish Ministry of Health, SAF2009-09711 and SAF2013-46161-R (to R.T.) from the Ministry of Science and Innovation of Spain and, PRI09A029 and grants to INPATT research group from the Junta de Extremadura (GRU10104) and from the University of Extremadura (to R.T.) and grants from the

Junta de Andalucia (to R.S.) cofinanced by the European Regional Development Fund (FEDER). The following reagent was obtained through the AIDS Reagent Program, Division of AIDS, NIAID, NIH: (human rIL-2) from Dr. Maurice Gately, Hoffmann–La Roche Inc.

References

1. Cooper MA, Fehniger TA, Caligiuri MA (2001) The biology of human natural killer-cell subsets. Trends Immunol 22:633–640

2. Poli A, Michel T, Theresine M, Andres E, Hentges F, Zimmer J (2009) CD56bright natural killer (NK) cells: an important NK cell subset. Immunology 126:458–465

3. Romagnani C, Juelke K, Falco M, Morandi B, D'Agostino A, Costa R, Ratto G, Forte G, Carrega P, Lui G, Conte R, Strowig T, Moretta A, Munz C, Thiel A, Moretta L, Ferlazzo G (2007) CD56bright. J Immunol 178: 4947–4955

4. Chan A, Hong DL, Atzberger A, Kollnberger S, Filer AD, Buckley CD, McMichael A, Enver T, Bowness P (2007) CD56bright human NK cells differentiate into CD56dim cells: role of contact with peripheral fibroblasts. J Immunol 179:89–94

5. Gayoso I, Sanchez-Correa B, Campos C, Alonso C, Pera A, Casado JG, Morgado S, Tarazona R, Solana R (2011) Immunosenescence of human natural killer cells. J Innate Immun 3:337–343

6. Solana R, Tarazona R, Gayoso I, Lesur O, Dupuis G, Fulop T (2012) Innate immunosenescence: effect of aging on cells and receptors of the innate immune system in humans. Semin Immunol 24:331–341

7. Solana R, Pawelec G, Tarazona R (2006) Aging and innate immunity. Immunity 24:491–494

8. Bjorkstrom NK, Riese P, Heuts F, Andersson S, Fauriat C, Ivarsson MA, Bjorklund AT, Flodstrom-Tullberg M, Michaelsson J, Rottenberg ME, Guzman CA, Ljunggren HG, Malmberg KJ (2010) Expression patterns of NKG2A, KIR, and CD57 define a process of CD56dim NK-cell differentiation uncoupled from NK-cell education. Blood 116:3853–3864

9. Lopez-Verges S, Milush JM, Pandey S, York VA, Arakawa-Hoyt J, Pircher H, Norris PJ, Nixon DF, Lanier LL (2010) CD57 defines a functionally distinct population of mature NK cells in the human CD56dimCD16+ NK-cell subset. Blood 116:3865–3874

10. Fauriat C, Just-Landi S, Mallet F, Arnoulet C, Sainty D, Olive D, Costello RT (2007) Deficient expression of NCR in NK cells from acute myeloid leukemia: evolution during leukemia treatment and impact of leukemia cells in NCRdull phenotype induction. Blood 109:323–330

11. Sanchez-Correa B, Gayoso I, Bergua JM, Casado JG, Morgado S, Solana R, Tarazona R (2012) Decreased expression of DNAM-1 on NK cells from acute myeloid leukemia patients. Immunol Cell Biol 90:109–115

12. Sanchez-Correa B, Morgado S, Gayoso I, Bergua JM, Casado JG, Arcos MJ, Bengochea ML, Duran E, Solana R, Tarazona R (2011) Human NK cells in acute myeloid leukaemia patients: analysis of NK cell-activating receptors and their ligands. Cancer Immunol Immunother 60:1195–1205

13. de Andrade LF, Smyth MJ, Martinet L (2014) DNAM-1 control of natural killer cells functions through nectin and nectin-like proteins. Immunol Cell Biol 92:237–244

14. Alter G, Malenfant JM, Altfeld M (2004) CD107a as a functional marker for the identification of natural killer cell activity. J Immunol Methods 294:15–22

15. Lahm HW, Stein S (1985) Characterization of recombinant human interleukin-2 with micromethods. J Chromatogr 326:357–361

Chapter 3

Flow Cytometric Identification of Fibrocytes in the Human Circulation

Xinyuan Hu, Erin M. DeBiasi, and Erica L. Herzog

Abstract

Because the incidence of organ fibrosis increases with age, various fibrosing disorders are projected to account for significant increases in morbidity, mortality, and healthcare costs in the years to come. Treatments for these diseases are scarce and better understanding of the immunopathogenesis of fibrosis and its relationship to aging are sorely needed. One area of interest in this field is the role that fibrocytes might play in the development of tissue remodeling and fibrosis. Fibrocytes are mesenchymal progenitor cells presumed to be of monocyte origin that possess the tissue remodeling properties of tissue resident fibroblasts such as extracellular matrix production and α-SMA-related contractile properties, as well as the immunologic functions typically attributed to macrophages including production of cytokines and chemokines, antigen presentation, regulation of leukocyte trafficking, and modulation of angiogenesis. Fibrocytes could participate in the development of age-related fibrosing disorders through any or all of these functions. This chapter presents methods that have been developed for the study of circulating human fibrocytes. Protocols for the quantification of fibrocytes in the human circulation will be presented along with discussion of the technical challenges that are frequently encountered in this field. It is hoped that this information will facilitate further investigation of the relationship between fibrocytes, aging, and fibrosis, and perhaps uncover new areas of study in these difficult-to-treat and deadly diseases.

Key words Aging, Collagen, Extracellular matrix, Fibrocyte, Fibrosis, Flow cytometry

1 Introduction

The incidence of many diseases characterized by chronic inflammation and fibrosis increases with age. Because these ailments are difficult to treat, the combined toll of end-organ fibrosis accounts for substantial morbidity, mortality, and healthcare costs [1]. Despite many years of research, precise identification of the cells and mediators driving these responses remain undefined [2, 3]. Current paradigms of fibrogenesis feature damage to structural cells followed by a chronic macrophage-rich inflammatory infiltrate and an aberrant fibroblast-driven wound repair response [2, 4]. Given the age-related nature of these diseases, it is possible that various forms of immunosenescence are involved. Identification of

Albert C. Shaw (ed.), *Immunosenescence: Methods and Protocols*, Methods in Molecular Biology, vol. 1343, DOI 10.1007/978-1-4939-2963-4_3, © Springer Science+Business Media New York 2015

age-related profibrotic immune responses has the potential to advance our understanding of the pathogenic mechanism(s) driving these diseases. Fibrocytes are a monocyte-derived population of mesenchymal progenitor cells possessing a remarkable array of pro-inflammatory and reparative functions [5]. Strong experimental evidence obtained in murine models and in primary human cells reveals enhanced concentrations of peripheral blood fibrocytes in many forms of solid organ fibrosis, as well as in normal aging, thereby suggesting that fibrocyte abnormalities might reflect a novel form of age-related immune dysregulation [6]. Therefore, the development of methods to accurately quantify fibrocytes in the human circulation has the potential to significantly advance the study of immunosenescence. This chapter will present the data linking fibrocytes with fibrosis and aging and will describe the factors regulating their function and trafficking. Methods for the accurate detection of fibrocytes in the circulation will be described, along with common technical challenges encountered in these studies. It is hoped that this information will facilitate novel investigation of the role that fibrocytes might play in age-related fibrosing disorders and perhaps uncover new areas of study related to immunosenescence in these difficult-to-treat and deadly diseases.

1.1 Fibrocytes: Disease Associations

Fibrocytes are an important area of interest in the immunopathogenesis of many diseases characterized by fibrosis and remodeling [6]. Identified by the co-expression of leukocyte markers such as CD45, extracellular matrix proteins such as Collagen-1α, and pluripotency markers such as CD34 [5], fibrocytes display an increasingly recognized association with a wide variety of diseases characterized by autoimmunity such as rheumatoid arthritis [7], autoimmune thyroiditis [8], amyopathic antisynthetase syndrome [9], and scleroderma [10, 11]. Quantitative and phenotypic abnormalities in circulating and parenchymal fibrocytes are also seen in chronic inflammatory disorders that are not classically thought of as autoimmune including idiopathic pulmonary fibrosis [12–14], asthma [15–17], nephrogenic systemic fibrosis [18], cardiovascular disease [19], and pulmonary hypertension [20]. In support of these studies, animal modeling implicates fibrocytes in the development of several forms of tissue fibrosis including those affecting the lungs [13, 14, 21, 22], liver [23], kidney [24, 25], heart [26–28], and vasculature [29]. When viewed in this light, it is particularly relevant that elevations in circulating fibrocytes are seen in the blood of aged but otherwise healthy individuals, and in several animal models of aging [30, 31], leading to speculation that fibrocytes might represent a form of abnormal immune activation related to aging. Additionally, fibrocytes are emerging as mediators of tumor metastasis [32–34]. For all of these reasons, the study of fibrocytes as it relates to immunosenescence has become both important and timely.

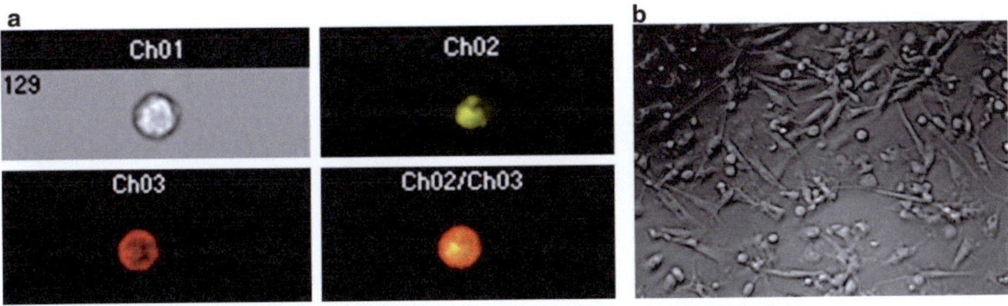

Fig. 1 Representative imaging of fibrocytes from an aged subject. Panel (**a**) shows an image of a fibrocyte obtained from the peripheral blood monocytes of a healthy but aged individual. This image was generated using Amnis image stream technology in which flow cytometry is combined with real-time confocal microscopy. *Top left*: brightfield; *top right*: FITC-detected Pro-Collagen Iα1 (Pro-Col Iα1, pseudocolored yellow here). *Bottom left*: PE-detected CD45, *bottom right*: merged image of CD45 and Pro-Col Iα1. (**b**) Brightfield image of cultured fibrocytes. The *spindle-shaped* cells demonstrate the typical morphology of fibrocytes

1.2 Identification of Fibrocytes in the Circulation

Flow cytometric identification of fibrocytes in the circulation employs the co-detection of characteristic cell surface markers and intracellular staining for collagens and/or other extracellular matrix components. Human fibrocytes express nonspecific hematopoietic markers such as CD45 [5] and leukocyte-specific protein-1 (LSP-1) [35] along with more specific markers of monocyte lineage and function (CD11b, CD11c, CD11d) [36], chemokine receptors (CXCR4) [13], host defense proteins and scavenger receptors (CD16/32, CD163) [36], antigen presentation (Major Histocompatibility Complex (MHC) I and II, CD80, and CD86) [37], and cell surface enzymes such as CD10 and CD13 [36]. Most sources agree that fibrocytes lack markers of lymphocyte origin [36, 38] though this may not be true in all cases. Circulating fibrocytes also express CD34 [5], a motility protein also found on certain populations of stem cell that is often used to distinguish fibrocytes from related cells such as macrophages and tissue resident fibroblasts [6]. In addition to these cell surface markers, fibrocytes also produce many extracellular matrix components including structural proteins and glycosaminoglycans (GAGs) [36, 38, 39]. Representative imaging of fibrocytes is shown in Fig. 1 and a complete listing of fibrocyte markers is compiled in Table 1.

1.3 Fibrocytes: Differentiation and Homing

Because human and murine fibrocyte precursors copurify with peripheral blood monocytes that express CD14 [40], fibrocytes are considered to be of monocytic origin, though lineage tracing studies will be required to definitively address this question. Enrichment for CD11b(+) CD115(+) Gr1(+) expression enhances fibrocyte outgrowth from cultured murine monocytes; these effects require direct contact with activated CD4+ lymphocytes and occur via an mTOR-PI3 kinase-dependent pathway [24]. Human and rodent fibrocyte precursors also express the Fcγ receptor [41], which responds to aggregated IgG by inducing fibrocyte outgrowth.

Table 1

Markers used to identify fibrocytes

Marker	Expression
Adhesion and motility	
CD9, CD11a, CD11b, CD11c, CD43	Intermediate to high
CD164, Mac2, LSP-1, CD29, CD44, CD81	Intermediate to high
ICAM-1, CD49 complex, CD34	Intermediate to high
Cell surface enzymes	
CD10, CD172a, FAP	Intermediate to high
CD13, Prolyl-4-hydroxylase	Intermediate to high
Scavenging receptors and host defense	
CD14, CD68, CD163, CD206, CD209, CD35, CD36	Conflicting reports
Fcγ receptors	
CD16, CD32a, CD32b, CD32c	Intermediate to high
Chemokine receptors	
CCR2, CCR5, CCR4, CCR7, CCR9	Intermediate to high
CXCR1, CXCR4, CXC3R1	Intermediate to high
Antigen presentation	
CD45, CD80, CD86, MHCI, MCHII	Low to intermediate
Extracellular matrix	
Collagen-I/III/IV, vimentin, tenascin	Low to intermediate
Fibronectin, α-SMA	Conflicting reports
Collagen V	High
Glycosaminoglycans	
Perlecan, Versican, Hyaluronan	Intermediate to high
Decorin	Low to intermediate
Miscellaneous	
Semaphorin 7a, CD115, Thy 1.1, CD105	Low to intermediate

These effects are opposed by exposure to the short pentraxin protein serum Amyloid P [21] via an ITIM-dependent mechanism [42]. In vitro studies of primary human cells also reveal that the monocyte to fibrocyte transition is inhibited by Th1 cytokines such as IFNγ, TNF, and IL-12, and by Th17 cytokines such as IL-17A [43]; this transition is augmented by Th2 cytokines including IL-4 and IL-13 [43, 44], as well as exposure to TGF-β1, and engagement of the β1 integrin subunit [11, 20]. The β1 integrin effects require Erk phosphorylation [20], though other signaling pathways might also be involved.

Recruitment of murine fibrocytes to injured tissue occurs via the chemokine receptors CCR2, CCR7, and CXCR4 [22, 45, 46]. Human fibrocytes express the chemokine receptors CCR3 (eotaxin receptor) and CCR5 (MCP-1 receptor) as well as CD29 and

Semaphorin 7a [47], and it is assumed that these receptors regulate in vivo trafficking though this assumption has not been confirmed. Despite the paucity of direct data regarding the mediators that affect fibrocyte recruitment in humans, our own work demonstrates an association between concentrations of soluble factors such as IL-4, IL-10, IL-13, MCP-1, and CCL18 in the blood of aged but otherwise healthy subjects, suggesting that fibrocytes might enter the circulation in response to one or more of these cytokines. In studies involving the bleomycin model of murine lung fibrosis, elevations in circulating and intrapulmonary fibrocytes and the soluble mediators TGF-β1 and Stromal-derived factor-1 (SDF-1) were seen in unchallenged mice with null mutations of the Senescence-Associated Mutation Prone gene which confers an enhanced fibrotic phenotype [30]. Similarly, in studies employing in vivo imaging of transgenic mice in which the luciferase gene is placed under control of the Col-Iα promoter, enhanced bone marrow egress of circulating fibrocytes is detected [31]. In humans, high levels of CXCL12, which binds to CXCR4, have been found in the lungs and blood of patients with idiopathic pulmonary fibrosis (IPF), and these levels correlate with circulating fibrocyte concentrations [13]. The blood of patients with scleroderma-associated lung fibrosis also demonstrates high level expression of Plexin C1, the cognate inhibitory receptor for Sema 7a [48]. Interestingly, in vitro knockdown of this receptor markedly promotes fibrocyte outgrowth, suggesting that Plexin C1 might serve as a counter-regulatory response. To date, these pathways have not been specifically assessed in fibrocytes obtained from aged but otherwise healthy individuals.

1.4 Fibrocytes: Functions

Fibrocytes possess an array of functions implicating them in the pathogenesis of chronic inflammatory conditions and fibrosis. For example, human fibrocytes respond to stimulation with interleukin-1 beta (IL-1β) by increasing secretion of the cytokines interleukin-6 (IL-6) and interleukin-8 (IL-8), the chemokines CCL2 and CCL3, and by upregulating expression of intercellular adhesion molecule-1 (ICAM-1) [49]. In the setting of Toll-Like Receptor stimulation and viral infections, porcine fibrocytes participate in antigen presentation and activation of cytotoxic CD8+ cells by increasing expression of Major Histocompatibility Complex I and II, and the costimulatory proteins CD80 and CD86 [50]. In addition to these proinflammatory activities, in some settings fibrocytes can also respond to IL-1β by increasing interleukin-10 (IL-10) production [49] which would be expected to reduce inflammation in part through recruitment of regulatory T cells. Fibrocytes might also participate in repair and remodeling through their ability to adopt the alpha-Smooth Muscle Actin (α-SMA)-expressing, contractile phenotype of activated myofibroblasts, and their participation in wound contraction has been demonstrated *ex vivo* in studies using wound chambers [5]. Normal human fibrocytes exhibit a pattern of ECM production that would be expected to recruit inflammatory cells and enact repair; this pattern includes robust expression of Collagen V, hyaluronan, and versican, and decorin [39].

In addition to direct production of ECM, fibrocytes might also participate in remodeling and fibrosis via secretion of soluble mediators such as platelet-derived growth factor (PDGF) and TGF-β1. These growth factors regulate transformation of cultured myofibroblasts. Fibrocytes are also involved in the regulation of angiogenesis via secretion of matrix metalloproteinases (MMPs), vascular endothelial growth factor (VEGF), PDGF-A, hepatocyte growth factor (HGF), granulocyte–macrophage colony stimulating factor (GM-CSF), basic fibroblast growth factor (b-FGF), IL-8 and IL-1β [51]. Additional immunoregulatory properties are suggested by fibrocyte expression of Semaphorin 7a ("Sema 7a" or CD108W) [11], a GPI-anchored membrane protein that can activate macrophages and dendritic cells, control T-cell activation and induce secretion of TGF-β1 [52].

Fibrocytes are also identified in certain human malignancies [32, 53, 54] and have in animal models been shown to facilitate tumor metastasis through several mechanisms. Fibrocytes can augment tumor growth by mediating immunosuppression via both active suppression of interferon-gamma (IFNγ) and tumor necrosis factor (TNF) [55] and production of indoleamine oxidase [32]. Fibrocytes recruit immunosuppressive monocytes via CCL2 to metastatic sites [34]. Additionally, murine fibrocytes contribute to the development of a premetastatic niche through regulation of cell migration via CCR5 and induction of MMP9 [33]. This array of functions frames fibrocytes as a pluripotent cell population that responds to the local inflammatory milieu by adopting diverse phenotypic characteristics involving varying degrees of inflammation and ECM production (Fig. 2). Any or all of these properties might participate in the immunopathogenesis and tissue remodeling responses seen in age-related pathologies.

The following protocol has been developed for the accurate detection of fibrocytes in the human circulation. The stepwise protocol is included along with detailed notes regarding the assiduous use of blocking agents and controls and commonly encountered technical challenges.

2 Materials

1. Kendall Monoject Blood Collection Tubes (Tyco/Healthcare, Mansfield, MA).
2. Histopaque (Sigma-Aldrich, St. Louis, MO).

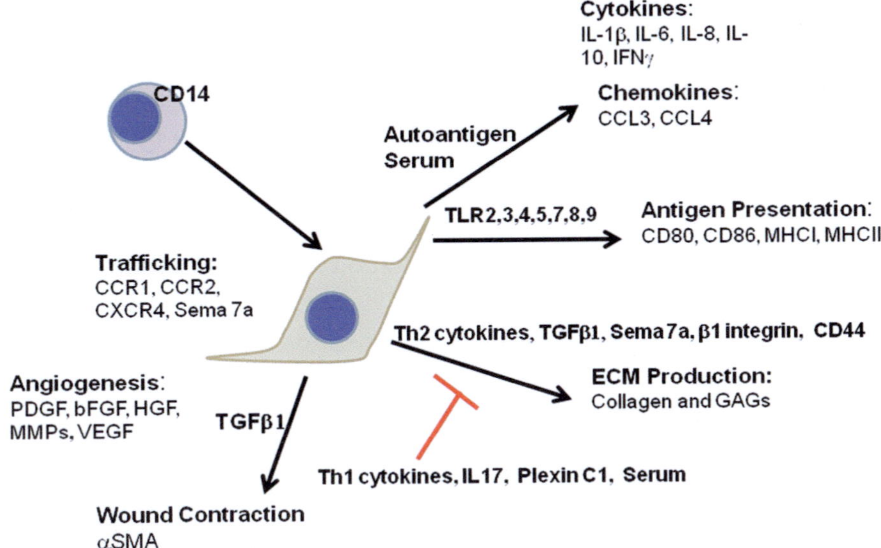

Fig. 2 Potential contributions of fibrocytes to the pathogenesis of age-related fibrosis. Fibrocyte precursors copurify with CD14+ monocytes and possess immunomodulatory functions including production of chemokines and cytokines, antigen presentation, extracellular matrix production, wound contraction, paracrine regulation of angiogenesis, and regulation of leukocyte trafficking. Any or all of these functions might contribute to the age-related immune abnormalities

3. PE-conjugated Anti-human CD45 (HI30, BD Biosciences, San Jose, CA).

4. IsoPE Mouse IgG1 (MOPC-21), Isointracellular Purified Rat IgG1 (R3-34) (BD Biosciences Pharmingen).

5. Alexa Fluor 488 conjugated Goat Anti-rat IgG (Invitrogen, Eugene, Oregon).

6. FCR Blocking Reagent Human (MACS Miltenyi Biotec).

7. Rat anti Human Pro-Collagen Iα1 (M-58, Millipore, Temecula, CA).

8. 10× Phosphate-buffered saline (PBS) pH 7.4: 1.4 M NaCl, 0.1 M phosphate, pH 7.4, 0.03 M KCl. Mixed with dH$_2$O to get 1× PBS (American Bioanalytical, Natick, MA).

9. Ethylenediaminetetraacetate (EDTA) pH 8.0 (American Bioanalytical, Natick, MA).

10. Fetal Bovine Serum (FBS).

11. FACS Buffer: PBS with 2 % FBS, 0.01 % NaN$_3$ and 1 mM EDTA/500 mL.

12. Paraformaldehyde (PFA) (JT Baker, Phillipsburg, NJ).

13. FACS Calibur (Becton Dickinson).

14. CellQuest (BD Biosciences).

15. FlowJo software.

16. 4 % Paraformaldehyde (see recipe).

3 Methods

The methods described here outline (a) human peripheral mononuclear cell collection and staining for identification of fibrocytes; (b) flow cytometry of stained samples; and (c) accurate analysis of flow cytometry data.

3.1 Human Peripheral Blood Mononuclear Cell Collection and Staining

3.1.1 Separation of Peripheral Blood Mononuclear Cells from Plasma

1. Collect peripheral blood in sterile sodium heparin tubes (10 mL draw).

2. Dilute blood with Phosphate-buffered Saline (PBS) 1:2 blood to PBS.

3. Layer diluted blood over histopaque: 1:3 histopaque to blood/PBS (typically 10 mL of histopaque to 30 mL blood/PBS) (*see* **Note 1**).

4. Centrifuge at $1240 \times g$ for 22 min at 12 °C with acceleration, deceleration curves at (1,1) (most gradual).

5. Remove peripheral blood mononuclear cells (PBMCs) in the buffy coat layer (layer between plasma and histopaque) with pipettor (*see* **Note 2**).

6. Wash with PBS twice, centrifuge at $500 \times g$ for 8 min at 4 °C with acceleration, deceleration curves at (9,9).

7. Count cells with hemocytometer and tryphan blue and re-suspend at one million cells/mL (*see* **Note 3**).

8. If needed, separate cells for RNA and DNA analysis prior to FACS staining.

9. One million cells/Eppendorf tube (Individual Eppendorfs for RNA and DNA).

10. One million cells/tube (For FACS).

11. RNA and DNA storage (non-sterile).

12. Centrifuge cells at $900 \times g$ for 3 min.

13. Pipette off supernatant.

14. Store DNA pellet at −80 °C.

15. Re-suspend RNA pellet in 350 μL of RLT + βME buffer (RNeasy kit, Qiagen) and store at −80 °C.

3.1.2 Staining of Cells for CD45 and Pro-Collagen-Iα1 Expression

1. Place approximately 1×10^6 cells/tube. Prepare the following tubes for CD45 and Pro-Collagen Iα1 staining (*see* **Note 4**):

    (a) No Stain.

    (b) CD45 PE (2 μL) + Intracellular isotype control + FITC labeled secondary antibody.

    (c) CD45 PE (2 μL), Rat Anti-human Procol-I and FITC labeled secondary antibody (1 μL).

2. Centrifuge cells at $250 \times g$ for 5 min at 4 °C with acceleration, deceleration curves at (9,9).

3. Re-suspend cells in 100 µL of 10 % normal goat serum (NGS) FACS Buffer and 5 µL/sample of FCR blocker (*see* **Note 5**).

4. Add appropriate antibodies (amount noted above) for extra-cellular staining.

5. Incubate at 4 °C for 30 min.

6. Wash with FACS Buffer twice, centrifuge at $250 \times g$ for 5 min at 4 °C with acceleration, deceleration curves at (9,9).

7. Add 100–200 µL of cytofix/cytoperm buffer (BD Biosciences) to remaining samples and incubate at 4 °C for 15 min (*see* **Note 6**).

8. Wash with PermWash buffer (P/W; BD Biosciences), centrifuge at $250 \times g$ for 5 min at 4 °C with acceleration, deceleration curves at (9,9).

9. Wash extracellular stains with FACS Buffer and intracellular stains with P/W, centrifuge at $250 \times g$ for 5 min at 4 °C with acceleration, deceleration curves at (9,9) (*see* **Note 7**).

10. Re-suspend intracellular samples in 100 µL of P/W and add 1 µL of Pro-collagen Iα1 antibody to all applicable samples and one 1 µL of isotype intracellular to all applicable samples (*see* **Note 8**).

11. Incubate covered at 4 °C for 30 min.

12. Wash all with P/W, centrifuge at $250 \times g$ for 5 min at 4 °C with acceleration, deceleration curves at (9,9).

13. Add 100 µL of Alexa Fluor 488 dilution (1:500 Alexa Fluor 488 to P/W) to all intracellular samples.

14. Incubate at 4 °C for 30 min.

15. Wash with P/W then wash with FACS Buffer, centrifuge at $250 \times g$ for 5 min at 4 °C with acceleration, deceleration curves at (9,9).

16. Fix all intracellular samples with 100–200 µL of 4 % PFA and store at 4 °C until flow cytometric analysis (*see* **Note 9**).

3.1.3 Flow Cytometry of Stained Samples

1. Open Cell Quest, connect to the cytometer and make sure the setup box is checked.

2. Voltages for the FACS Calibur are set using the non-stain control.

    (a) Adjust the Forward Scatter (FSC) (controls lateral movement of events on graph if FSC is *x*-axis) and Side Scatter (SSC) (controls vertical tilt if SSC is *y*-axis) to record as many of the cells of interest as possible.

(b) Using histograms of each of the channels (FL1, FL3) or a dot plot, adjust voltages so that the majority of events occur between 0 and 10^1.

3. Compensations for the FACS Calibur are set using the single color controls.

(a) Using the FITC control, adjust the compensation so that the majority of events occur in the FITC channel (it will bleed into PE).

(b) Using the PE control, adjust the compensations so that the majority of events occur in the PE channel (it will bleed into FITC and APC).

4. Uncheck the setup box, set the location to record all samples to, and acquire all samples (including controls).

3.2 Analysis of Flow Cytometry Data

1. Open the flow cytometry analysis software (in this case, FlowJo).

3.2.1 FACS Analysis for Fibrocytes

2. First a gate is set for all of the live cells based on the FSC and SSC and applied to all samples (Fig 3a, *see* **Note 10**).

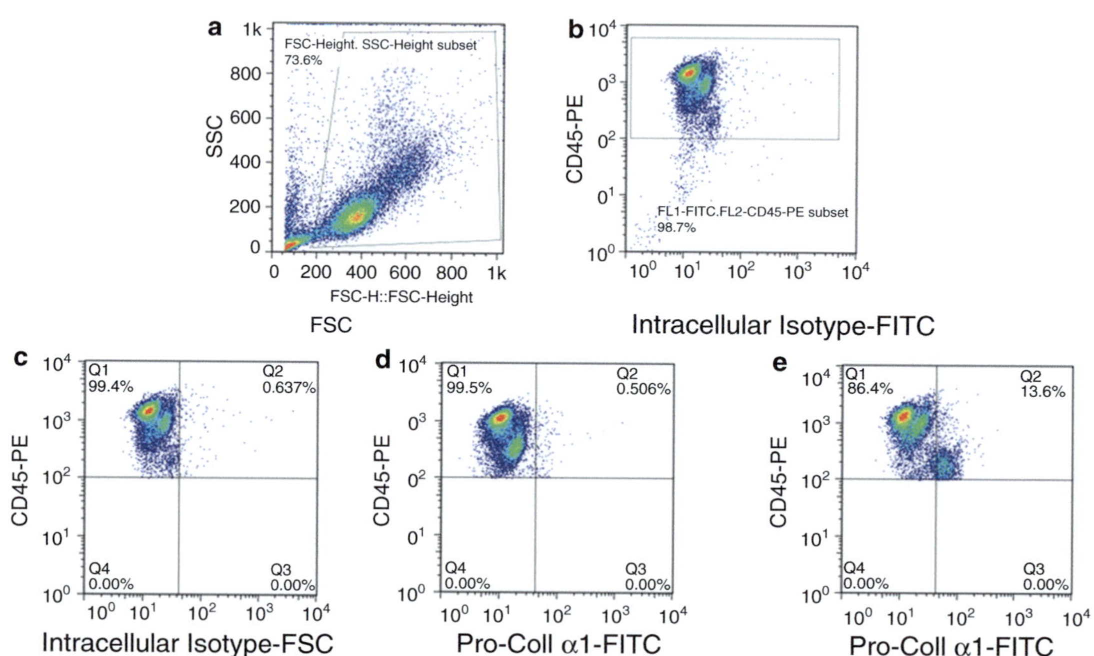

Fig. 3 FACS-based identification of fibrocytes in human PBMCs. (**a**) The live cell gate is set based on forward (FSC) vs. side scatter (SSC). (**b, c**) FITC-detected intracellular isotype control (*X* Axis) vs. Anti-CD45-PE (*Y* axis). The negative gate for PE is set (**b**). PE-stained CD45+ve cells are selected and the negative gate for intracellular FITC staining is chosen (**c**). (**d**) This gate is then applied to the sample stained with FITC-detected Pro-Collagen- Iα1 (*X* Axis) vs. Anti-CD45-PE. The dual positive cells in the right upper quadrant represent fibrocytes. The proportion of dual positive cells in the *right upper quadrant* in the negative control (**c**) is subtracted from the proportion of dual positive cells in the sample stained with Pro-Collagen-Iα1 in a young (**d**) or aged (**e**) subject to determine the overall percentage of double positive cells

3. The negative gate for fibrocyte analysis is determined by staining a CD45-stained sample with intracellular isotype control and secondary antibody (Fig. 3b).

4. Once the negative gate for Col-I staining of CD45+ cells is established, this gating strategy should be applied to the sample(s) of interest (Fig. 3c) (*see* **Note 11**).

4 Notes

1. Red blood cell lysis is also sometimes performed using brief exposure to a hypotonic solution such as deionized water. This approach has not been validated for detection of fibrocytes and as such is not recommended.

2. The buffy coat will appear as a pale yellow layer of cells at the interface between the plasma and blood layers. It is important to avoid pipetting red blood cells into this layer as the presence of red blood cells will make flow cytometry difficult.

3. If starting material is limited and there are not enough cells, scale down all reagents as needed.

4. The combination of hematopoietic cell surface marker expression such as CD45, LSP-1, or CXCR4 combined with intracellular staining detecting production of ECM components such as collagen, vimentin, or prolyl-4 hydroxylase is considered sufficient for the detection of circulating fibrocytes. While CD45 and Procollagen co-expression has been classically used to define fibrocytes, these other markers are acceptable as well and the protocols described in this unit can be easily modified for these markers.

5. The goat serum helps block nonspecific staining and is a critical aspect of performing this protocol properly.

6. The initial permeabilization is an absolute necessity due to the intracellular nature of the collagen staining. If permeabilization is not achieved the protocol will not work and fibrocytes will not be detected.

7. From here on, all antibodies should be diluted in perm/wash solution to maintain a permeabilized membrane.

8. It is critical that an intracellular isotype antibody be included as a control. The permeabilization step causes a pronounced increase in autofluorescence that may be incorrectly interpreted as collagen staining if the correct control is not included.

9. If flow cytometry is not performed immediately, cells should be maintained in fixation solution such as paraformaldehyde, at 4 ° C in the dark. The fluorescence of cells increases when samples are stored in this manner so in order to avoid detection

artifact, all controls and experimental tubes should be fixed and stored identically.

10. Selection of live cells based on FSC vs. SSC is critical. Dead or dying cells demonstrate increased autofluorescence and inclusion of these cells in the gating strategy will cause increased overall brightness that might be erroneously captured as actual staining.

11. It is crucial that consistent populations be analyzed for each sample. Thus it is recommended that rather than manually applying the CD45/Pro-Col$I\alpha$1 gate to each sample, that the gate be established on the CD45/isotype intracellular control and automatically applied to the subsequent sample.

12. The most commonly encountered challenge is the inherent autofluorescence of unstained cells in subjects with undiagnosed inflammatory disease. While in normal individuals the inherent autofluorescence of the unstained cells will be low, some subjects may exhibit increased baseline autofluorescence, which is likely due to alterations in the phenotypes of circulating leukocytes. When this challenge is encountered, use of an isotype control stain prepared from the diseased individual can be helpful. Otherwise this shift in autofluorescence may be incorrectly interpreted as intracellular staining.

13. Fibrocyte quantities are reported as the percentage of total PBMCs or as concentrations (fibrocytes per mL of blood). The former is calculated by using the gating strategy shown in Fig. 3 and subtracting CD45/intracellular isotype from CD45/ Pro-Col $I\alpha$1 staining. The latter is calculated by dividing the Post-Ficoll cell count by the input mLs of blood to derive cells per mL. Then this value is multiplied by the percentage of cells in the live cell gate based on FSC vs SSC, and then by the CD45/ Pro-Col $I\alpha$1 subtracted CD45/intracellular isotype staining.

14. The extracellular matrix proteins used to identify fibrocytes are intracellular stains requiring fixation and permeabilization. Therefore, in vitro functional studies are impossible to perform on fibrocytes detected in this manner. For detailed methods allowing the isolation and characterization of live human fibrocytes, the reader is referred to reference [56].

15. Most reagents are prepared as stock solutions, stored at 4 or at −80 °C, and used in aliquots. Reagents stored in a −20 °C frost free freezer may be damaged due to recurrent freeze–thaw cycles.

Acknowledgements

This work was supported in part by grants R01 HL109033, U01 HL112702-01 (both to E.L.H) from the National Institutes of Health.

References

1. Murray PJ, Wynn TA (2011) Protective and pathogenic functions of macrophage subsets. Nat Rev Immunol 11:723–737

2. Murray LA, Rubinowitz A, Herzog EL (2012) Interstitial lung disease: is interstitial lung disease the same as scleroderma lung disease? Curr Opin Rheumatol 24:656–662

3. Homer RJ, Elias JA, Lee CG et al (2011) Modern concepts on the role of inflammation in pulmonary fibrosis. Arch Pathol Lab Med 135:780–788

4. Gross TJ, Hunninghake GW (2001) Idiopathic pulmonary fibrosis. N Engl J Med 345:517–525

5. Bucala R, Spiegel LA, Chesney J et al (1994) Circulating fibrocytes define a new leukocyte subpopulation that mediates tissue repair. Mol Med 1:71–81

6. Reilkoff RA, Bucala R, Herzog EL (2011) Fibrocytes: emerging effector cells in chronic inflammation. Nat Rev Immunol 11:427–435

7. Galligan CL, Siminovitch KA, Keystone EC et al (2009) Fibrocyte activation in rheumatoid arthritis. Rheumatology (Oxford) 49:640–651

8. Douglas RS, Afifiyan NF, Hwang CJ et al (2009) Increased generation of fibrocytes in thyroid-associated ophthalmopathy. J Clin Endocrinol Metab 95:430–438

9. Peng X, Mathai SK, Murray LA et al (2011) Local apoptosis promotes collagen production by monocyte-driven cells in transforming growth factor β1-induced lung fibrosis. Fibrogenesis Tissue Repair 4:12–25

10. Mathai SK, Gulati M, Peng X et al (2010) Circulating monocytes from systemic sclerosis patients with interstitial lung disease show an enhanced profibrotic phenotype. Lab Invest 90:812–823

11. Gan Y, Reilkoff RA, Peng X et al (2011) Role of semaphorin 7a signaling in transforming growth factor β1-induced lung fibrosis and scleroderma-related interstitial lung disease. Arthritis Rheum 63:2484–2494

12. Moeller A, Gilpin SE, Ask K et al (2009) Circulating fibrocytes are an indicator for poor prognosis in idiopathic pulmonary fibrosis. Am J Respir Crit Care Med 179:588–594

13. Mehrad B, Burdick MD, Zisman DA et al (2006) Circulating peripheral blood fibrocytes in human fibrotic interstitial lung disease. Biochem Biophys Res Commun 353:104–108

14. Mehrad B, Burdick MD, Strieter RM (2009) Fibrocyte cxcr4 regulation as a therapeutic target in pulmonary fibrosis. Int J Biochem Cell Biol 41:1708–1718

15. Schmidt M, Sun G, Stacey MA et al (2003) Identification of circulating fibrocytes as precursors of bronchial myofibroblasts in asthma. J Immunol 171:380–389

16. Wang CH, Huang CD, Lin HC et al (2008) Increased circulating fibrocytes in asthma with chronic airflow obstruction. Am J Respir Crit Care Med 178:583–591

17. Nihlberg K, Larsen K, Hultgardh-Nilsson A et al (2006) Tissue fibrocytes in patients with mild asthma: A possible link to thickness of reticular basement membrane? Respir Res 7:50

18. Vakil V, Sung JJ, Piecychna M et al (2009) Gadolinium-containing magnetic resonance image contrast agent promotes fibrocyte differentiation. J Magn Reson Imaging 30:1284–1288

19. Falk E (2006) Pathogenesis of atherosclerosis. J Am Coll Cardiol 47:C7–C12

20. Nikam VS, Wecker G, Schermuly R et al (2011) Treprostinil inhibits adhesion and differentiation of fibrocytes via camp and rap dependent erk inactivation. Am J Respir Cell Mol Biol 45:692–703

21. Murray LA, Chen Q, Kramer MS et al (2010) Tgf-beta driven lung fibrosis is macrophage dependent and blocked by serum amyloid p. Int J Biochem Cell Biol 43:154–162

22. Phillips RJ, Burdick MD, Hong K et al (2004) Circulating fibrocytes traffic to the lungs in response to cxcl12 and mediate fibrosis. J Clin Invest 114:438–446

23. Kisseleva T, Uchinami H, Feirt N et al (2006) Bone marrow-derived fibrocytes participate in pathogenesis of liver fibrosis. J Hepatol 45:429–438

24. Niedermeier M, Reich B, Gomez RM et al (2009) Cd4+ t cells control the differentiation of gr1+ monocytes into fibrocytes. Proc Natl Acad Sci U S A 106:17892–17897

25. Katebi M, Fernandez P, Chan ES et al (2008) Adenosine a2a receptor blockade or deletion diminishes fibrocyte accumulation in the skin in a murine model of scleroderma, bleomycin-induced fibrosis. Inflammation 31:299–303

26. Haudek SB, Cheng J, Du J et al (2010) Monocytic fibroblast precursors mediate fibrosis in angiotensin-ii-induced cardiac hypertrophy. J Mol Cell Cardiol 49:499–507

27. Haudek SB, Xia Y, Huebener P et al (2006) Bone marrow-derived fibroblast precursors mediate ischemic cardiomyopathy in mice. Proc Natl Acad Sci U S A 103:18284–18289

28. Haudek SB, Trial J, Xia Y et al (2008) Fc receptor engagement mediates differentiation of

cardiac fibroblast precursor cells. Proc Natl Acad Sci U S A 105:10179–10184

29. Buday A, Orsy P, Godo M et al (2010) Elevated systemic tgf-beta impairs aortic vasomotor function through activation of nadph oxidase-driven superoxide production and leads to hypertension, myocardial remodeling, and increased plaque formation in apoe(−/−) mice. Am J Physiol Heart Circ Physiol 299:H386–H395

30. Xu J, Gonzalez ET, Iyer SS et al (2009) Use of senescence-accelerated mouse model in bleomycin-induced lung injury suggests that bone marrow-derived cells can alter the outcome of lung injury in aged mice. J Gerontol A Biol Sci Med Sci 64:731–739

31. Scholten D, Reichart D, Paik YH et al (2011) Migration of fibrocytes in fibrogenic liver injury. Am J Pathol 179:189–198

32. Zhang H, Maric I, DiPrima MJ, Khan J, Orentas RJ, Kaplan RN, Mackall CL (2013) Fibrocytes represent a novel MDSC subset circulating inn patients with metastatic cancer. Blood 122:1105–1113

33. Van Deventer HW, Wu PQ, Bergsstralh DT, Davis BD, O'Connor BP, Ting J, Serody JS (2008) C-C chemokine receptor 5 on pulmonary fibrocytes facilitates migration and promotes metastasis via matrix metalloproteinase 9. Am J Pathol 173:253–264

34. Van Deventer HW, Palmieri DA, Ping Q, McCook EC, Serody JS (2013) Circulating fibrocytes prepare the lung for cancer metastasis by recruiting Ly-6C+ monocytes via CCL2. J Immunol 190:4861–4867

35. Yang L, Scott PG, Giuffre J et al (2002) Peripheral blood fibrocytes from burn patients: identification and quantification of fibrocytes in adherent cells cultured from peripheral blood mononuclear cells. Lab Invest 82:1183–1192

36. Pilling D, Fan T, Huang D et al (2009) Identification of markers that distinguish monocyte-derived fibrocytes from monocytes, macrophages, and fibroblasts. PLoS One 4:e7475

37. Chesney J, Bacher M, Bender A et al (1997) The peripheral blood fibrocyte is a potent antigen-presenting cell capable of priming naive t cells in situ. Proc Natl Acad Sci U S A 94:6307–6312

38. Bellini A, Mattoli S (2007) The role of the fibrocyte, a bone marrow-derived mesenchymal progenitor, in reactive and reparative fibroses. Lab Invest 87:858–870

39. Bianchetti L, Barczyk M, Cardoso J et al (2012) Extracellular matrix remodeling properties of human fibrocytes. J Cell Mol Med 3:483–495

40. Abe R, Donnelly SC, Peng T et al (2001) Peripheral blood fibrocytes: differentiation pathway and migration to wound sites. J Immunol 166:7556–7562

41. Pilling D, Buckley CD, Salmon M et al (2003) Inhibition of fibrocyte differentiation by serum amyloid p. J Immunol 171:5537–5546

42. Castano AP, Lin SL, Surowy T, Nowlin BT et al (2009) Serum amyloid p inhibits fibrosis through fc gamma r-dependent monocyte-macrophage regulation in vivo. Sci Transl Med 1:5ra13

43. Bellini A, Marini MA, Bianchetti L et al (2011) Interleukin (il)-4, il-13, and il-17a differentially affect the profibrotic and proinflammatory functions of fibrocytes from asthmatic patients. Mucosal Immunol 5:140–149

44. Shao DD, Suresh R, Vakil V et al (2008) Pivotal advance: Th-1 cytokines inhibit, and th-2 cytokines promote fibrocyte differentiation. J Leukoc Biol 83:1323–1333

45. Moore BB, Murray L, Das A et al (2006) The role of ccl12 in the recruitment of fibrocytes and lung fibrosis. Am J Respir Cell Mol Biol 35:175–181

46. Sakai N, Wada T, Yokoyama H et al (2006) Secondary lymphoid tissue chemokine (slc/ccl21)/ccr7 signaling regulates fibrocytes in renal fibrosis. Proc Natl Acad Sci U S A 103:14098–14103

47. Quan TE, Cowper S, Wu SP et al (2004) Circulating fibrocytes: Collagen-secreting cells of the peripheral blood. Int J Biochem Cell Biol 36:598–606

48. Lazova R, Gould Rothberg BE, Rimm D et al (2009) The semaphorin 7a receptor plexin c1 is lost during melanoma metastasis. Am J Dermatopathol 31:177–181

49. Chesney J, Metz C, Stavitsky AB et al (1998) Regulated production of type i collagen and inflammatory cytokines by peripheral blood fibrocytes. J Immunol 160:419–425

50. Balmelli C, Alves MP, Steiner E et al (2007) Responsiveness of fibrocytes to toll-like receptor danger signals. Immunobiology 212:693–699

51. Hartlapp I, Abe R, Saeed RW et al (2001) Fibrocytes induce an angiogenic phenotype in cultured endothelial cells and promote angiogenesis in vivo. FASEB J 15:2215–2224

52. Sultana H, Neelakanta G, Foellmer HG et al (2012) Semaphorin 7a contributes to west nile virus pathogenesis through tgf-beta1/smad6 signaling. J Immunol 189:3150–3158

53. Barth PJ, Ebrahimsade S, Hellinger A et al (2002) Cd34+ fibrocytes in neoplastic and inflammatory pancreatic lesions. Virchows Arch 440:128–133

54. Barth PJ, Koster H, Moosdorf R (2005) Cd34+ fibrocytes in normal mitral valves and myxomatous mitral valve degeneration. Pathol Res Pract 201:301–304

55. Kraman M, Bambrough PJ, Arnold JN et al (2010) Suppression of antitumor immunity by stromal cells expressing fibroblast activation protein-alpha. Science 330:827–830

56. Quan TE, Bucala R (2007) Culture and analysis of circulating fibrocytes. Methods Mol Med 135:423–434

Chapter 4

Experimental Approaches to Tissue Injury and Repair in Advanced Age

Aleah L. Brubaker, Stewart R. Carter, and Elizabeth J. Kovacs

Abstract

Cutaneous wound healing is a complex physiological process. This process can be altered by multiple physiological and pathological factors. Multiple pathophysiological disturbances act to impair resolution of cutaneous wound injury, including obesity, diabetes, peripheral vascular disease, and advanced age. As our longevity increases without a concomitant increase in healthy living years, it is plausible to assume that problematic wound closure will continue to consume a large portion of our health care resources. Furthermore, advanced age is associated with numerous alterations in the innate and adaptive immune responses that complicate outcomes following cutaneous injury, trauma, or infection. Thus, models that examine the impact of advanced age on cutaneous wound repair will be of great benefit to the development of potential therapeutics that target age-related aberrancies in tissue repair. Herein, we detail two animal models of tissue injury, excisional wound injury and burn injury, that can be used to evaluate wound healing in the context of advanced age. We also describe modifications of these methods to examine wound infection following either excisional or burn injury. Lastly, we discuss methods of subsequent tissue analysis following injury. Models described below can be further adapted to genetically engineered murine strains to study the effects of aging and other co-morbidities on wound healing.

Key words Wounding healing, Animal model, Aging, Excisional biopsy, Burn injury, Infection

1 Introduction: Aging and Cutaneous Wound Healing

Cutaneous wound healing is a complex physiological process comprised of three primary phases: the inflammatory, proliferative, and remodeling phases [1, 2]. The inflammatory phase begins immediately following tissue injury. Platelets at the wound site act to aid in hemostasis and degranulate to release a host of pro-inflammatory mediators. Simultaneously, antimicrobial peptides released from cutaneous keratinocytes help to provide direct bactericidal activity following tissue injury. These mediators, alongside the cytokines and chemokines released from damaged keratinocytes and resident tissue leukocytes, aid in recruitment of innate immune cells to help prevent microorganism contamination and infection [3]. Early in the inflammatory phase, neutrophils predominate, helping

Albert C. Shaw (ed.), *Immunosenescence: Methods and Protocols*, Methods in Molecular Biology, vol. 1343,
DOI 10.1007/978-1-4939-2963-4_4, © Springer Science+Business Media New York 2015

phagocytose pathogens and debris [4]. Macrophages then enter the wound bed to aid in phagocytosis, eventually undergoing a phenotypic shift in order to facilitate the transition to the proliferative phase [5]. During the proliferative phase, keratinocytes aid in re-epithelialization by migrating over the open wound bed to restore the epidermis. Concurrent deposition of immature collagen by fibroblasts and angiogenesis help to restore the dermal architecture and vascularity of the injured tissue, creating a provisional extracellular matrix [6, 7]. Over time, the proliferative phase gives way to the remodeling phase, where the initial type III collagen is replaced with type I collagen, which improves the tensile strength of the wound [2]. Additionally, the developing vasculature is pruned to form an efficient vascular network. Timely progression through these phases is required for efficient wound healing. Alterations in any of these phases of wound healing can impair wound closure, resulting in a range of clinical complications from infection to chronic wounds to excessive scar formation.

Currently, it is estimated the U.S. health care system spends 25 billion dollars treating chronic wounds and related complications [8]. Multiple pathophysiological disturbances act to impair resolution of cutaneous wound injury, including obesity, diabetes, peripheral vascular disease, and advanced age [8–10]. Of note, the average human lifespan continues to lengthen, with a growing number of individuals greater than 65. Moreover, the aforementioned co-morbidities are on the rise, compromising healthy living years in this aging population [11]. As our longevity increases without a concomitant increase in healthy living years, it is plausible to assume that problematic wound closure will continue to consume a large portion of our health care resources. Furthermore, advanced age is associated with numerous alterations in the innate and adaptive immune responses that complicate outcomes following cutaneous injury, trauma or infection [12, 13]. Thus, models that examine the impact of advanced age on cutaneous wound repair will be of great benefit to the development of potential therapeutics that target age-related aberrancies in tissue repair.

Herein, we detail two animal models of tissue injury, excisional wound injury and burn injury, that can be used to evaluate wound healing in the context of advanced age. These models were selected based on clinical reports of impaired wound healing, increased wound dehiscence and worse outcomes following burn trauma in elderly patients [8, 9, 14, 15]. We also describe modifications of these methods to examine wound infection following either excisional or burn injury. Lastly, we discuss methods of subsequent tissue analysis following injury. Models described below can be further adapted to genetically engineered murine strains to study the effects of aging and other co-morbidities on wound healing.

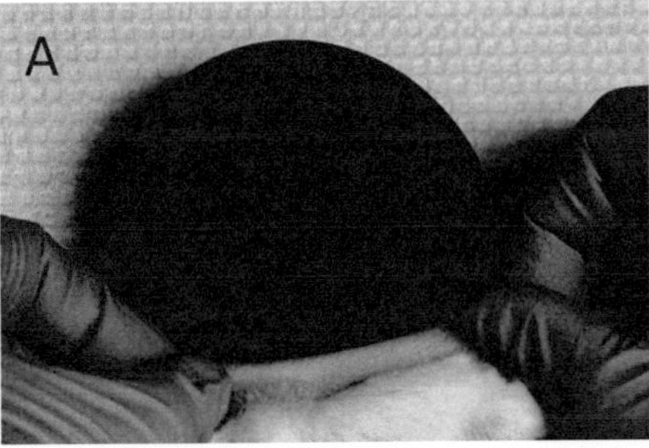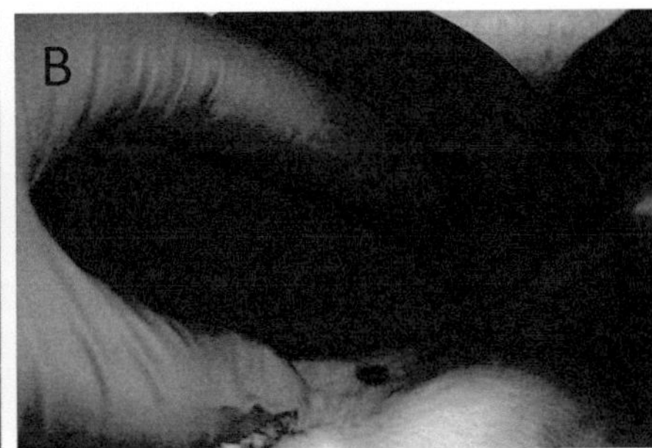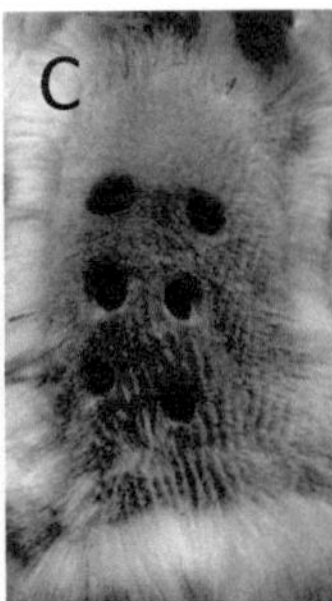

Fig. 1 Excisional wound by punch biopsy. Lift the skin in the mid-dorsal line and fold over a hockey puck (**a**). Push the punch biopsy tool through the folded skin, such that the puck is visible on the other side. This will create a wound on each side of the dorsal midline (**b**). Repeat this procedure for the desired number of wounds (**c**)

1.1 Excisional Wound Healing

Excisional wound injury models allow for evaluation of the phases of wound healing outlined above. In these models, a full thickness, cutaneous injury results in removal of the murine epidermis, dermis, hypodermis and the smooth muscle layer known as the panniculus carnosus. Depending on the interest of the researchers, the number and size of wounds can be varied using a standard dermal punch biopsy. Briefly, young and aged mice of the desired strains and age ranges are anesthetized and the fur is removed either by shaving with an electric animal clipper, hair removal cream or plucking. The skin is then lightly cleansed with ethanol, and the wounds are induced by lifting the murine skin in the dorsal midline and folding it over a hockey puck. Then 2–6 wounds, from 3 to 8 mm in diameter, can be created using dermal punch biopsies, allowing for symmetrical and identical sized wounds on either side of the dorsal midline (Fig. 1). This method also allows for full excision of the epidermis, dermis, hypodermis, and panniculus carnosus as mentioned above. Mice can then be sacrificed at early (3 h–3 days), mid (5–10 days), or late (14 days onward) time points to evaluate the different phases of wound repair described above [1, 2]. At sacrifice, wounds are removed with a larger punch biopsy than used to injure the animal to allow for consistent removal of intact skin around the wound margin (Fig. 2). During dissection of the pelt of the mouse, it is important to carefully remove the tissue around the wound site to ensure removal of the entire wound matrix. This requires special attention during the early phases of wound repair when the granulation tissue is easily disrupted. After removal of the tissue, the wounds can be analyzed as detailed later in the chapter.

1.2 Burn Wound Healing

Similar to perturbations in excisional or incisional cutaneous injury with aging, advanced age is also associated with worse outcomes following burn trauma. Though improvements in clinical management over the past few decades have improved the mortality

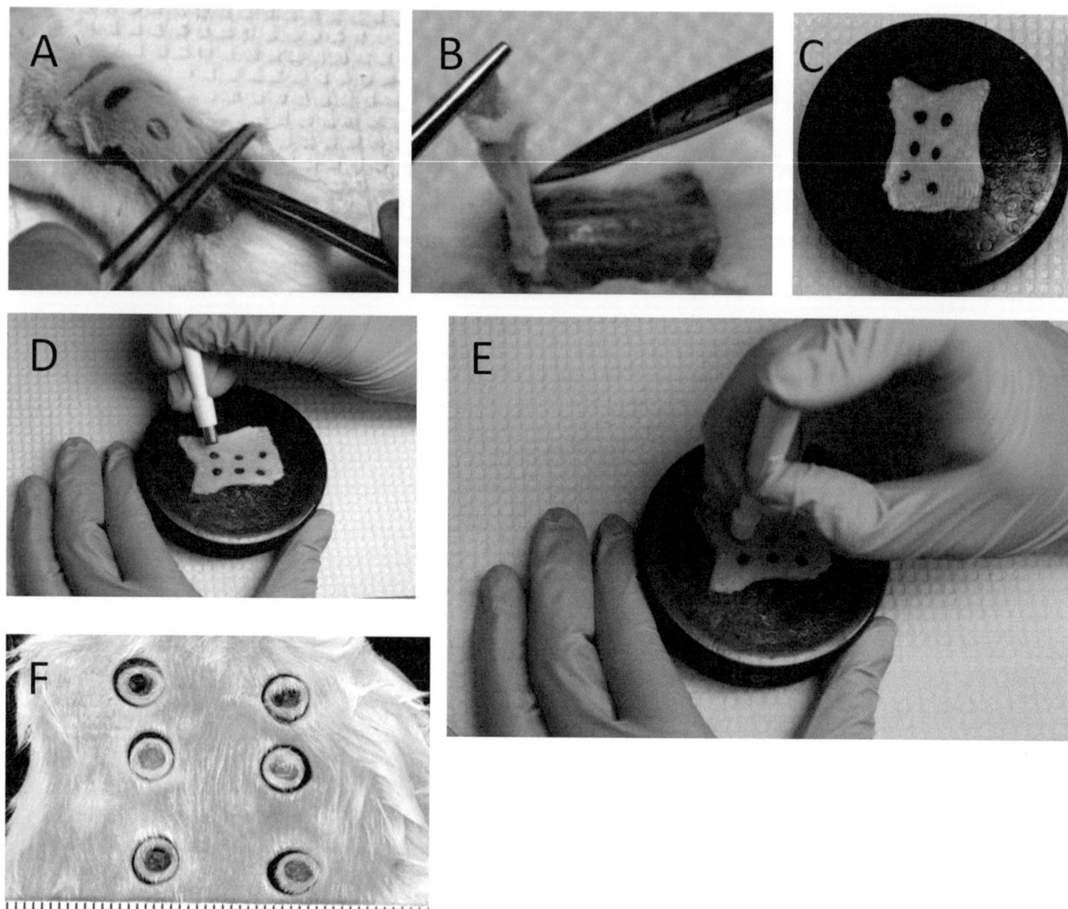

Fig. 2 Wound harvesting. Carefully dissect the dorsal pelt from the mouse using scissors and forceps (**a**). Using scissors, cut around the wound site to ensure inclusion of all granulation tissue. Using forceps, provide counter traction while cutting directly on top of the muscular layer to include epidermis, dermis, hypodermis, and panniculus carnosa (**b**). Place the excised specimen on a hockey puck (**c**). Using a punch biopsy 2 mm larger than the size used to inflict the wounds, remove the wound tissue and surrounding wound margins (**d–e**)

following burn injury in elderly patients over 65, clinical outcomes are still mediocre compared to young counterparts [14, 16]. In addition to direct cutaneous insult, burn injury also results in significant systemic inflammation and subsequent pulmonary complications, such as pneumonia and acute respiratory distress syndrome, which are particularly devastating in the elderly patient [17–19]. Thus, the model described within not only allows for direct comparison of burn wound healing with age, but also allows for evaluation of the systemic complications associated with burn trauma and aging. Briefly, young and aged mice of the age ranges delineated previously are anesthetized and the fur is removed as mentioned above. The mice are weighed and then placed in a burn template (Fig. 3) that represents ~12–15 % of their total body

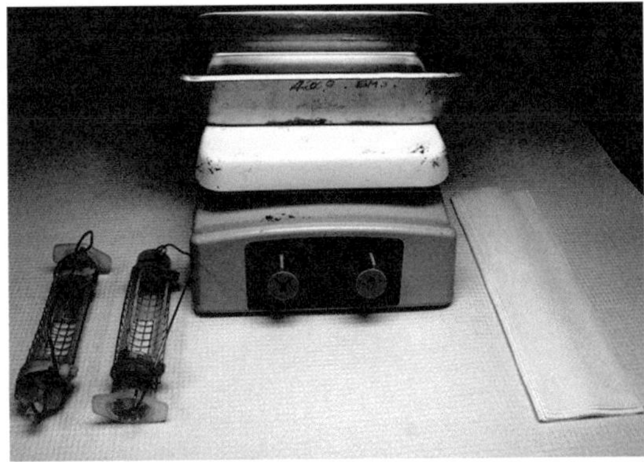

Fig. 3 Scald burn apparatus and burn template. The apparatus consists of a metal container for water, heating plate, templates, and paper towels for drying mice after burn injury. The template is selected based on mouse weight in order to achieve a 12–15 % total body surface area burn. The inferior surface of the template has a portion removed that corresponds to the needed size. Hardware cloth is used to reinforce the bottom of the template

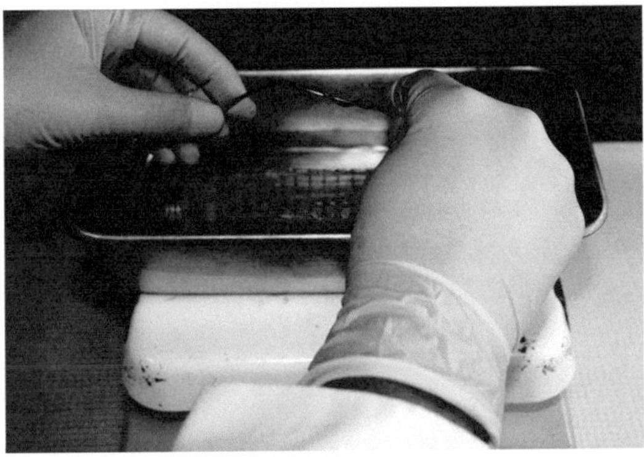

Fig. 4 Scald burn administration. Immerse the dorsum, template lined area of the mouse in the water bath for 8 s. Push gently on the abdomen to ensure the dorsum of the animal is flush with the burn template. The tail should remain out of the template and above the water

surface area (TBSA). The mice are then immersed in a 90–92 °C water bath to produce a ~12–15 % TBSA full thickness, scald injury (Fig. 4). Using this method, the damage encompasses the epidermis, dermis, hypodermis, and the murine panniculus carnosa. Mice can be sacrificed at similar time points as those used for excisional wound healing to evaluate the wound closure, as well as systemic inflammation and complications associated with burn trauma. It is important to note that in the absence of excisional debridement and grafting, the wound will heal significantly by contracture and fibrosis. At sacrifice, wounds are removed with an 8 mm punch biopsy which encompasses half of the burn wound tissue and half of the uninjured tissue just proximal to the burn site.

2   Materials

2.1 Prototypical Animal Strains in Aging Studies

1. BALB/c: Young 10–16 weeks, Aged 18–22 months [20, 21].
2. C57BL/6: Young 8–14 weeks, Aged 25–32 months [22].
3. CBA: Young 8–14 weeks, Aged 25–27 months [23].

2.2 Excisional Wound Injury and Isolation of Wound Tissue

1. Anesthesia solution: Ketamine (100 mg/mL solution), xylazine (100 mg/mL) and sterile saline. Prior to injury, combine 1 mL of stock ketamine, 0.2 mL of stock xylazine and 3.8 mL of sterile, 0.9 % normal saline in a sterile 15 mL polypropylene conical tube. Mix by inverting the tube.
2. Sterile, 0.9 % normal saline, warmed to 37 °C.
3. Sterile alcohol prep pads.
4. Electric animal hair clippers with #40 blade.
5. Single-use, sterile, 25 G, 1 mL tuberculin syringes.
6. 3 mm punch biopsy for wounding (Acuderm Inc., Fort Lauderdale, FL).
7. Hockey puck.
8. Scissors and forceps.
9. 5 mm punch biopsy for removal of wounds and adjacent tissue from dorsal skin pelt (Acuderm Inc., Fort Lauderdale, FL).
10. Analytical balance and weigh boats.
11. Single use, straight edge razors (Personna America Safety Razor Co., Verona, VA).
12. Paper towels.
13. Examination gloves.
14. Heating pads.

2.3 Burn Wound Injury and Isolation of Wound Tissue

1. Anesthesia solution: Ketamine (100 mg/mL solution), xylazine (100 mg/mL) and sterile saline. Prior to injury, combine 1 mL of stock ketamine, 0.2 mL of stock xylazine and 3.8 mL of sterile, 0.9 % normal saline in a 15 mL polypropylene conical tube. Mix by inverting the tube.
2. Sterile 0.9 % normal saline, warmed to 37 °C (Hospira Inc., Lake Forest, IL).
3. Electric animal hair clippers (*see* Subheading 2.2).
4. Hot plate.
5. Thermometer.
6. Two Metal pans with lid (1 quart, ~21.5 × 11.5 cm pans, Fisher Scientific, Pittsburgh, PA).
7. Deionized water.

8. Single-use, sterile, 1 mL tuberculin syringes with 25 G needles Burn injury template (Fig. 3).

9. 8 mm punch biopsy for removal of burn tissue and adjacent tissue from dorsal skin pelt (Acuderm Inc., Fort Lauderdale, FL).

10. Analytical balance and weigh boats.

11. Single use straight edge razors (Personna America Safety Razor Co., Verona, VA).

12. Paper towels.

13. Examination gloves.

14. Stop watch or timer.

15. Heating pads.

16. Blunt dissecting scissors.

17. Forceps.

2.4 Subsequent Tissue Analysis: Excisional Wounds and Burn Wounds

Bacterial colonization

1. 5 mL polypropylene, round bottom tubes.

2. Sterile PBS.

3. Rotor-stator homogenizer.

4. Agar plates for desired bacteria (i.e., MSA for *S. aureus* and centrimide for *P. aeruginosa*).

5. Sterile plate spreaders.

6. Incubator.

2.5 Preparation for Measurement of Wound Closure by Pixels

1. Digital Canon EOS SLR Camera.

2. Camera stand.

3. Metric ruler.

4. Hockey puck.

5. Adobe Photoshop Version 7.0 (Adobe Systems Inc., San Jose, CA).

2.6 Preparation for Wound Cell Isolation for Flow Cytometry

1. 24-well tissue culture dishes.

2. Dispase Solution: 5 mL of RPMI 1640 culture media containing 10 % fetal bovine serum (FBS), 2 mM L-glutamine, 1 % penicillin/streptomycin, 3 mL of dispase II at 1 mg/mL (Roche Diagnostics, Indianapolis, IN), 2 mL of gentamicin sulfate at 10 mg/mL.

3. Plate shaker at 4 °C.

2.7 RNA Isolation from Wound Tissue

1. Liquid nitrogen.

2. 1.7 mL Eppendorf tubes.

3. RNA Easy Kit (Qiagen, Valencia, CA).

2.8 Protein Isolation from Wound Tissue	1. Liquid nitrogen. 2. 1.7 mL Eppendorf tubes. 3. 5 mL polypropylene tubes (BD Falcon, Bedford, MA). 4. Acrodisc filter, 1.2 mm, 32 mm (Utech Products, Schenectady, NY). 5. 1 mL sterile tuberculin syringes with 25 G needle. 6. BioRad Lysis Buffer (Lysis Buffer, Factor 1 and Factor 2; BioRad, Hercules, CA). 7. Ice and dry ice.
2.9 OCT Embedding of Wound Tissue	1. Tissue-Tek O.C.T compound (Sakura Finetek, Torrance, CA). 2. Straight edge razor (Personna America Safety Razor Co., Verona, VA). 3. Disposable base molds, 15 mm × 15 mm × 5 mm (Fischer HealthCare, Houston, TX).
2.10 Formalin Fixation of Wound Tissue	1. 10 % formalin. 2. Tissue-Tek Uni-cassette (Sakura Finetek, Torrance, CA). 3. Straight Edge Razor (Personna America Safety Razor Co., Verona, VA).
2.11 Immunofluorescent Staining of Wound Tissue	1. Superfrosted PLUS slides (Fischer Scientific, Pittsburgh, PA). 2. PAP pen (Sigma-Aldrich, St. Louis, MO). 3. 4 % paraformaldehyde (PFA) in sterile PBS, filtered, 37 °C Sterile PBS, filtered. 4. Normal Goat Serum (NGS, Jackson ImmunoResearch, West Grove, PA), or serum that is appropriate given the speciation of the secondary antibody in use. 5. Bovine Serum Albumin (BSA, Sigma-Aldrich, St. Louis, MO). 6. Primary and secondary antibodies of interest. 7. VectaShield Hard Set Mounting Media with DAPI (Vector Labs, Burlingame, CA). 8. Coverslips.

3   Methods

All animal procedures and protocols must be reviewed and approved by the Institutional Animal Care and Use Committee (IACUC) in the investigator's home institution and researchers must be appropriately trained and qualified to carry out the procedures below.

3.1 Excisional Wound Injury and Isolation of Wound Tissue

1. Prepare anesthesia mixture fresh prior to use as described (*see* Subheading 2.2 above) and load into a single use syringe. Weigh the mice. For a 20–25 g mouse, 100 µL of solution will result in 100 mg/kg ketamine/10 mg/kg xylazine as desired.

2. Grasp the mouse at the nape of the neck and tail. Tilt the head of the mouse downwards. Inject desired volume of anesthetic *intraperitoneally* (*i.p.*) in the left lower quadrant based on the weight of the animals to achieve 100 mg ketamine/10 mg xylazine as desired.

3. Following injection of the anesthesia, inject 1 mL of warmed, sterile saline *i.p.* in the left lower quadrant. This promotes distribution of the anesthetic and prevents dehydration as the full effects of anesthesia can last upwards of 3 h. Return the mouse to a clean cage and allow for the anesthesia to take effect, ~5 min.

4. Once the mouse no longer responds to firm pressure applied to the hind limb, shave the dorsum with animal clippers. Alternate methods of hair removal mentioned above can be used but will not be discussed here.

5. Cleanse the shaved area with an alcohol prep pad. Be sure to cleanse the entire area but do not douse the mouse in ethanol as excessive ethanol can perturb the epidermal barrier. Allow the ethanol to evaporate.

6. Lift the skin in the mid-dorsal line and fold over a hockey puck (Fig. 1a). Using a 3 mm (or size desired) dermal punch biopsy, push punch biopsy tool through the folded skin, such that a wound on each side of the dorsal midline is created (Fig. 1b). Repeat this procedure for the desired number of wounds (Fig. 1c). With 3–5 mm dorsal punch biopsies, we suggest creating 4–6 wounds per mouse. We recommend limiting larger wounds, 6 mm or greater, to two wounds per mouse dorsum.

7. Return the mice to clean cages on heating pads and allow for recovery from anesthesia (~3–4 h). Given that these studies involve the evaluation of the inflammatory stages of wound healing, no analgesics are given as they can interfere with the inflammatory immune process.

8. Sacrifice mice by CO_2 inhalation at desired time point to evaluate the various phases of wound healing: Inflammatory (3 h to 3 days), Proliferative (3–14 days), Remodeling (14 days and onwards). These time delineations will be variable to a certain degree depending on the initial size of the wound.

9. To harvest the wounds, carefully dissect the dorsal pelt from the mouse using scissors and forceps (Fig. 2a, b). Ensure that when removing tissue around the wound site to include all granulation tissue. This requires patience particularly at early

time points when the granulation tissue and wound matrix is still delicate.

10. Place the pelt on a hockey puck (Fig. 2c). Then, use a punch biopsy 2 mm larger than the size used to inflict the wounds to remove the wound tissue and surrounding wound margins (Fig. 2d, e). If evaluating wound size, photograph the pelt at a fixed distance with a metric ruler in the plane of the photo. Process the tissue as described below.

3.2 Burn Wound Injury and Isolation of Wound Tissue

1. Prepare anesthesia mixture prior to use on day of injury as described in Subheading 3.1 and load into single use syringe. Weigh the mice. For a 20–25 g mouse, 100 μL of solution will result in 100 mg/kg ketamine/10 mg/kg xylazine as desired.

2. Grasp the mouse at the nape of the neck and tail. Tilt the head of the mouse downwards. Inject desired volume of anesthetic *i.p.* in the left lower quadrant based on the weight of the animals to achieve 100 mg ketamine/10 mg xylazine as desired.

3. Prepare the water bath by filling two metal containers with deionized water. Heat one container to 90–92 °C for scald burn injury. Keep the thermometer in the water bath at all times to ensure the temperature remains tightly controlled from mouse to mouse. The second container will be maintained at ambient temperature for sham injury (Fig. 3).

4. Once the mouse no longer responds to firm pressure applied to the hind limb, shave the dorsum with an electric clipper. Be sure to shave over the entire area of anticipated injury, from the nape of the neck to the tail. Shave beyond where the injury itself will be placed, as skin will contract after burn. Alternate methods of hair removal mentioned above can be used but will not be discussed here.

5. Based on the animal's weight, select the appropriate burn template to give a 12–15 % total body surface area (TBSA) burn (Fig. 3). When placing the mouse in the burn template, ensure that the dorsum of the animal is flush with the burn template by gently pushing on the abdomen. Ensure the tail remains out of the template and above the water.

6. Immerse the dorsum, template lined area of the mouse in the water bath for 8 s (Fig. 4). Watch the timer carefully to ensure the time in the water is a constant 8 s for each mouse. We recommend this temperature and timing to ensure a full thickness burn.

7. Immediately remove the mouse and blot the dorsal scald area with a paper towel to prevent continued scald injury.

8. Resuscitate the mouse by injecting 1 mL of warmed, sterile saline *i.p.* in the left lower quadrant.

9. Return the mouse to a clean cage and place the cages on heating pads for 3–4 h, or until the mice are aroused from anesthesia. Given that these studies involve evaluation the inflammatory stages of wound healing, no analgesics are given as they can interfere with the inflammatory immune process.

10. Sacrifice mice by CO_2 inhalation at desired time point to evaluate the various phases of wound healing as delineated above.

11. To harvest the wounds, carefully dissect the dorsal pelt from the mouse. Remove an extra 4 mm of tissue from the margin of the burn wound to include all granulation tissue.

12. Place the pelt on a hockey puck. Use a 5–8 mm punch biopsy to remove the burn tissue at the wound margin, such that half of the punch biopsy contained burn wound and the remaining half contains intact skin from the wound margin.

13. Process the tissue as described below.

3.3 Models of Combined Wound Injury and Infection: Excisional Wound Injury and Staphylococcus aureus Infection

1. Follow the steps above under Subheading 3.1 through **step 6**.

2. Immediately after injury, pipette desired CFU/mL in 10 µL directly into each open wound bed. Be sure to change pipette tips between each wound on a given mouse.

   (a) *S. aureus* growth and inoculation: *S. aureus* of the desired strain can be grown overnight in tryptic soy broth (TSB) at 37 °C under constant agitation. The next day, 1 mL of *S. aureus* in TSB is resuspended in 2 mL fresh TSB and incubated at 37 °C for 2 h under constant agitation to ensure mid-logarithmic growth at the time of application to cutaneous wounds. Bacterial concentration (CFU/mL) is then determined by absorbance at 600 nm and the final inoculum confirmed by back-plating on mannitol salt agar (MSA; BD Diagnostics, Sparks, MD).

3. Resume the protocol under Subheading 3.1 at **step 7**. Evaluation of bacterial colonization at the time of sacrifice is described below.

3.4 Burn Wound Injury and Topical Pseudomonas aeruginosa Infection

1. Follow the steps above under Subheading 3.2 through **step 8**.

   (a) *P. aeruginosa* growth and inoculation: *P. aeruginosa* of the desired strain can be grown overnight on centrimide agar plates (BD Diagnostics, Sparks, MD) at 37 °C. The next day, inoculate sterile saline with one loop of *P. aeruginosa* from centrimide agar plate. Bacterial concentration (CFU/mL) is then determined by absorbance at 600 nm and the final inoculum confirmed by back-plating on centrimide agar plates (BD Diagnostics, Sparks, MD).

2. After towel drying the mouse to prevent further scald injury, slowly pipette desired bacteria concentration in CFU/mL in

100 μL directly onto the burn wound surface. (*Note*: A larger volume is used in the burn injury protocol secondary to the larger surface are of injury as compared to the individual wounds in the cutaneous punch biopsy model). Be sure to change pipette tips between each wound on a given mouse.

3. Resume the protocol under Subheading 3.2 at **step 9**. Evaluation of bacterial colonization at the time of sacrifice is described below.

3.5 Subsequent Tissue Analysis: Excisional Wounds and Burn Wounds Bacterial Colonization

1. Prior to euthanizing animals, place 1 mL of sterile PBS in each tube, with one tube per animal. Place tube on ice.

2. After harvesting the wounds from individual animals, place one wound in a 1 mL saline-filled tube. Maintain the tube on ice until all harvesting is complete.

    (a) Note: You may choose to weigh each wound as to express your final data as CFU/gm of tissue. If you do not weigh your tissue, you will express your data as CFU/mL or CFU/wound.

3. Using the rotor-stator homogenizer, homogenize the wound in saline. Maintain the tube on ice during homogenization.

4. Directly plate 20 μL of homogenate onto agar plates in duplicate. Spread with sterile plate spreaders.

5. Next create 1:10 serial dilutions of the homogenate. The number of serial dilutions created will depend on the initial bacterial inoculum and expected growth. We recommend creating 8 serial dilutions of 1:10 for your initial experiments.

6. Plate each serial dilution in duplicate.

7. Incubate plates for 24–48 h depending on the bacterial species utilized.

8. Following incubation, count the colonies on each agar plate. Be sure to multiply the colony count on a given plate by the dilution factor. Average these colony counts to obtain the CFU/20 μL and then multiply this by a factor of 50 to obtain the CFU/mL (or per wound). If expressing the data as per gram of tissue, multiply by the gram weight of the wound measured (*see* **Note 1**).

3.6 Measurement of Wound Closure by Digital Photography and Image Analysis

1. Attach the digital camera onto the camera stand at a fixed distance above the height of the hockey puck. We recommend a fixed distance of 20 cm.

2. Remove the dorsal pelt as described above in Subheading 3.2.

3. Place the pelt flat on the hockey puck. Align a metric ruler with the wounds in the frame of the photograph.

4. Photograph the pelt including all wounds in a single image.

5. Using Adobo Photoshop 7.0 (Adobe Systems Inc., San Jose, CA) determine the number of pixels in the open wound area using the magic wand tool, with zoom at 100 % and a tolerance setting of 60.

6. As controls, a separate set of animals should be sacrificed immediately following wound injury and wound size determined to represent day 0.

7. Each wound area at each time point is then compared with average pixels of day 0 wounds such that: [(individual wound pixels at day greater than day 0)/(averaged pixels of day 0 wounds) × 100] is used to determine the percent open wound area at each time point.

8. The individual wounds of each animal are then averaged to give one value for the open wound area for the animal. Example: If an animal has six wound sites, the % open area of each wound would be calculated as above, and then the wounds from that animal would be calculated as the average of the % open area of all six wounds (sum of % open wound are of six wounds divided by 6). Thus, the average of six wounds is an N of one individual animal.

3.7 Wound Cell Isolation for Flow Cytometry

A detailed procedure for isolation and staining of wound cells can be found in our previously published manuscript [24]. The procedure below only details the initial processing for tissue for flow cytometry following wound excision. Details of subsequent processing and staining can be carried out as described [24].

1. Prepare "Dispase Solution."

2. Remove dorsal pelt and excise wounds from mice at desired time-points following excisional cutaneous injury as described above. Be sure to not use any ethanol in washing of the pelt as ethanol may disrupt the cell membrane and promote lysis. If you wish to wash the pelt, do so in sterile PBS.

3. Collect 2–3 wounds per animal and determine weight of samples in grams.

4. Mince wounds into small pieces (<2 mm × 2 mm) with a straight razor.

5. Place wound pieces into a 24-well culture plate (1 well/animal) filled with 15.4 mL "Dispase Solution"/gram of tissue (*see* **Note 2**).

6. Incubate plate overnight at 4 °C on a rotating shaker at a gentle setting.

7. Follow remaining step as outlined [24].

3.8 RNA Isolation from Wound Tissue

1. Immediately following removal of the wound tissue, add 1–2 wounds to a 1.7 mL Eppendorf tube and snap freeze in liquid nitrogen.

2. Store at –80 °C until ready to process tissue for RNA.

3. Using the RNA Easy Kit (Qiagen), isolate RNA as per the manufacturer's instructions (*see* **Note 3**).

3.9 Protein Isolation from Wound Tissue

1. Prepare Lysis Buffer: 9.9 mL BioRad Lysis Buffer, 40 µL BioRad Factor I, 20 µL BioRad Factor 2, and 40 µL PMSF.

2. Place frozen tissue samples on dry ice.

3. Add 1 mL of Lysis Buffer to each polypropylene tube and keep on wet ice.

4. Using forceps, remove tissue and place in polypropylene tube and homogenize for 30 s until no tissue bits are left. Return to ice bucket.

5. Spin the polypropylene tubes at $300 \times g$ at 4 °C for 5 min.

6. Transfer the supernatant to 1.7 mL Eppendorf tubes.

7. Sonicate samples at a 30 % setting for 10 s.

8. Centrifuge at 4 °C for 10 min at $2655 \times g$ (5000 rpm using an Eppendorf centrifuge 5417 R, Eppendorf, Hamburg, Germany).

9. Remove the supernatant, avoiding the pellet, with a 1 mL single-use syringe.

10. Filter the supernatant through a 25 µM single use syringe filter into a clean 1.7 mL Eppendorf tube. Maintain tube on ice.

11. Aliquot sample into fresh 1.7 mL Eppendorf tubes.

12. Snap freeze in liquid nitrogen and store at –80 °C until use.

3.10 OCT Embedding of Wound Tissue

1. Place a small amount of OCT compound into the Tissue Tray. Allow to lightly cover the bottom of the cassette.

2. Using the straight razor, cut the outer 1/3 of wound.

3. Place the wound so the straight edge is flush with edge of tissue cassette.

4. Cover the tissue with OCT, avoiding bubbles.

5. Freeze immediately by placing cassette on dry ice.

6. Store at –80 °C until use.

3.11 Formalin Fixation of Wound Tissue

1. Fill a plastic container with 10 % formalin.

2. Using the straight razor, cut the outer 1/3 of the wound.

3. Place the wound in the tissue cassette.

4. Place the tissue cassette in the formalin bath.

5. Store at room temperature until use.

3.12 Immunofluorescent Staining of Wound Tissue

1. Remove stored frozen tissue in OCT.

2. Section wound tissue at 3–8 μm onto Superfrosted Plus slides. We recommend sectioning tissue at 5 μm.

3. Place sections in a humidified chamber at room temperature for 2 h.

4. Encircle sections with PAP pen.

5. Fix tissue sections in 4 % PFA (filtered, 37 °C) for 15 min. Tap off PFA.

6. Wash with sterile PBS three times for 5 min, tapping off PBS between washes (*see* **Note 4**).

7. Block with 10 % BSA and 3 % Normal Goat Serum (or normal serum of the species of the secondary antibody) in sterile PBS for 1 h at room temperature.

8. Tip slides to remove blocking solution. Do not wash the tissue sections after removal of the blocking solution.

9. Gently add ~100 μL of the primary antibody diluted in PBS to each tissue section. Note it will be important to titrate the primary antibody to an appropriate concentration (*see* **Note 5**). Incubate the slide in the primary antibody overnight at 4 °C. Be sure to include appropriate positive and negative controls.

10. Tap off the primary antibody. Wash the tissue sections three times with sterile PBS for 5 min each, tapping of PBS between each wash.

11. Incubate with secondary antibody diluted in PBS (titrated to the desired concentration) for 1 h at room temperature (*see* **Note 6**). Protect the slides from direct light.

12. Tap off the secondary antibody. Wash the slides three times for 5 min each in sterile PBS, tapping off PBS between washes.

13. Let slides air dry and then place 2–4 drops of VectaShield Mounting Media with DAPI nuclear stain on the slide and cover slip. Avoid air bubbles. Seal cover slip to slide with clear nail polish. Once completely dried, store samples at 4 °C.

14. Visualize tissue with fluorescent microscope of choice.

---

4   Notes

1. This calculation can be confusing without additional explanation. The wound is homogenized in 1 mL of sterile saline. 20 μL of this solution is then plated following 1:10 serial dilutions. As an example, say 40 colonies grew on the 10^3 serial dilution—thus, 40×1000 would be 4×10^4 CFU/20 μL. Multiplying this value by 50 will transform this in CFU/mL or 2×10^6 CFU/mL.

2. Again this calculation can be confusing without further explanation. The average 3 mm wound with a 5 mm excision perimeter weight from 0.015 to 0.025 g per wound. As an example, assume all wounds weigh 0.02 g and multiple this value by the number of wounds that are used per isolation, for example three wounds, and this yields 0.06 g of tissue. Extending the calculation, if using the concentrations given above, then 15.4 mL of the dispase solution per gram of tissue is 15.4×0.06 results in 924 µL.

3. We recommend using two wounds for RNA analysis to ensure enough RNA is isolated for subsequent PCR analysis. We also recommend homogenizing the tissue with a rotor-stator homogenizer, taking care to rinse the homogenizer between each sample with ethanol.

4. We recommend performing all the washes with PBS with the slides horizontal position, such that you gentle pipette the PBS on and gently tap it off, rather than in a vertical position as you would if they were to wash the slides in Coplin jars. We found that this results in better retention of tissue on the Superfrosted plus slides.

5. Antibody titration will be dependent of the antibody and manufacturer. However, in our experience, the recommended concentration by the manufacturer tends to result in significant non-specific binding and high background. We recommend starting at half the concentration recommended by the manufacturer and then performing a 1:2 serial dilution.

6. Of note, it is important to have three control slide: (a) tissue that was blocked but received no antibody, (b) tissue that was blocked and stained with the primary antibody only, and (c) tissue that was blocked and stained with the secondary antibody only. The first two serve as negative controls as no fluorescent signal should be detected, the third allows you to determine the specificity of the secondary antibody for the primary antibody and the amount of background staining that is not specific. Significant signal on the third slide suggests: (a) poor blocking by the blocking solution, (b) poor affinity of the secondary antibody for the primary antibody, or (c) too high of a concentration of the secondary antibody.

Acknowledgements

The authors thank Jessica Palmer for her critical review and discussion of this manuscript. This work was supported by NIH R21 AI073987 (E.J.K.), R01 AG018859 (E.J.K.), T32 AG031780 (P.L.W.), T32 GM008750 (R.L.G.) and by the Dr. Ralph and Marian C. Falk Medical Research Trust (E.J.K.).

References

1. Singer AJ, Clark RA (1999) Cutaneous wound healing. N Engl J Med 341:738–746
2. Reinke JM, Sorg H (2012) Wound repair and regeneration. Eur Surg Res 49:35–43
3. Gillitzer R, Goebeler M (2001) Chemokines in cutaneous wound healing. J Leukoc Biol 69:513–521
4. Kim MH, Liu W, Borjesson DL et al (2008) Dynamics of neutrophil infiltration during cutaneous wound healing and infection using fluorescence imaging. J Invest Dermatol 128:1812–1820
5. Daley JM, Brancato SK, Thomay AA et al (2010) The phenotype of murine wound macrophages. J Leukoc Biol 87:59–67
6. Nissen NN, Polverini PJ, Koch AE et al (1998) Vascular endothelial growth factor mediates angiogenic activity during the proliferative phase of wound healing. Am J Pathol 152:1445–1552
7. Swift ME, Kleinman HK, DiPietro LA (1999) Impaired wound repair and delayed angiogenesis in aged mice. Lab Invest 79:1479–1487
8. Sen CK, Gordillo GM, Roy S et al (2009) Human skin wounds: a major and snowballing threat to public health and the economy. Wound Repair Regen 17:763–771
9. Kaye KS, Anderson DJ, Sloane R et al (2009) The effect of surgical site infection on older operative patients. J Am Geriatr Soc 57:46–54
10. Vowden KR, Vowden P (2009) The prevalence, management and outcome for patients with lower limb ulceration identified in a wound care survey within one English health care district. J Tissue Viability 18:13–19
11. Christensen K, Doblhammer G, Rau R et al (2009) Ageing populations: the challenges ahead. Lancet 374:1196–1208
12. Brubaker AL, Palmer JL, Kovacs EJ (2011) Age-related dysregulation of inflammation and innate immunity: lessons learned from rodent models. Aging Dis 2:346–360
13. Panda A, Arjona A, Sapey E et al (2009) Human innate immunosenescence: causes and consequences for immunity in old age. Trends Immunol 30:325–333
14. Slater H, Gaisford JC (1981) Burns in older patients. J Am Geriatr Soc 29:74–76
15. Linn BS (1980) Age differences in the severity and outcome of burns. J Am Geriatr Soc 28:118–123
16. Clayton MC, Solem LD, Ahrenholz DH (1995) Pulmonary failure in geriatric patients with burns: the need for a diagnosis-related group modifier. J Burn Care Rehabil 16:451–454
17. Ely EW, Wheeler AP, Thompson BT et al (2002) Recovery rate and prognosis in older persons who develop acute lung injury and the acute respiratory distress syndrome. Ann Intern Med 136:25–36
18. Dancey DR, Hayes J, Gomez M et al (1999) ARDS in patients with thermal injury. Intensive Care Med 25:1231–1236
19. Le HQ, Zamboni W, Eriksson E et al (1986) Burns in patients under 2 and over 70 years of age. Ann Plast Surg 17:39–44
20. Nomellini V, Brubaker AL, Mahbub S et al (2012) Dysregulation of neutrophil CXCR2 and pulmonary endothelial ICAM-1 promotes age-related pulmonary inflammation. Aging Dis 3:234–247
21. Birjandi SZ, Ippolito JA, Ramadorai AK et al (2011) Alterations in marginal zone macrophages and marginal zone B cells in old mice. J Immunol 186:3441–3451
22. Zook EC, Krishack PA, Zhang S et al (2011) Overexpression of Foxn1 attenuates age-associated thymic involution and prevents the expansion of peripheral CD4 memory T cells. Blood 118:5723–5731
23. Bhattacharyya TK, Thomas JR (2004) Histomorphologic changes in aging skin: observations in the CBA mouse model. Arch Facial Plast Surg 6:21–25
24. Brubaker AL, Schneider DF, Palmer JL, Faunce DS, Kovacs EJ (2011) Wound cell isolation for flow cytometric and functional analysis neutrophils and natural killer T cells as negative regulators of wound healing. J Immunol Methods 373:161–166

Chapter 5

Multicolor Digital Flow Cytometry in Human Translational Immunology

Samit R. Joshi, Subhasis Mohanty, and Albert C. Shaw

Abstract

By facilitating the simultaneous analysis of parameters from diverse cell lineages and biological pathways, multicolor flow cytometry is integral to many studies in human immunology—particularly those in older individuals—where sample amounts may be limiting. Studies in human cohorts require particular attention to fluorochrome panel design and procedures to standardize instrument performance; reproducible instrument conditions (over time and between centers) are crucial to accurate comparisons and conclusions in the analysis of heterogeneous groups of human subjects. Here, we describe procedures for multicolor digital flow cytometry, our experience in flow cytometry panel design and our approach in standardizing instrument performance using BD Biosciences hardware and software (BD Biosciences, San Jose, CA). These techniques allow for the generation of accurate and precise data in a variety of settings.

Key words Multicolor flow cytometry, Translational immunology, Application settings, Flow cytometry standardization, Flow cytometry panel design

1   Introduction

Multicolor digital flow cytometry expands the opportunities for investigators to conduct translational immunological studies particularly in the context of limited samples (commonly encountered with human samples in general and with samples in studies of aging in particular). An increasing number of fluorochromes and antibodies, and advances in instrumentation/software have facilitated a growing number of applications; however, experimental design remains complex because of the need to maintain sample resolution in the context of controlling spillover in complex compensation matrices [1]. Thus, the optimal antibody panel for a given application depends upon variables such as: cytometer configuration, the type of sample (and the types/numbers of cells), and availability of flurochrome-conjugated antibodies [2].

Albert C. Shaw (ed.), *Immunosenescence: Methods and Protocols*, Methods in Molecular Biology, vol. 1343,
DOI 10.1007/978-1-4939-2963-4_5, © Springer Science+Business Media New York 2015

Here, we describe techniques our laboratory uses routinely, such as in the study of innate immune system parameters in freshly isolated PBMCs stimulated ex-vivo from patients. Specifically, we describe flow cytometry experimental design and processes for standardizing instrument performance using our center's experience with BD Biosciences hardware and software (BD Biosciences, San Jose, CA). We will not discuss sample preparation and staining which have been described in detail elsewhere [2, 3]. Rather, we focus on several practical "highlights" of this tool. Many of the techniques described below were utilized in several manuscripts and can be adapted for use in other applications [4, 5]. Ultimately, accurate and standardized data generated using these techniques are important in conducting large-scale (multicenter) translational studies.

2 Methods

2.1 Selection of Color Matrix

1. The investigator should identify the specific cytometer, available lasers, and installed filters at their institution. This information can be entered into an online spectral viewer allowing for an approximation of the spectral overlap between wavelengths (e.g.   http://www.bdbiosciences.com/research/multicolor/ spectrum_viewer/index.jsp). In our experience, employing more than 8–9 colors can lead to an increase in spectral overlap and subsequent difficulties in compensation. However, others have developed 15-color panels with success [6]. Consider that even though an instrument may support n colors, given the need to maintain resolution of populations, optimal panel design may only employ a portion of the available colors (e.g. $n-2$). Sufficient time should be dedicated to panel design to optimize results (*see* **Note 1**).

2.2 Selection of Antibodies

1. After identifying available fluorochromes, determine antibodies for the desired cell surface and intracellular markers of interest; the investigator should note which markers are relatively more important to their desired application than others. Some investigators advocate factoring in antigen density (number of molecules/cell) and whether the antigen is distinct or has a range of expression. One can consider prioritizing bright fluorochromes (e.g. PE or APC) on dim antigens (and more dim fluorochromes such as FITC or Alexa-700 paired with more abundant antigens) [7]. Consider using a site (e.g. http://www.biocompare.com) to conduct a screen of available antibodies for a given antigen. Keeping cost and antibody quality in mind, creating a matrix of fluorochromes and various cellular markers can aid in experimental design and maximize

the number of interrogated cellular targets (*see* **Note 2**). Arrive at a final list of cell surface and/or intracellular antibodies and obtain trial sizes of the desired antibodies from the manufacturers.

2.3 Optimizing Antibody Concentration for Staining

1. While all antibody manufacturers suggest a working dilution of antibody, the investigator should always take the opportunity to optimize antibody concentration for their application. For each new antibody, one can try several dilutions (e.g. 1:10, 1:50, 1:100) on the cells of interest (*see* **Note 3**). For cellular targets with relatively low baseline expression (e.g. inflammatory cytokines), consider using conditions similar to your experimental protocol. For example, our experimental timeline for interrogating dendritic cells requires 2 h of stimulation with TLR ligands followed by the addition of Brefeldin A and 4 additional hours of incubation [4]. Accordingly, when optimizing our intracellular antibody concentration for assessing production of a given pro-inflammatory cytokine, we will conduct the antibody concentration optimization trial following the same experimental conditions. Additionally, the optimal dilution should be tested on approximately the same number of cells that will be present in the experimental sample. Consider using the dilution at which the Mean Fluorescence Intensity plateaus (on a histogram plot) (*see* **Note 4**).

2. Once optimal antibody concentrations have been developed, carry out a trial experiment using experimental conditions with the full antibody panel to evaluate panel performance and identify, in the early stages, possible refinements to the steps above [6] (*see* **Note 5**).

2.4 Create Application Settings

1. Since many institutions, including our own, use BD Flow Cytometers (BD Biosciences, San Jose, CA), we will take this opportunity to briefly describe key features in BD FACSDiva v6.0 software. Like many others, our center utilizes Cytometer Setup and Tracking (CST) beads for reproducible instrument setup and tracking of performance on a daily basis. We find this leads to decreased variability and improved data quality. Using the information gathered from the CST baseline cytometer support, Application settings can be established for a particular assay. We find the use of Application settings allows for consistent settings, less spillover, higher resolution, and more reproducible data by automatically adjusting Photomultiplier Tube (PMT) voltages based upon daily instrument performance. In our experience, the use of both Application settings and CST beads will keep a consistent Mean Fluorescence Intensity (MFI) for a particular parameter over time despite any potential minor variations in instrument performance. This is particularly

Detector Settings (Continued)

Laser	Detector	Parameter	Linearity Min Channel	Linearity Max Channel	Slope	Intercept	Electronic Noise Robust SD	Qr	Br
Blue	FSC	FSC	N/A	N/A	0.0038	3.4	N/A	N/A	N/A
Blue	C	SSC	N/A	N/A	6.1987	-9.9	N/A	N/A	N/A
Blue	B	Alexa Fluor 488	117	238677	7.6572	-16.3	14.5	0.126	251
Blue	A	PerCP	648	237031	7.8299	-16.9	14.5	0.0607	19
Red	C	APC	41	235762	7.5226	-15.5	17.8	0.1529	0
Red	B	Alexa Fluor 680	71	234323	7.5239	-15.9	20.5	0.0154	1733
Red	A	APC-Cy7	47	235799	7.6689	-15.7	15.8	0.0167	5230
Violet	C	Cascade Blue	55	235614	7.5658	-15.2	21.5	0.124	5156
Violet	B	AmCyan	34	247762	7.5371	-15.5	20.7	0.0042	75370
Violet	A	Qdot 655	29	237684	7.6880	-16.2	22.2	0.0564	169

Fig. 1 Sample cytometer baseline report. *Red arrows* indicate baseline maximum linearity and electronic noise rSD for each respective parameter, respectively. The operator should calculate one-half the maximum linearity and 2.5–3× the rSD (this can be done separately on paper or using computer software)

important for data accuracy and consistency when frequently running clinical samples over a long period of time or between multiple centers (*see* **Note 6**).

2. First, using information gathered from the cytometer baseline report (*see* Fig. 1), separately calculate 2.5–3× the baseline robust standard deviation of the electronic noise (rSD) and one-half of the baseline maximum linearity for each desired parameter. This will optimize resolution by keeping the negative population above the background electronic noise and the positive population below the maximum of the range in which the relation between MFI and PMT voltage is linear.

3. For our experiments, we prepare freshly isolated unstained human PBMCs and also stain (with one color) PBMCs with anti-CD8 antibodies. For most fluorochromes (including Alexa 700, FITC, APC-Cy7, PerCP, and APC) we use 10 μl of stock antibody. However, for PE and PE-Cy7 we use a 5 μl 1:10 dilution (in PBS alone) and for PE-Texas Red we prefer a 5 μl 1:100 dilution (in PBS alone) (*see* **Note 7**).

4. Next, we create a new experiment with all of the desired parameters (adding or deleting as necessary). For human PBMCs, we prefer to set the Forward Scatter (FSC) threshold to 10,000 (see Inspector—Cytometer settings, Thresholds tab). In Fig. 2, the global worksheet is arranged with a scatter plot gating on the lymphocyte population (P1). This population (P1) will be used to evaluate the unstained and stained (for CD8+) PBMCs through histograms and related statistics. Create one table of statistics for rSD that will be later used when recording unstained cells (Fig. 3).

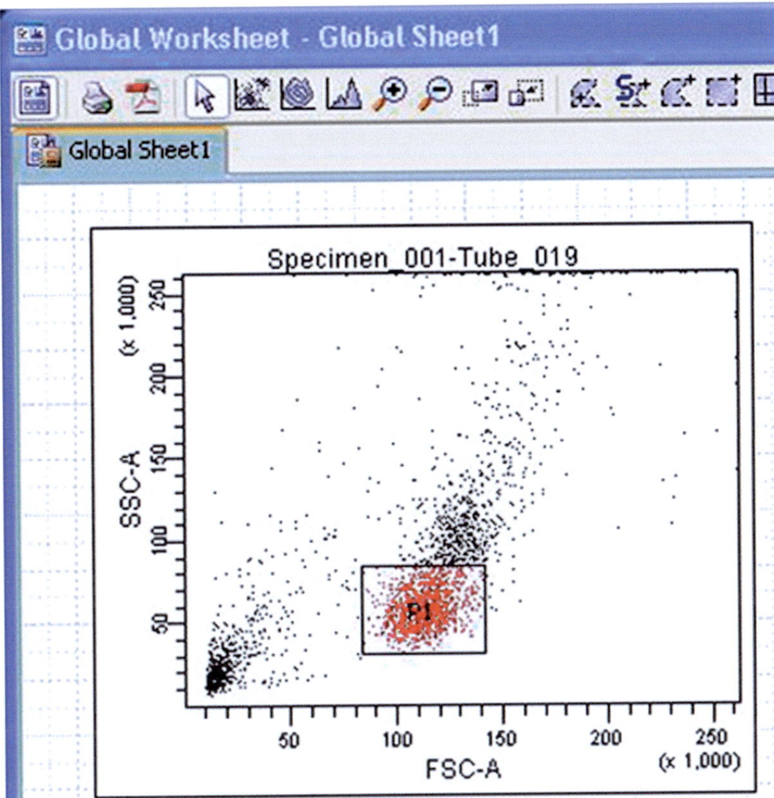

Fig. 2 Lymphocyte gate (P1) in global worksheet. Note adjustments using FSC, SSC, and actual gate can be adjusted when acquiring PBMCs

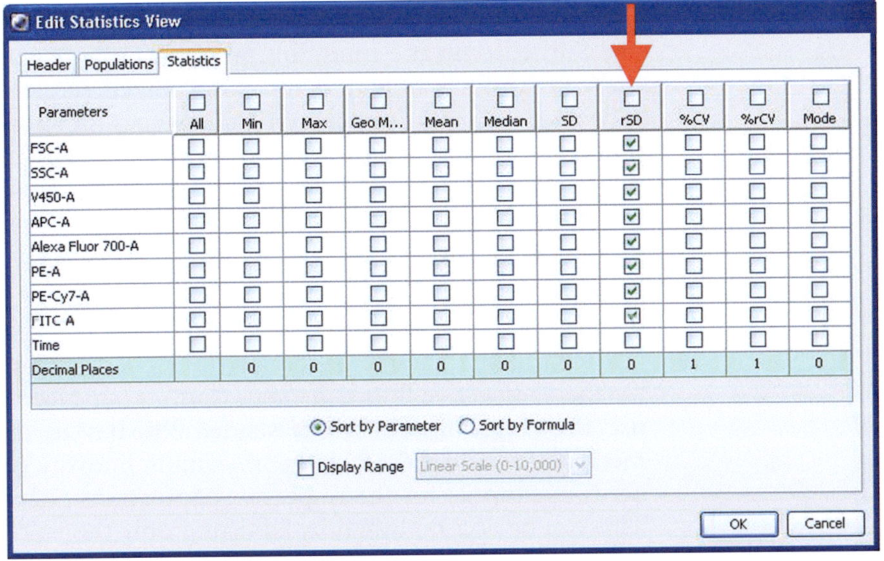

Fig. 3 Table of statistics (rSD). Creation of a table of statistics only with rSD values (*red arrow*). Notice how our sample experiment only uses six flurochromes

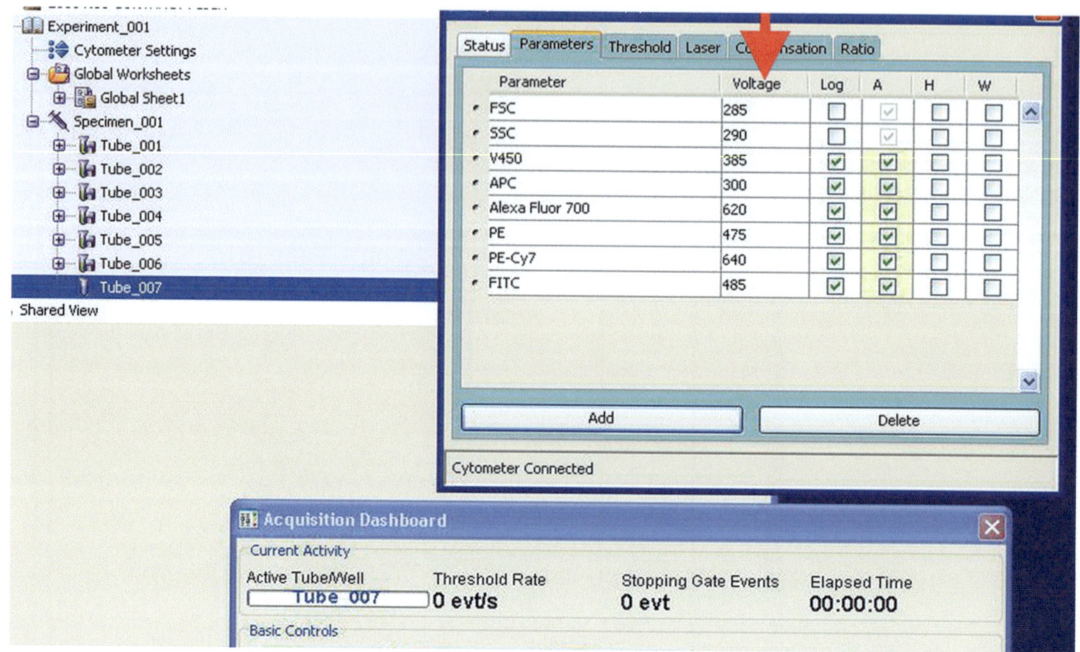

Fig. 4 Adjust parameter voltage. While recording events, the voltage of each parameter can be adjusted individually (*red arrow*)

5. Use unstained PBMCs to record approximately 2000 events. Adjust the voltage of each flurochrome (Fig. 4) to ensure the rSD statistic for that flurochrome in P1 (the lymphocyte gate) is inside a range of 2.5–3× the baseline standard deviation of the electronic noise value (calculated above in **step 2**). On a practical note, it is easier for the operator to focus on one flurochrome at a time; this process can be repeated when the voltage for any parameter is optimized (creating a new tube after each adjustment) until all voltages for all parameters reflect their respective rSD to be within a range of 2.5–3× the baseline standard deviation of the electronic noise (Fig. 5) (*see* **Note 8**).

6. Create another table of statistics for medians (Fig. 6) and a histogram for each parameter (showing the P1 population) with an interval gate located on the bright (CD8+) population (P2 for the first parameter, P3 for the second parameter, etc.) for their respective fluorochromes (Fig. 7) (*see* **Note 9**). Next, use the single fluorochrome-stained PBMCs to ensure the median is one-half the baseline maximum linearity (calculated above in **step 2**) for the respective populations (P2, P3, etc.). This can be accomplished by adjusting only the voltage of the parameter corresponding to the actively recorded single fluorochrome-stained PBMCs for CD8+. For example, if using v450-stained CD8+ PBMCs, only adjust the v450 voltage to

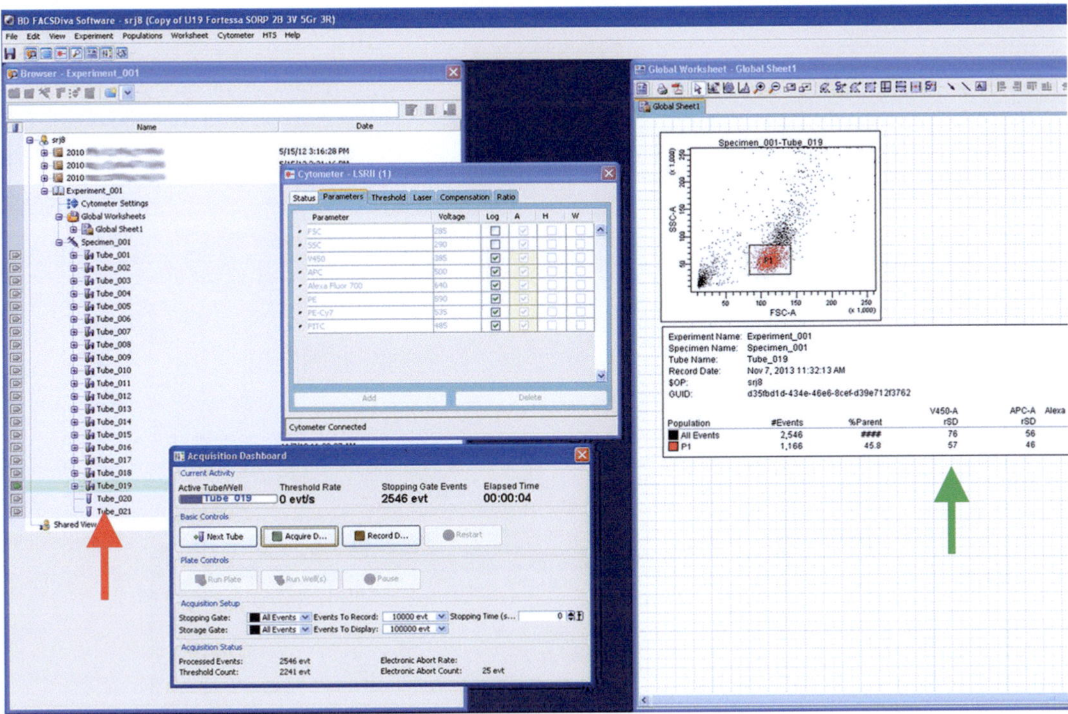

Fig. 5 Using unstained PBMCs to optimize voltage based on 2.5–3× the baseline rSD. A new tube (*red arrow*) is created after each adjustment of the voltage for the respective parameter's rSD (in this case V450, *green arrow*) to be within 2.5–3× the baseline value

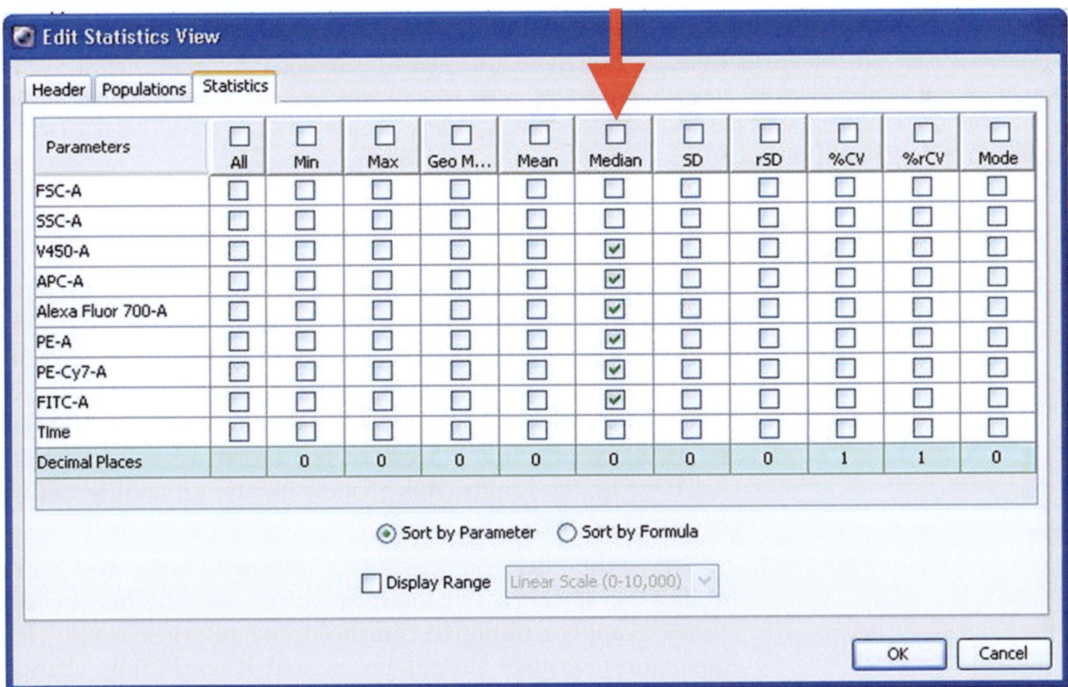

Fig. 6 Table of statistics (median) creation of a new table of statistics only with median values (*red arrow*)

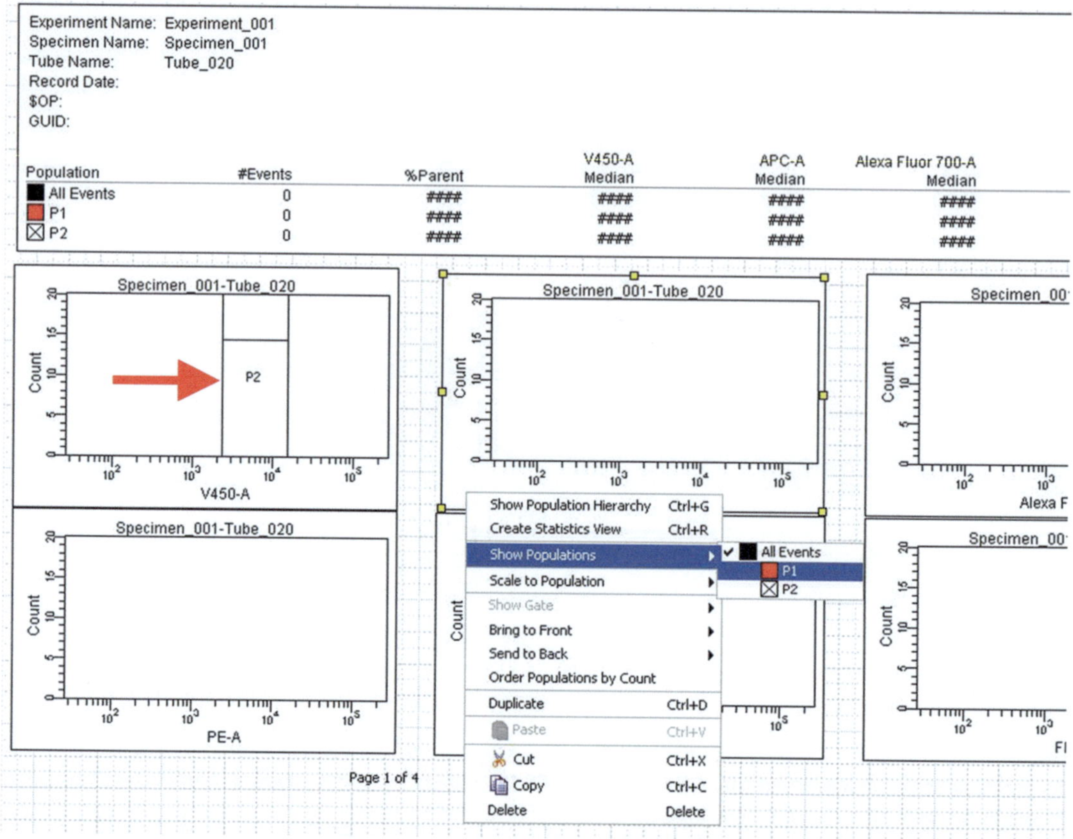

Fig. 7 Creation of individual histograms. Creation of individual histograms for each respective parameter (each with their own gate on their own bright population) showing only the P1 population (in our case PBMCs stained for CD8 using a v450-conjugated antibody, *red arrow*). *Note*: prior to running the single flurochrome stained PBMCs, this is a reasonable estimate of where the bright CD8$^+$ population will be. This can be modified during acquisition of the PBMCs (*see* Fig. 8)

ensure the median statistic of the PBMC CD8$^+$ v450 population is within one-half the baseline maximum linearity for the relative population (i.e. P2, Fig. 8). If using APC-stained CD8$^+$ PBMCs, adjust only the APC voltage to ensure the PBMC CD8$^+$ APC population median statistic is within one-half the baseline maximum linearity for the relative populations (i.e. P3, Fig. 9). Repeat this process for the remaining fluorochromes (*see* **Note 10**).

7. Finally, right click on cytometer settings, save, and name Application settings. The instrument may ask whether the user wishes to apply a modified threshold; our response is yes. New Application settings should be created if conditions change, such as: a new instrument baseline is obtained, new CST bead

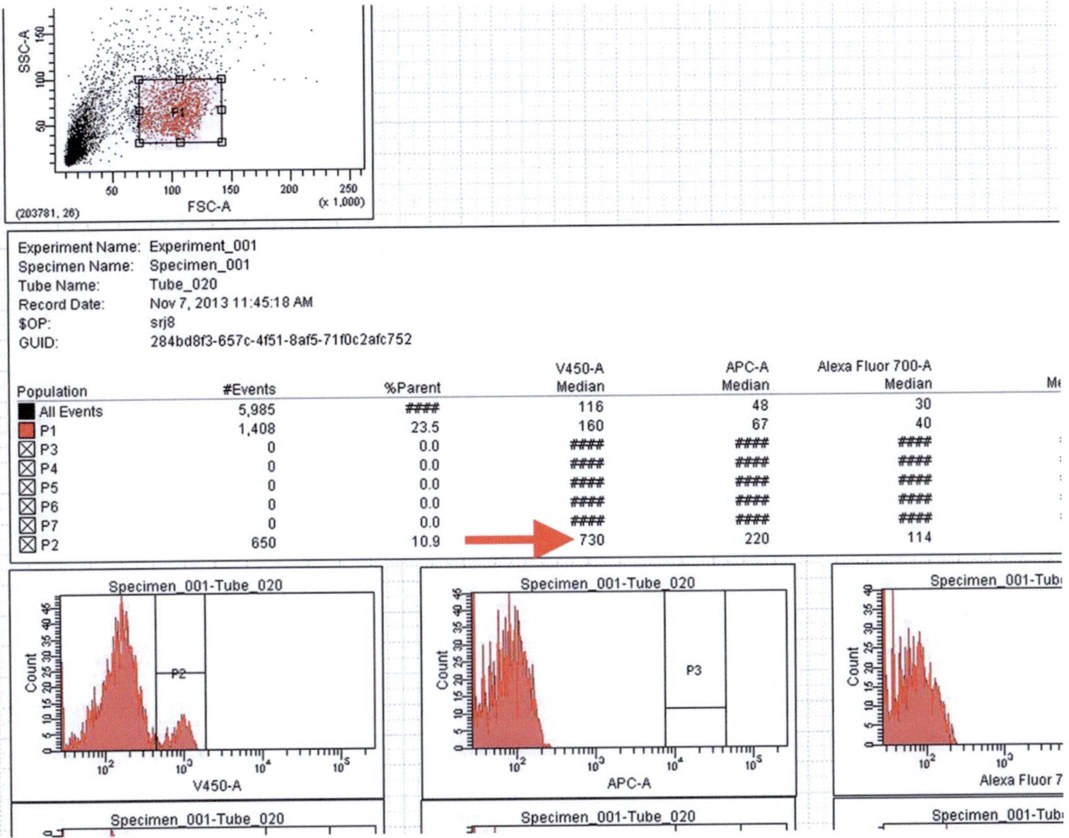

Population	#Events	%Parent	V450-A Median	APC-A Median	Alexa Fluor 700-A Median	M...
All Events	5,985	####	116	48	30	
P1	1,408	23.5	160	67	40	
P3	0	0.0	####	####	####	
P4	0	0.0	####	####	####	
P5	0	0.0	####	####	####	
P6	0	0.0	####	####	####	
P7	0	0.0	####	####	####	
P2	650	10.9	730	220	114	

Fig. 8 Individual histogram when recording PBMCs stained with a v450-conjugated CD8+ antibody. The table of statistics shows the Median (P2 gate) of PBMCs stained for CD8 using a v450-conjugated antibody, *red arrow*. Notice how the initial position of the P2 gate has changed from Fig. 7 to the actual position of the bright population

lot is used, or hardware (lasers/filters) is changed. Running CST beads on a routine basis will inform the operator whether the cytometer is performing optimally.

2.5 Run Compensation

1. When conducting a new experiment, first apply the Application settings to the experiment by right clicking on cytometer settings and then clicking on Application settings. The optimized voltages (created above) will be imported.

2. Use unstained PBMCs and single color stained CompBeads (BD Biosciences, San Jose, CA) to create a compensation matrix. With the designated Application settings, we find we do not need to further adjust our PMT voltages and subsequent spectral overlap should be optimized. With low spillover the operator should achieve the best resolution possible. Finally, the operator can record their experiment.

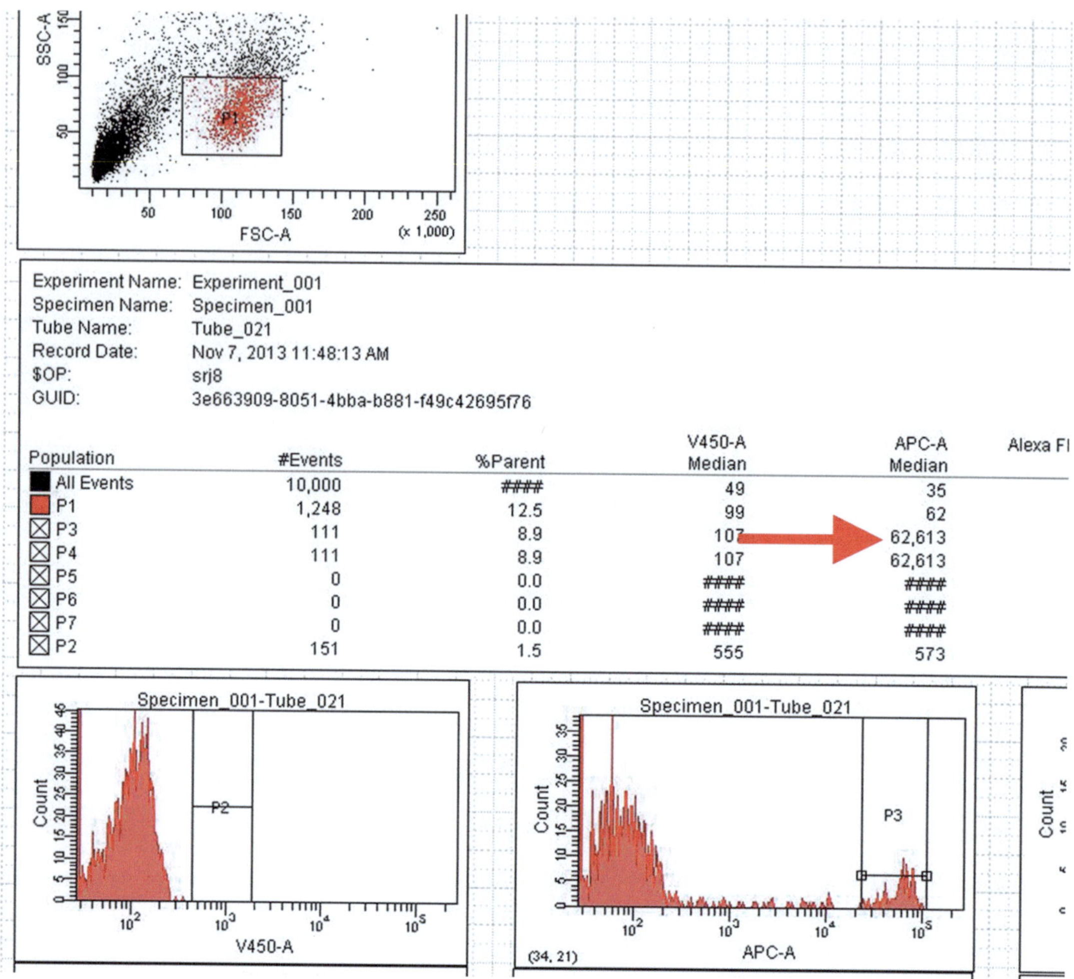

Fig. 9 Individual histogram when recording PBMCs stained with APC-conjugated CD8+ antibody. The table of statistics shows the Median (P3 gate) of PBMCs stained for CD8 using a APC-conjugated antibody, *red arrow*. Again, notice how the P3 gate is on the bright population

3   Notes

1. The operator may need to revisit this critical planning step if subsequent difficulties in population resolution are found in the planned experimental conditions. If in doubt and assuming enough sample is available, a conservative number of parameters should be chosen.

2. Our experiments utilize a relatively fixed number of PBMCs isolated. Thus in order to maximize our data output, we use the matrix to plan for a panel of extracellular targets and a separate panel for intracellular targets using the same experimental conditions.

3. We generally find relatively bright fluorochromes require greater dilution (for example with PE-Texas red we use a 1:100 dilution).

4. This can be accomplished by staining a fixed number of cells of interest in various dilutions of a single fluorochrome. When performing this evaluation, we do not apply Application settings or a compensation matrix.

5. Although we could follow standard manufacturer recommendations for antibody dilution, these usually call for a vast excess in antibody. While in theory excess unbound antibody can be washed away, we have found on occasion that such concentrations result in fluorescence that is beyond the linear range. Consequently, we carry out our own titrations for each antibody and repeat them for new lots of the same antibody clone.

6. We have applied some of these techniques to achieve accuracy and precision across two highly similar instruments within our institution. Generally, using guidance from BD Biosciences, we identified the highest rSD and lowest maximum linearity for matched parameters between instruments; next we used these numbers for calculating 2.5–3× the rSD and one-half the maximum linearity (*see* Subheading 2.4, **step 2**). We ultimately found our experimental results to be reproducible across the two instruments. In theory this approach could be used to reproduce settings across remote locations. However, we recommend expert guidance from the instrument manufacturer since a variety of factors need to be considered (e.g. model, filters, lasers, etc.).

7. The unstained PBMCs will be used for adjusting parameter voltage based on rSD and the stained PBMCs will be used for adjusting parameter voltage based on maximum linearity. Most of our procedures are conducted in 96-well round bottom plates. To be efficient, we plate 1×10^6 PBMCs/well, centrifuge, and then flick out the supernatant. Our antibody staining is then conducted on re-suspended cells within the well in antibody cocktails. For antibodies where we do not dilute, we directly pipette antibody from the manufacturer's tube to the cells in the well.

8. This important step again highlights the need to have an ample number of unstained PBMCs available. Also, it is expected that the rSD values of already optimized parameters may slightly change from tube to tube. This is acceptable as long as the subsequent values are still within 2.5–3× the baseline value.

9. The operator can change the position of the respective interval gates once the precise location of the bright peaks are known when running the single color stained PBMCs.

10. If substantial changes are made to the voltage of a particular parameter when using the single colored PBMCs, consider re-running unstained PBMCs to ensure that the rSD continues to remain with 2.5–3× the baseline value. On very rare occasions we have made the observation that the optimal voltage for such a parameter must balance between the voltage settings for these two individual variables.

Acknowledgements

Work in Dr. Shaw's laboratory is supported, in part, by U19 AI089992, NIAID contract 272201100019C-3-0-1, K24 AG042489, and the Yale Claude D. Pepper Older Americans Independence Center (P30AG021342). Additional support (to S.J.) was from NIA T32 AG019134 and NIAID T32 AI007517.

References

1. Sugar IP, Gonzalez-Lergier J, Sealfon SC (2011) Improved compensation in flow cytometry by multivariable optimization. Cytometry A 79(5):356–360. doi:10.1002/cyto.a.21062

2. Kalina T, Flores-Montero J, van der Velden VH, Martin-Ayuso M, Bottcher S, Ritgen M, Almeida J, Lhermitte L, Asnafi V, Mendonca A, de Tute R, Cullen M, Sedek L, Vidriales MB, Perez JJ, te Marvelde JG, Mejstrikova E, Hrusak O, Szczepanski T, van Dongen JJ, Orfao A (2012) EuroFlow standardization of flow cytometer instrument settings and immunophenotyping protocols. Leukemia 26(9):1986–2010. doi:10.1038/leu.2012.122

3. Maino VC, Picker LJ (1998) Identification of functional subsets by flow cytometry: intracellular detection of cytokine expression. Cytometry 34(5):207–215

4. Panda A, Qian F, Mohanty S, van Duin D, Newman FK, Zhang L, Chen S, Towle V, Belshe RB, Fikrig E, Allore HG, Montgomery RR, Shaw AC (2010) Age-associated decrease in TLR function in primary human dendritic cells predicts influenza vaccine response. J Immunol 184(5):2518–2527. doi:10.4049/jimmunol.0901022

5. van Duin D, Allore HG, Mohanty S, Ginter S, Newman FK, Belshe RB, Medzhitov R, Shaw AC (2007) Prevaccine determination of the expression of costimulatory B7 molecules in activated monocytes predicts influenza vaccine responses in young and older adults. J Infect Dis 195(11):1590–1597. doi:10.1086/516788

6. Mahnke YD, Roederer M (2007) Optimizing a multicolor immunophenotyping assay. Clin Lab Med 27(3):469–485. doi:10.1016/j.cll.2007.05.002, v

7. Edinger M (2009) Multicolor flow cytometry—principles of panel design. http://www.bd.com/videos/bdb/webinars/multicolor_flow_principals_of_panel_design/. Accessed 21 Feb 2013

Chapter 6

Flow Cytometry-Based Methods to Characterize Immune Senescence in Nonhuman Primates

Christine Meyer*, Kristen Haberthur*, Mark Asquith*, and Ilhem Messaoudi

Abstract

Flow cytometry is an invaluable technique that can be used to phenotypically and functionally characterize immune cell populations ex vivo. This technology has greatly advanced our ability to gain critical insight into age-related changes in immune function, commonly known as immune senescence. Rodents have been traditionally used to investigate the molecular mechanisms of immune senescence because they offer the distinct advantages of an extensive set of reagents, the presence of genetically modified strains, and a short lifespan that allows for longevity studies of short duration. More recently, nonhuman primates (NHPs), and specifically rhesus macaques, have emerged as a leading translational model to study various aspects of human aging. In contrast to rodents, they share significant genetic homology as well as physiological and behavioral characteristics with humans. Furthermore, rhesus macaques are a long-lived outbred species, which makes them an ideal translational model. Therefore, NHPs offer a unique opportunity to carry out mechanistic studies under controlled laboratory conditions (e.g., photoperiod, temperature, diet, and medications) in a species that closely mimics human biology. Moreover similar techniques (e.g., activity recording and MRI) can be used to measure physiological parameters in NHPs, making direct comparisons between NHP and human data sets possible. In addition, the outbred genetics of NHPs enables rigorous validation of research findings that goes beyond proof of principle. Finally, self-selection bias that is often unavoidable in human clinical trials can be completely eliminated with NHP studies. Here we describe flow cytometry-based methods to phenotypically and functionally characterize innate immune cells as well as T and B lymphocyte subsets from isolated peripheral blood mononuclear cells (PBMC) in rhesus macaques.

Key words Flow cytometry, Lymphocyte, B cell, T cell, Regulatory T cell, Rhesus macaque, Age, Proliferation, Cytokine, Dendritic cell, Monocyte, Natural killer cell, Pattern recognition receptor

1 Introduction

The immune system can be broadly divided into two branches: innate and adaptive. The innate immune system is poised to respond rapidly to infection and is composed of several cell types including monocytes/macrophages, dendritic cells (DC), natural killer (NK) cells, and granulocytes. Adaptive immunity is mediated primarily by T and B lymphocytes that require several days

---

*These authors made equal contributions to this work.

Albert C. Shaw (ed.), *Immunosenescence: Methods and Protocols*, Methods in Molecular Biology, vol. 1343,
DOI 10.1007/978-1-4939-2963-4_6, © Springer Science+Business Media New York 2015

to generate responses tailored specifically for each pathogen. The main distinguishing characteristic of these two branches of the immune response is antigen recognition. Innate immunity relies on germline-encoded receptors to sense the presence of pathogens, whereas adaptive immunity utilizes a highly diverse set of receptors generated through somatic mutation and gene recombination. The second major defining and unique characteristic of the adaptive immune system is the development of immunological memory that manifests itself as increased functionality and frequency of responding cells upon reexposure to the same antigen.

Aging results in several structural and functional changes in the immune system that affect both innate and adaptive immunity. These changes lead to a dysregulation of immune function and increased vulnerability to infection. These complex changes are grouped under the umbrella term "immune senescence". In recent years, the use of rhesus macaques in gerontology research has increased dramatically. Several studies have shown that rhesus macaques experience immune senescence in a similar fashion as described for humans, thereby providing a robust translational model to further our understanding of the mechanisms and impact of immune senescence. In this chapter, we first outline several staining protocols to allow: (1) discrimination of monocyte and dendritic cells subpopulations as well as NK cells in peripheral blood; (2) measurement of cytokine production by innate immune cells; (3) delineation of major T and B cell subsets; (4) assessment of the magnitude and kinetics of T and B cell proliferation; and (5) measurement of the frequency of antigen-specific T cells.

2   Materials

1. RP10: RPMI 1640 medium (1×) supplemented with 10 % fetal bovine serum and penicillin/streptomycin/L-glutamine (100 U/ml penicillin, 100 μg/ml streptomycin/2 mM L-glutamine).

2. 1× phosphate buffered saline.

3. Fixation buffer (containing 4 % paraformaldehyde; BioLegend).

4. PermWash 10× buffer (BioLegend): dilute to 1× (contains 0.1 % saponin) in diH$_2$O.

5. Superperm: 1× PermWash buffer supplemented with 10 % DMSO.

6. Antibodies (Tables 1, 2, 3 for a complete list of antibodies, clones, and vendors).

7. Toll-like receptor (TLR) agonists: *Escherichia coli* K12 Lipopolysaccharide (LPS, 2 ng/ml) and Imiquimod (10 mg/ml) (Invivogen).

Table 1
Innate cell antibody information for use in rhesus macaques

Marker	Clone	Manufacturer
AQUA Live/Dead	–	Invitrogen
CD3 Pacific Blue	UCHT1	BD Biosciences
HLA-DR APC-Cy7	L243	BioLegend
CD14 Alexa Fluor 700	HCD14	BioLegend
CD8α PeCy5	B9.11	Beckman Coulter
CD16 PeCy7	3G8	BD Biosciences
CD20 ECD	B9E9	BD Biosciences
CD123 PerCyP-Cy5.5	6H6	BioLegend
CD11c Alexa Fluor 647	3.9	BioLegend

Table 2
Intranuclear and intracellular antibody information
for use in rhesus macaques

Marker	Clone	Manufacturer
Ki67 FITC	B56	BD Pharmingen
IFNy PeCy7	4S.B3	eBioscience
TNFα APC	MAb11	eBioscience
IL-2 Alexa Fluor 700	MQ1-17H12	BioLegend
IL-17 Alexa Fluor 647	BL168	BioLegend
IL-6 APC	MQ2-13A5	eBioscience
MIP-1β PE	D21-1351	BD Pharmingen
IFNα FITC	MMHA-11	PBL interferon source

8. Brefeldin A (BFA, Sigma).

9. Dimethyl sulfoxide solution (DMSO).

10. 96-well tissue-culture-treated round bottom plate (BD Falcon).

11. Microtiter tubes.

12. Flow cytometer (LSRII or similar instrument).

13. Analytic software (e.g., FlowJo (TreeStar)).

Table 3
Rhesus macaque B and T cell antibody panel

B cell panel	Clone	Manufacturer
CD3 Pacific Blue	SP34-2	BD Biosciences
CD20 ECD	B9E9	Beckman Coulter
CD27 APC	O323	BioLegend
IgD Biotin[a]	Pooled antisera from goats hyperimmunized with human IgD paraproteins	SouthernBiotech
T cell panel		
CD4 PerCp-Cy5.5	RPA-T4	BioLegend
CD8β ECD	2ST8.5H7	Beckman Coulter
CD25 APC-Cy7	BC96	BioLegend
CD28 PE	CD28.2	BioLegend
CD95 Pacific Blue	DX2	BioLegend
CD127 A647	A019D5	BioLegend
CCR7 PE-Cy7	3D12	BD Biosciences

[a]Requires addition of secondary antibody conjugated to a fluorophore Streptavidin-BD Horizon V500 (BD biosciences)

3   Methods

3.1   Delineating Innate Immune Cells by Flow Cytometry

The innate immune system is the first line of defense against pathogens and its action is mediated by several immune cell subsets that include granulocytes (e.g., neutrophils), natural killer (NK) cells, dendritic cells (DC), and monocytes/macrophages. Because little information is available for rhesus macaque granulocytes, they are not discussed here.

1. Add 2×10^6 peripheral blood mononuclear cells (PBMC) per well in a 96-well round bottomed plate (*see* **Notes 1** and **2**). Rhesus PBMC are isolated from whole blood by centrifugation over Ficoll (density 1.077) exactly as described for human blood. PBMC yields per milliliter blood are also comparable between rhesus and humans.

2. Add 150 µl of PBS to each well (washing step) and spin down plate at $900 \times g$ for 3 min. Discard the supernatant and briefly vortex the plate (*see* **Notes 3** and **4**).

3. Repeat **step 2** with 200 µl of PBS.

4. Add surface antibody cocktail described in Table 1 diluted to 50 µl of PBS (*see* **Note 5**) resuspend, and incubate for 20 min at 4 °C in the dark.

5. Add 150 µl of PBS to each well and spin down plate at $900 \times g$ for 3 min at 4 °C. Discard supernatant, and briefly vortex plate.

6. Repeat **step 5** with 200 µl of PBS.

7. Resuspend cells in 100 µl fixation buffer. Incubate for 30 min at 4 °C (*see* **Note 6**).

8. Add 100 µl of PBS to each well, spin down at $900 \times g$ for 3 min at 4 °C, discard supernatant, and briefly vortex pellet. Repeat this wash step with 200 µl of PBS.

9. Resuspend cells in 100 µl of PBS and transfer to microtiter tubes for acquisition on flow cytometer. Samples may be stored at 4 °C for up to 48 h until they can be acquired.

10. Acquire samples on LSR II or similar instrument and analyze data using FlowJo or comparable software. Since monocytes represent 3–5 % and DC 1–2 % of the PBMC, it is important to acquire at least 1×10^6 events.

11. Following acquisition by flow cytometer, samples can be analyzed as depicted in Fig. 1: First, exclude AQUA LIVE/ DEAD+ cells (dead), CD3 (T cells), and CD20 (B cells) to define the live "non-lymph" population. From here, classical monocytes are defined as CD14^{hi}CD16$^-$ cells, whereas nonclassical monocytes are defined as CD14^{lo}CD16$^+$ cells [1]; DCs are defined as HLA-DR$^+$CD14$^-$ cells and can be further subdivided using CD123 and CD11c markers into CD123$^+$ plasmacytoid DCs (pDCs) and CD11c$^+$ myeloid DCs (mDCs) [2]; NK cells are defined as CD14$^-$HLA-DR$^-$CD8α$^+$ and can be subdivided into a major CD16+ cytolytic population and a minor CD16- cytokine-producing population. Two major differences between human and rhesus macaque NK cells should be noted here: (1) rhesus macaque NK cells, but not human NK cells, express high-levels of CD8α [3]; and (2) human but not rhesus macaque NK cells express CD56. CD56 is expressed by monocytes in rhesus macaques [4].

3.2 Analysis of Innate Immune Cell Cytokine Production

Functional changes in cytokine production by innate immune cells can also be examined by flow cytometry [5]. Here we outline a protocol for examining cytokine production by monocytes and dendritic cell subsets following stimulation with the Toll-Like Receptor (TLR) agonists LPS (TLR4) and Imiquimod (TLR7) to model stimulation with bacterial (TLR4) and viral (TLR7) pathogen associated molecular patterns (PAMPs), respectively [6].

1. Maintain sterile conditions by using a tissue culture hood and fresh media to avoid microbial contamination of cell cultures.

2. Add 2×10^6 PBMC in 200 µl of RP10 into a 96-well round bottomed plate (*see* **Note 2**). For each sample aliquot three

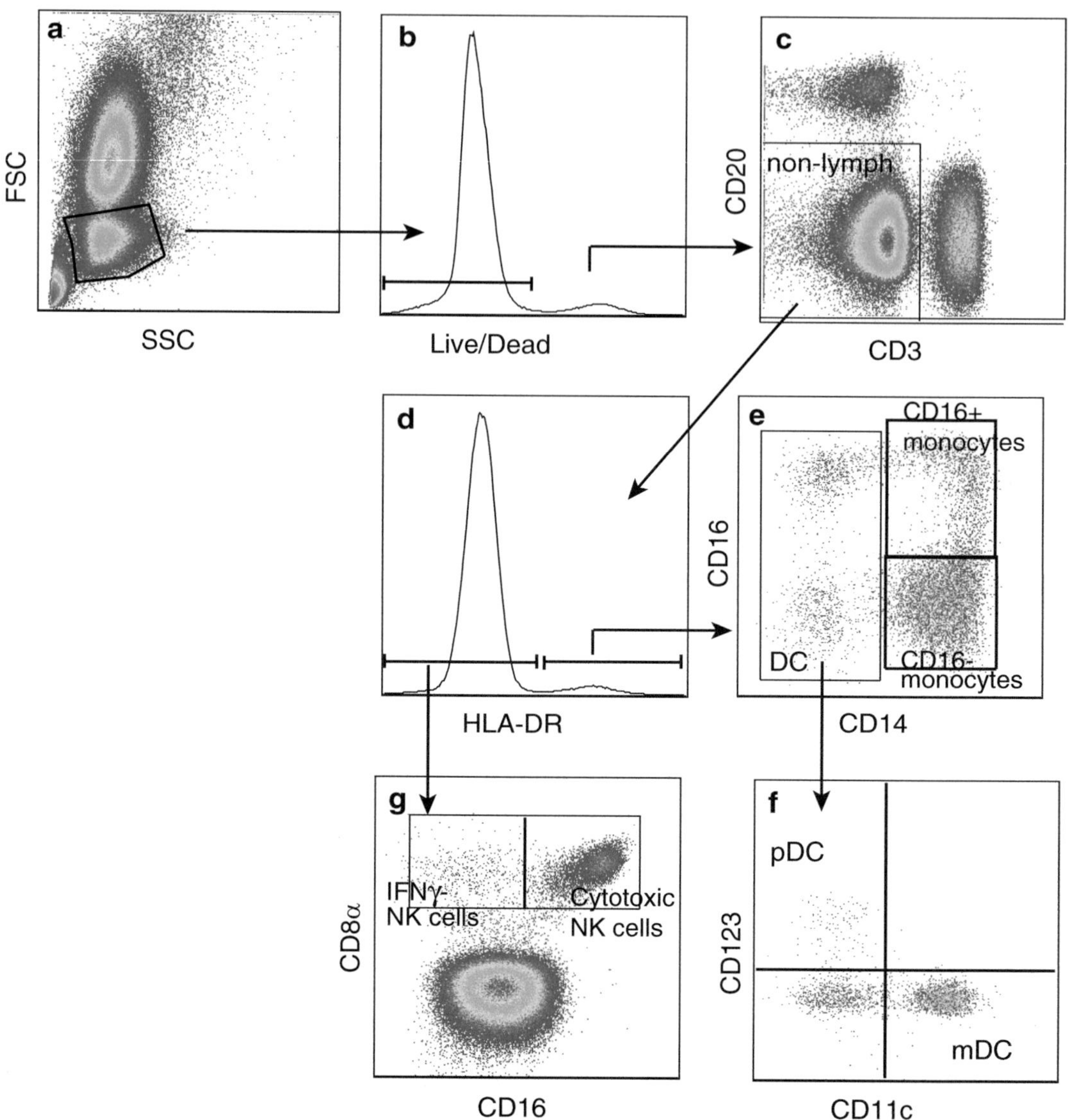

Fig. 1 Delineation of innate immune cells using flow cytometry. Live PBMCs are discriminated by forward scatter (FSC) and side scatter (SSC) measuring size and granularity, respectively (**a**), and Live/Dead gating (**b**). CD3 to CD20− cells are identified as non-lymph cells (**c**). Monocytes and DCs are HLA-DR+ (**d**). CD14 and CD16 co-staining can be used to delineate major monocyte/macrophage subpopulations (**e**). HLA-DR+ CD14− cells can be gated to delineate DCs (**e**), which are further subdivided into CD123+ plasmacytoid DC (pDC) and CD11c+ myeloid DCs (mDC) (**f**). NK cells are identified as HLA-DR− cells that are CD8α+ and are subdivided into a major CD16+ cytotoxic subset and a minor CD16− IFNγ-producing subset (**g**)

wells (LPS, Imiquimod, and unstimulated control). Spin the plate at $900 \times g$ for 3 min. Discard supernatant and briefly vortex plate (*see* **Note 4**).

3. Resuspend cells in 200 μl of either RP10/LPS solution, RP10/ Imiquimod solution, or RP10 alone. Incubate for 1 h in a humidified incubator at 37 °C and 5 % CO_2 (*see* **Notes 7** and **8**).

4. Add 2 μl of Brefeldin A stock solution (500 μg/ml) to all wells (*see* **Note 9**).

5. Incubate for an additional 5 h in a humidified incubator at 37 °C and 5 % CO_2.

6. Spin down cells at $900 \times g$ for 3 min. Discard supernatant and vortex plate.

7. Add 200 μl of PBS to all wells. Spin down at $900 \times g$ for 3 min. Discard supernatant and vortex plate.

8. Repeat **step 7** with 200 μl of PBS.

9. Add surface antibody cocktail described in Table 1 diluted to 50 μl of PBS (*see* **Note 5**) and incubate at 4 °C for 20 min in the dark.

10. Add 150 μl of PBS to all wells. Spin down at $900 \times g$ for 3 min at 4 °C. Discard supernatant and vortex plate.

11. Repeat wash **step 10** with 200 μl PBS.

12. Resuspend cells in 100 μl of fixation buffer (*see* **Note 6**). Incubate for 30 min at 4 °C.

13. Add 150 μl Perm/Washbuffer to all wells and spin plate at $900 \times g$ for 3 min at 4 °C. Discard supernatant and vortex plate.

14. Repeat **step 13** with 200 μl PermWash buffer.

15. Resuspend cells in 50 μl of intracellular cytokine antibody panel in PermWash buffer (Table 2). Incubate at 4 °C in the dark for 20 min or overnight.

16. Add 150 μl of Perm/Wash to all wells. Spin plate at $900 \times g$ for 3 min at 4 °C. Discard supernatant and vortex plate.

17. Repeat **step 16** with 200 μl of PBS.

18. Resuspend cells in 100 μl of PBS and transfer to microtiter tubes for acquisition on flow cytometer. Samples may be stored at 4 °C for up to 48 h until they can be acquired.

19. Acquire samples on LSR II or similar instrument and analyze data using FlowJo or comparable software.

20. Once acquired, cells can be gated as depicted in Fig. 2. First, exclude AQUA LIVE/DEAD⁺, CD3⁺ and CD20⁺ cells to gate on live, non-lymph cells. You can then gate on specific populations such as monocytes and DC subsets as described in Fig. 1. The frequency of TNFα⁺, IL-6⁺, and IFNα⁺ cells can be determined using the unstimulated control sample to adjust/subtract for background fluorescence (Fig. 2).

3.3 Delineating Lymphocyte Subpopulations by Flow Cytometry

The adaptive immune branch is composed of B and T lymphocytes, which unlike cells of the innate immune system can generate responses tailored to specific pathogens. Specificity is acquired through the expression of diverse, clonally distributed antigen receptors. Aging results in disturbances in lymphocyte homeostasis. Here we discuss how to delineate T and B cell subsets.

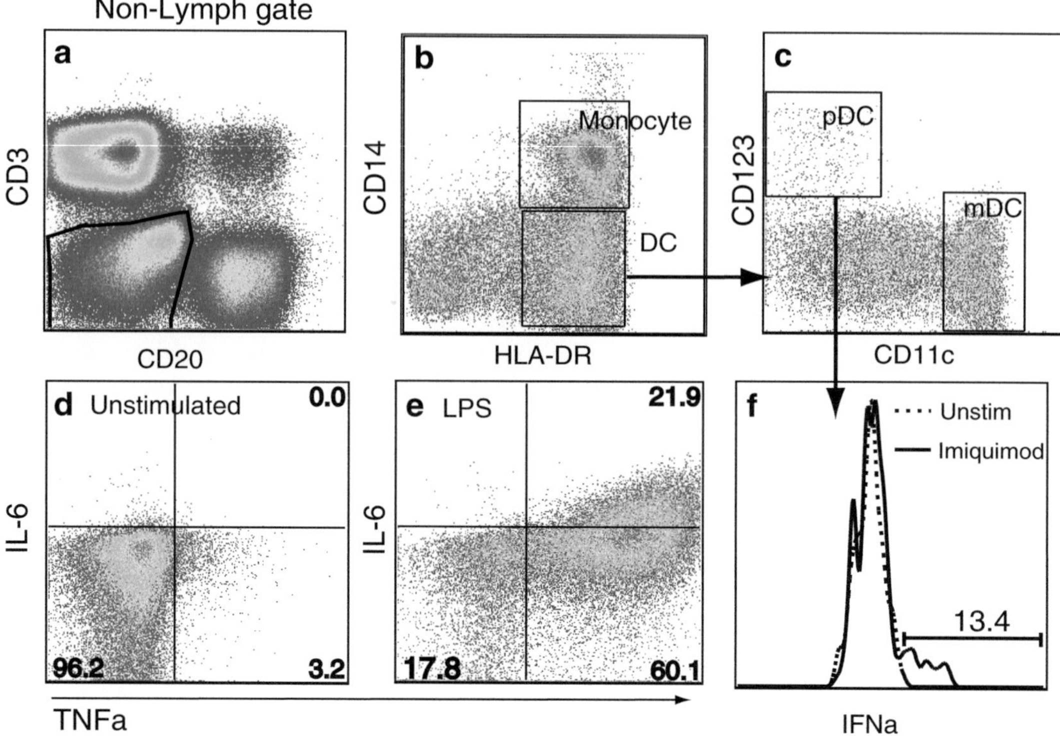

Fig. 2 Cytokine production by innate immune cells. PBMC were incubated for 6 h with either RP-10 alone ("unstimulated"), or in the presence of LPS or Imiquimod. Non-lymph cells are identified as CD3 to CD20− cells (**a**). Cells were then stained for surface markers to delineate monocytes (HLA-DR+ CD14+ cells) or DCs (HLA-DR+ CD14−) (**b**), with CD123 and CD11c used to delineate pDC and mDC respectively (**c**). Cells were stained intracellularly for TNFα, IL-6, and IFNα. Representative TNFα/IL-6 costaining by monocytes unstimulated (**d**) or incubated with LPS (**e**) and representative IFNα staining by pDCs unstimulated or stimulated with Imiquimod (**f**)

1. Add 1×10^6 PBMCs per well into a 96-well plate (*see* **Note 6**, Table 3).

2. Spin plates at $900 \times g$ for 3 min. Discard supernatant and vortex plate (*see* **Note 3**).

3. Add surface antibodies described in Table 3 in 50 μl of PBS per well and incubate in the dark at 4 °C for 30 min.

4. Wash plate with 150 μl of PBS, spin for 3 min at $900 \times g$ at 4 °C. Discard supernatant and vortex plate.

5. Repeat **step 4** with 200 μl of PBS.

6. If staining panel requires a secondary antibody (*see* **Note 10**) dilute in 50 μl of PBS per well and incubate plate in dark for 20 min at 4 °C.

7. Add 150 μl of PBS to the wells and spin for 3 min at $900 \times g$ at 4 °C. Discard supernatant and vortex plate.

8. Repeat **step 7** using 200 μl of PBS.

9. Add 100 µl fixation buffer and incubate in dark for 20 min at 4 °C.

10. Wash plate with 100 µl of PBS and spin for 3 min at $900 \times g$ at 4 °C. Discard supernatant and vortex plate.

11. Repeat **step 10** with 200 µl of PBS.

12. Resuspend cells in 100 µl PBS and transfer to microtiter tubes for acquisition on flow cytometer. Samples may be stored at 4 °C for up to 48 h until they can be acquired.

13. Acquire samples on LSR II or similar instrument and analyze data using FlowJo or comparable software. Since CD4 T cells account for 30–40 %, CD8 T cells account for 15–25 % and CD20 B cells account for 10–20 % of PBMC, acquiring 5×10^5 events is sufficient.

14. Once acquired, samples can be analyzed as depicted in Figs. 3 and 4. B cells can be identified in rhesus macaques based on the expression of CD20 and can then be subdivided into four subsets based on the expression of IgD and CD27 (Fig. 3): (1) naïve B cells express surface bound IgD and lack expression of CD27; (2) antigen-experienced memory B cells are defined as IgD⁻CD27⁺; (3) a transitional subset referred to as marginal zone-like (MZ-like) B cells, are identified as IgD⁺CD27⁺; and (4) a minor exhausted highly differentiated memory subset is defined as IgD⁻CD27⁻ [7, 8].

Rhesus macaque CD4 and CD8 T cells can be subdivided into naïve, central memory (CM), and effector memory (EM) subsets based on expression of CD28 (co-stimulatory molecule) and CD95 (FAS receptor) (Fig. 4) [9]. Naïve T cells are identified as CD95⁻CD28⁺, CM T cells are identified as CD95⁺CD28⁺, and EM T cells are identified as CD95⁺CD28⁻. This differentiation can be further refined based on the expression of the chemokine receptor CCR7, which allows cells to circulate through blood and lymphoid organs. The expression of CCR7 together with CD28 allows

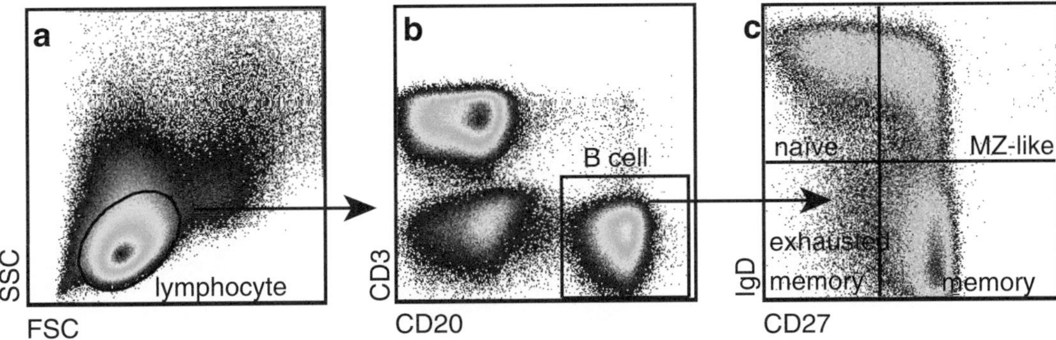

Fig. 3 Flow-cytometric gating strategy to delineate B cell populations. Live PBMC are delineated as previously described (**a**). B cells are identified as CD3− CD20+ (**b**). Naïve B cells are IgD+ CD27−, marginal zone-like (MZ-like) B cells are IgD+ CD27+, and memory B cells are IgD− CD27+ (**c**)

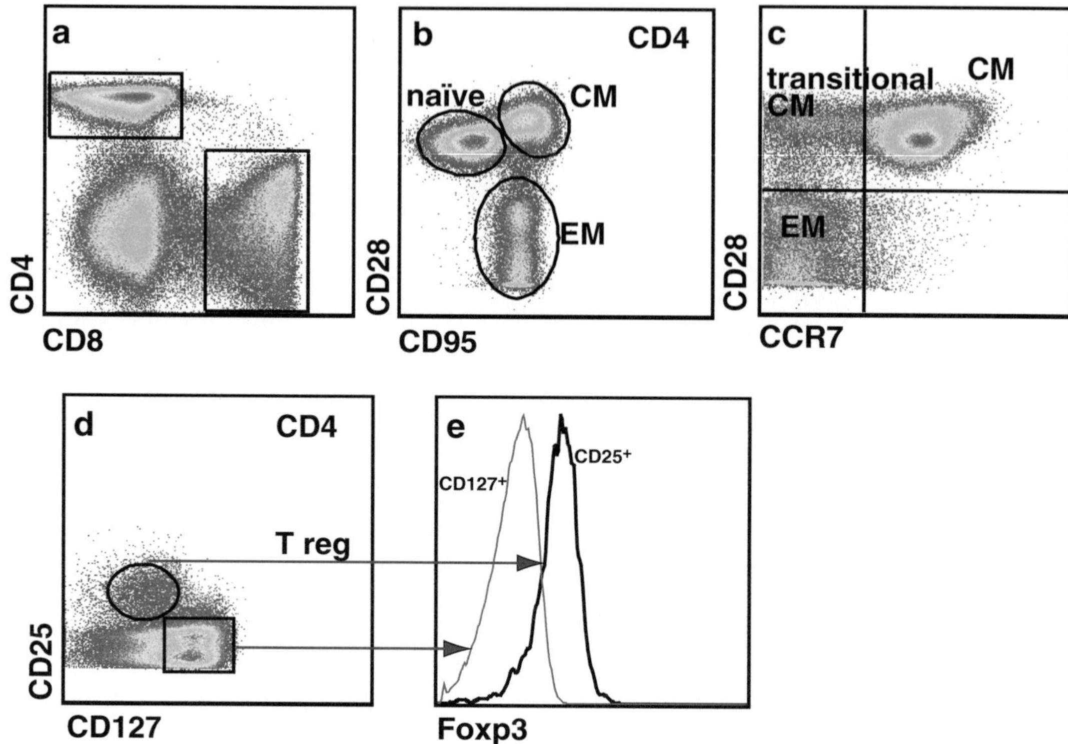

Fig. 4 Flow-cytometric gating strategy to delineate T cell populations. Lymphocytes are separated into CD4+ and CD8+ T cells (**a**). CD4 T and CD8 T cells are subdivided into naïve CD95− CD28+, central memory (CM, CD95+ CD28+) and effector memory (EM, CD95+ CD28−) T cells (**b**). The addition of CCR7 allows further subdivision of the memory CD95+ T cells population and the identification of transitional CM T cells CD95+ CD28+ CCR7− (**c**). T regulatory (T reg) cells are defined as CD4+ CD25+ CD127− (**d**). Confirmation is provided by the expression of Foxp3+ in this population (**e**)

the identification of fourth subset called transitional CM T cells that are CD95$^+$CD28$^+$CCR7$^-$, whereas terminally differentiated EM T cells are CD95$^+$CD28$^-$CCR7$^-$ and CM T cells are CD95$^+$CD28$^+$CCR7$^+$ (Fig. 4) [10]. As described for humans, aging is accompanied by a loss of naïve T cells and the accumulation of EM CD8 T cells and CM CD4 T cells in the rhesus macaque [5]. Regulatory T (Treg) cells are important mediators of immune tolerance and are classically defined based on expression of CD4, CD25, and the transcription factor FoxP3. Additionally, in the RM, the IL-7 receptor or CD127 can be alternatively used to identify Treg cells as CD4$^+$CD25$^+$CD127$^-$ (Fig. 4).

3.4 Monitoring Immune Cell Proliferation Through the Detection of Ki67 Expression

One of the hallmarks of the adaptive immune response is a robust proliferative burst. Ki67 is a nuclear protein that is upregulated during the G2–S phase of the cell cycle [11], and is an excellent marker for determining kinetics and magnitude of a proliferative burst. Rhesus macaques are an outbred population with a complex

MHC locus that remains incompletely understood. Consequently, very few tetramers have been designed and all are specific for Simian Immunodeficiency Virus (SIV). Therefore, Ki67 expression is used to determine the kinetics and magnitude of the proliferative burst instead, which reliably assesses the adaptive immune response quantitatively and qualitatively.

1. Add 1×10^6 PBMC per well of a 96-well plate.

2. Spin plate for 3 min at $900 \times g$. Discard supernatant and vortex plate.

3. Add surface antibodies to cells diluted in 50 μl PBS. This staining can be easily combined with that described in Subheading 3.1 or 3.3 to measure proliferation within a variety of immune cells.

4. Incubate plate in dark at 4 °C for 30 min.

5. Add 150 μl PBS, spin for 3 min at $900 \times g$ at 4 °C. Discard supernatant and vortex plate.

6. Repeat **step 5** with 200 μl PBS.

7. If staining panel requires a secondary antibody, add it diluted in 50 μl of PBS per well and incubate plate in dark for 20 min at 4 °C. If not continue with **step 10**.

8. Add 150 μl PBS, spin for 3 min at $900 \times g$ at 4 °C. Discard supernatant and vortex plate.

9. Repeat **step 8** with 200 μl PBS.

10. Add 100 μl l fixation buffer to each well. Incubate in dark for 20 min at 4 °C.

11. Add 100 μl Perm/Wash buffer, spin for 3 min at $900 \times g$ at 4 °C. Discard supernatant and vortex plate.

12. Repeat **step 11** with 200 μl Perm/Wash buffer.

13. Add 100 μl superperm buffer to each well. Incubate in dark for 20 min at 4 °C.

14. Add 100 μl Perm/Wash buffer, spin for 3 min at $900 \times g$ at 4 °C. Discard supernatant and vortex plate.

15. Repeat **step 14** with 200 μl Perm/Wash buffer.

16. Add Ki67 antibody (Table 2) diluted in 50 μl of 1× PermWash buffer to each well. Incubate in dark for 4 h or overnight at 4 °C.

17. Add 150 μl PermWash buffer, spin for 3 min at $900 \times g$ at 4 °C. Discard supernatant and gently vortex plate.

18. Repeat **step 17** with 200 μl PermWash buffer.

19. Wash plate in 200 μl 1× PBS. Spin for 3 min at $900 \times g$ at 4 °C. Discard supernatant.

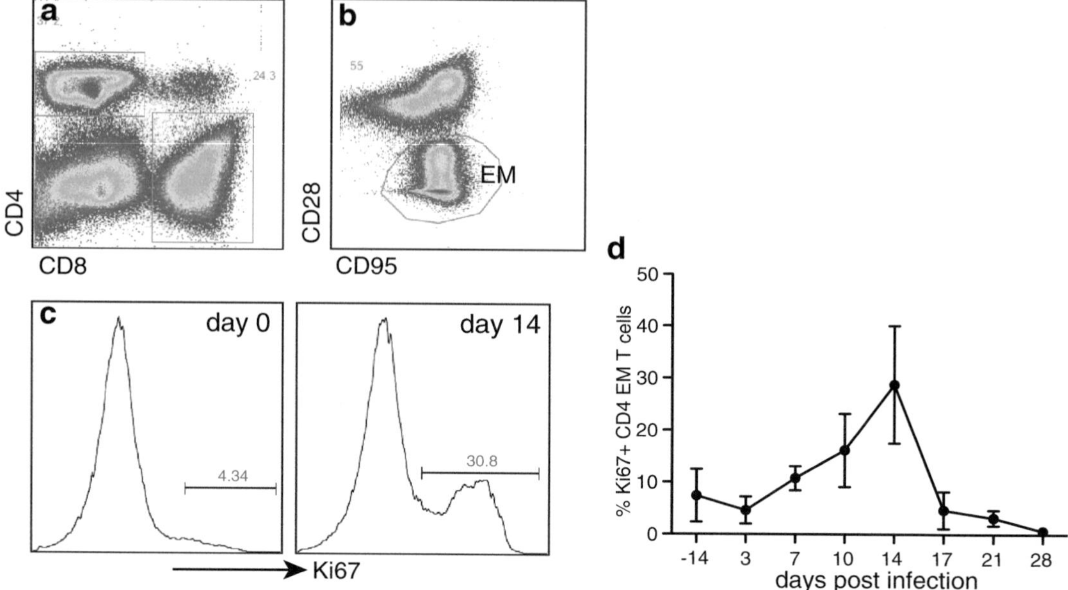

Fig. 5 Measuring T cell proliferation via analysis of Ki67 expression. Lymphocytes are separated into CD4+ and CD8+ T cells (a). CD4 EM T cell subsets are delineated based on CD28 and CD95 expression (b). Ki67+ expression in CD4 EM T cells increases dramatically 14 days post-infection with simian varicella virus (SVV) compared to day 0 post-infection (c). Representative example of CD4 EM T cell proliferative burst following SVV infection (average values of six animals, d)

20. Resuspend samples in 100 µl 1× PBS and transfer to microtiter tubes for running on the flow cytometer. Store at 4 °C for up to 48 h until they can be acquired.

21. Acquire samples on LSR II instrument or similar instrument and analyze data using FlowJo or comparable software.

22. To analyze the samples, first follow instructions provided above in Figs. 3 and 4 to gate on the lymphocyte population of choice. The percentage of Ki67+ cells can be obtained using a histogram as depicted in Fig. 5 for CD4 EM T cells.

3.5 Monitoring the Frequency of Antigen-Specific T Cells by Intracellular Cytokine Staining (ICS)

Antigen recognition by T cells results in the production of cytokines such as IFNγ and TNFα. Detection of these can be accomplished through the use of intracellular cytokine staining (ICS), a widely used flow cytometry-based assay that takes advantage of the protein transport inhibitory effects of Brefeldin A. Briefly, samples are (1) stimulated with a specific antigen in the presence of Brefeldin A, (2) stained with the appropriate cell surface antibodies, (3) fixed and permeabilized, (4) stained with antibodies directed against cytokines of choice such as IFNγ and TNFα, and (5) analyzed via flow cytometry.

1. Add 1×10^6 cells in 100 µl of RP10 per well into a 96-well plate. Aliquot at least three wells for each sample.

2. Add the following to each of the wells: (1) experimental antigen (*see* **Note 11**); (2) positive control (*see* **Note 12**); and (3) negative control (*see* **Note 13**).

3. Incubate at 37 °C for 1 h.

4. Add 2 µl per well of Brefeldin A. Incubate in a humidified incubator 5 % CO_2 at 37 °C overnight (9–14 h).

5. Spin plate for 3 min at $900 \times g$ at 4 °C. Discard supernatant and vortex plate.

6. Wash plate with 200 µl 1× PBS. Spin for 3 min at $900 \times g$ at 4 °C. Discard supernatant and vortex plate.

7. Add T cell surface antibodies to cells diluted in 50 µl PBS (*see* **Note 14**).

8. Incubate plate in dark at 4 °C for 20 min.

9. Add 150 µl PBS, spin for 3 min at $900 \times g$ at 4 °C. Discard supernatant and vortex plate.

10. Repeat **step 9** with 200 µl PBS buffer

11. Add 100 µl fixation buffer to each well. Incubate in dark for 20 min at 4 °C.

12. Add 100 µl Perm/Wash buffer, spin for 3 min at $900 \times g$ at 4 °C. Discard supernatant and gently vortex plate.

13. Repeat **step 12** with 200 µl PermWash buffer.

14. Add the cytokine-specific antibodies (Table 2) diluted in 50 µl of 1× PermWash buffer to each well. Incubate in dark for 4 h or overnight at 4 °C.

15. Add 150 µl PermWash buffer, spin for 3 min at $900 \times g$ at 4 °C. Discard supernatant and vortex plate.

16. Repeat **step 15** with 200 µl PermWash buffer.

17. Add 200 µl 1× PBS. Spin for 3 min at $900 \times g$ at 4 °C. Discard supernatant and vortex plate.

18. Resuspend samples in 100 µl 1× PBS and transfer to microtiter tubes for acquisition on a flow cytometer. Store at 4 °C until needed.

19. Acquire samples on LSR II or comparable instrument and analyze data using FlowJo or similar software.

20. Samples can be analyzed by gating on either total CD4 or CD8 T cells or specific memory subsets as delineated in Subheading 3.3 (*see* **Note 14**). An example of CD4 cytokine production following Simian Varicella Virus (SVV) infection is depicted in Fig. 6.

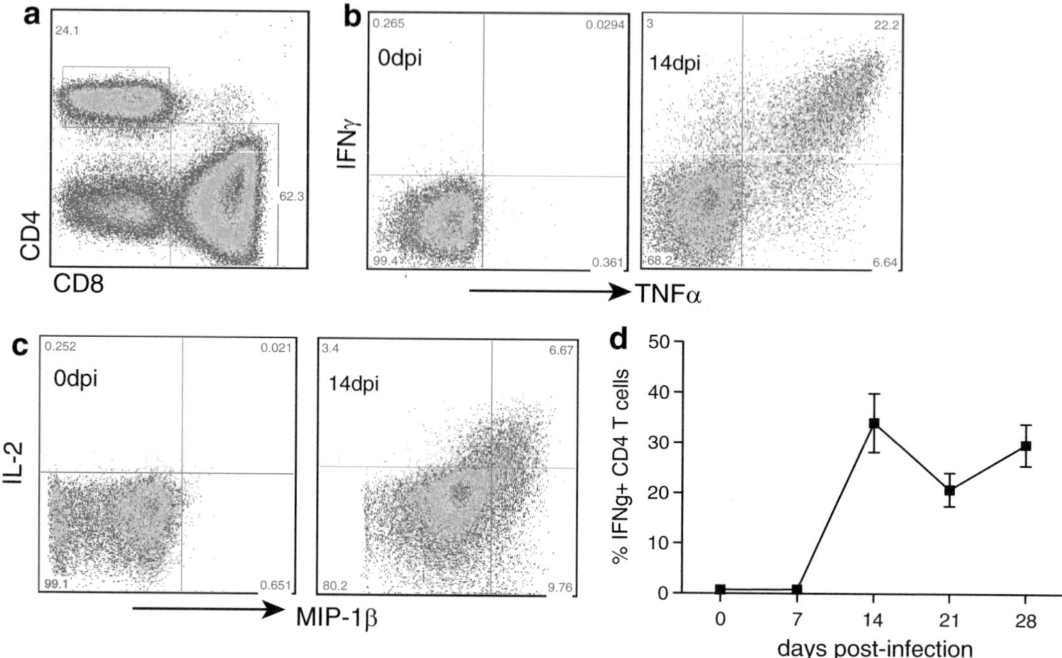

Fig. 6 Measuring frequency of antigen-specific T cells using intracellular cytokine production by flow cytometry. Lymphocytes are separated into CD4+ and CD8+ T cells (**a**). Representative examples of the frequency of IFNγ/TNFα− producing (**b**) and IL-2/MIP-1β− producing (**c**) CD4 T cells at 0 and 14 days post-infection with simian varicella virus (SVV) following ex vivo stimulation with SVV lysate are shown. Frequency of antigen-specific T cells can be reliably monitored over the course of SVV infection using ICS as demonstrated in panel **d** with the monitoring of the frequency of IFNγ+ CD4 T cells (average of six animals)

4   Notes

1. The number of PBMC to use depends on the frequency of target cell of interest. Some cells (e.g., plasmacytoid DC) are infrequent in peripheral blood and will require the acquisition of more total events to obtain a reliable population size.

2. Since innate immune cells are frequently adherent, use non-adherent tissue-culture-treated plates to improve cell yields. The plate material will also modulate the activation state of CD14+ cells.

3. After centrifugation, flick the supernatant into a waste container in a fast downward motion. Do not allow the supernatant to contaminate the adjacent wells.

4. When carrying out wash steps under sterile conditions, use a 200 μl pipette to slowly remove supernatant and discard supernatant. To ensure the pellet is not disrupted, it may help to angle the 96-well plate towards yourself.

5. For up to date information regarding cross-reactivity data please visit http://nhpreagents.bidmc.harvard.edu/NHP/reagentlist.aspx. Fluorochrome choices should be based on the instrument and laser configuration. Those suggested in the tables were optimized for a BD LSRII instrument. Use the antibodies at the amount recommended by the manufacturer. To titrate antibodies for which a recommended amount is not known or available, we recommend beginning with 1 µg and testing dilutions of the antibody in twofold increments. Run all dilutions on the flow cytometer and determine the concentration of antibody that best delineates the population of interest.

6. Fully resuspend cells immediately in fixation buffer, as this helps to limit clumping of cells. Use pipetting instead of vortexing to increase the efficiency of this step.

7. The bioactivity of TLR agonists is highly variable depending on manufacturer. We recommend careful titration of all TLR agonists to optimize stimulation conditions.

8. Make small aliquots of TLR agonists to avoid freeze-thawing and loss of bioactivity. Carefully follow manufacturer's storage specifications and expiration date.

9. Addition of Brefeldin A results in the accumulation of proteins (in this case, the proteins of interest are cytokines) within the endoplasmic reticulum [12]. To look at global PBMC cytokine production (rather than on a per cell basis), cells can be incubated in the absence of Brefeldin A for 6 h and supernatants harvested for subsequent analysis of cytokines (e.g., by ELISA or cytometric bead assay).

10. If one of the primary antibodies is labeled with biotin and not fluorescently conjugated, you will need to add the secondary antibody streptavidin conjugated to a fluorophore.

11. The reagents that can be used to stimulate T cell cytokine production are varied. When assessing antigen specific responses, one can use viral or bacterial lysate generated by disrupting infected cells. Alternatively purified viral or bacterial preps can also be used at a multiplicity of infection of typically 1–3. If the immunodominant antigens are known, then purified protein or overlapping peptide libraries can be also be used. The optimal stimulation conditions are determined specifically for each experimental system.

12. Positive controls are essential to ensure that the assay has worked. Polyclonal mitogens (that can stimulate a majority of T cells regardless of their antigen-specificity) are often used. The options include but are not limited to: CD3, PMA, PMA/ionomycin, superantigens, and ConA.

13. It is important that negative controls receive the same media/buffer that the experimental antigen was prepared in. For instance, if you were stimulating with viral lysate the negative control would be disrupted non-infected cells. Similarly, if you are using peptides, the negative control wells should receive the solution the peptides were reconstituted in (usually DMSO).

14. One can add anti-CD4 and CD8 antibodies only or together with CD28, CD95, and CCR7 if the goal is to delineate the exact subset of T cells producing cytokines. Naïve T cells are antigen inexperienced and typically do not produce cytokines following short term ex vivo stimulation.

References

1. Passlick B, Flieger D, Ziegler-Heitbrock HW (1989) Identification and characterization of a novel monocyte subpopulation in human peripheral blood. Blood 74:2527–2534

2. Coates PT, Barratt-Boyes SM, Zhang L et al (2003) Dendritic cell subsets in blood and lymphoid tissue of rhesus monkeys and their mobilization with Flt3 ligand. Blood 102:2513–2521

3. Ramothea L, Webster RPJ (2005) Delineation of multiple subpopulations of natural killer cells in rhesus macaques. Immunology 115:206–214

4. Carter LL, Murphy KM (1999) Lineage-specific requirement for signal transducer and activator of transcription (Stat)4 in interferon gamma production from CD4(+) versus CD8(+) T cells. J Exp Med 189:1355–1360

5. Asquith M, Haberthur K, Brown M et al (2012) Age-dependent changes in innate immune phenotype and function in rhesus macaques (*Macaca mulatta*). Pathobiol Aging Age Relat Dis. doi:10.3402/pba.v2i0.18052

6. Kawai T, Akira S (2011) Toll-like receptors and their crosstalk with other innate receptors in infection and immunity. Immunity 34:637–650

7. Bar-Or A, Oliveira EM, Anderson DE et al (2001) Immunological memory: contribution of memory B cells expressing costimulatory molecules in the resting state. J Immunol 167:5669–5677

8. Weller S, Braun MC, Tan BK et al (2004) Human blood IgM "memory" B cells are circulating splenic marginal zone B cells harboring a prediversified immunoglobulin repertoire. Blood 104:3647–3654

9. Pitcher CJ, Hagen SI, Walker JM et al (2002) Development and homeostasis of T cell memory in rhesus macaque. J Immunol 168:29–43

10. Picker LJ, Reed-Inderbitzin EF, Hagen SI et al (2006) IL-15 induces CD4 effector memory T cell production and tissue emigration in nonhuman primates. J Clin Invest 116:1514–1524

11. Gerdes J, Lemke H, Baisch H et al (1984) Cell cycle analysis of a cell proliferation-associated human nuclear antigen defined by the monoclonal antibody Ki-67. J Immunol 133:1710–1715

12. Fujiwara T, Oda K, Yokota S et al (1988) Brefeldin A causes disassembly of the Golgi complex and accumulation of secretory proteins in the endoplasmic reticulum. J Biol Chem 263:18545–18552

Chapter 7

Multiparameter Phenotyping of Human PBMCs Using Mass Cytometry

Michael D. Leipold, Evan W. Newell, and Holden T. Maecker

Abstract

The standard for single-cell analysis of phenotype and function in recent decades has been fluorescence flow cytometry. Mass cytometry is a newer technology that uses heavy metal ions, rather than fluorochromes, as labels for probes such as antibodies. The binding of these ion-labeled probes to cells is quantitated by mass spectrometry. This greatly increases the number of phenotypic and functional markers that can be probed simultaneously. Here, we review topics that must be considered when adapting existing flow cytometry panels to mass cytometry analysis. We present a protocol and representative panels for surface phenotyping and intracellular cytokine staining (ICS) assays.

Key words Mass cytometry, CyTOF, Immunophenotyping, Panel design

---

1 Introduction

Flow cytometry has become the method of choice in immunology for phenotypic and functional analysis of single cells, owing to its high throughput and ability to analyze multiple parameters in combination (up to 15 or so with advanced instruments). Still, the enormous complexity of immune cells makes even this degree of multiplexed readouts limiting. While it is possible to do single-cell analysis of gene expression across the entire genome [1], no technology has allowed a similar degree of comprehensive probing of proteins at the single-cell level.

By replacing fluorescent labeling of probes for flow cytometry with heavy metal ion labels, the potential for higher multiplexing is greatly enhanced. Unlike the highly overlapping emission spectra of typical fluorochromes, the readout of atomic masses by mass spectrometry is very discrete, and can span a wide mass window. Thus, the use of ion-labeled probes and mass spectrometry as a readout for flow cytometry (i.e., mass cytometry) is a conceptually attractive approach [2, 3].

Albert C. Shaw (ed.), *Immunosenescence: Methods and Protocols*, Methods in Molecular Biology, vol. 1343,
DOI 10.1007/978-1-4939-2963-4_7, © Springer Science+Business Media New York 2015

The development of mass cytometry as a viable research tool for multiparameter analysis of immune cells was greatly facilitated by the availability of a commercial mass cytometer (CyTOF, DVS Sciences, Toronto; hereafter referred to as mass cytometer), along with software for conversion of the mass spectrometry signals to conventional flow cytometry standard (fcs) files. At least two laboratories have since exploited this technology to examine the heterogeneity of human immune cells in unprecedented detail [4–7].

Among the theoretical advantages of mass cytometry are (1) increased numbers of simultaneous probes that can be used, without loss of sensitivity and (2) lack of spillover between mass channels. In fluorescence flow cytometry, the number of simultaneous probes one can use is limited not only by the optical spectrum, but also by the availability of sufficiently bright fluorophores. Similarly, optical spillover between fluorochromes requires the application of compensation matrices to fluorescence flow cytometry data, increasing the complexity of analysis and the chances for errors of interpretation. Here we will address the degree to which these factors are in fact resolved by mass cytometry, and the considerations that remain.

One important difference between fluorescence flow cytometers and a mass cytometer is that there is no mass cytometer analog to either forward scatter or side scatter. Therefore, there is a strict requirement for metal-labeling to discriminate cell types, or to identify cell events at all. If a cell is not labeled with at least one metal in the mass range of the mass cytometer, it will not be counted, adversely affecting percent-of-parent statistics. This is commonly addressed by labeling all cells containing DNA using iridium-containing intercalators (Atomic mass, AM 191, 193). Similarly, live-dead stains must also contain appropriate metal ions to be counted. Molecules containing both a chelator and maleimide moiety [5], or cisplatin [8] have been used as viability stains in mass cytometry. *See* Fig. 1 for an example of gating on iridium intercalator, viability stain, and monocytes vs. lymphocytes using CD14 and CD33.

The collection of pulse height and area (or width) information in fluorescence flow cytometers allows for reasonably efficient discrimination of cell aggregates, which differ from single cells in the ratio of these parameters. This is obviously not possible on a mass cytometer, and hence positive identification of single-cell events is more difficult. The use of the "cell length" parameter, or the amount of time over which a cell event is detected, during gating analysis only partially eliminates cell aggregates (*see* Fig. 1). Slowing the acquisition rate by diluting the sample reduces doublets at the cost of increased time per sample. More complex strategies can be undertaken, such as "cell barcoding" [6], followed by gating out of events that contain more than a single barcode. This strategy can be effective if the majority of aggregation occurs after the stage of barcode labeling.

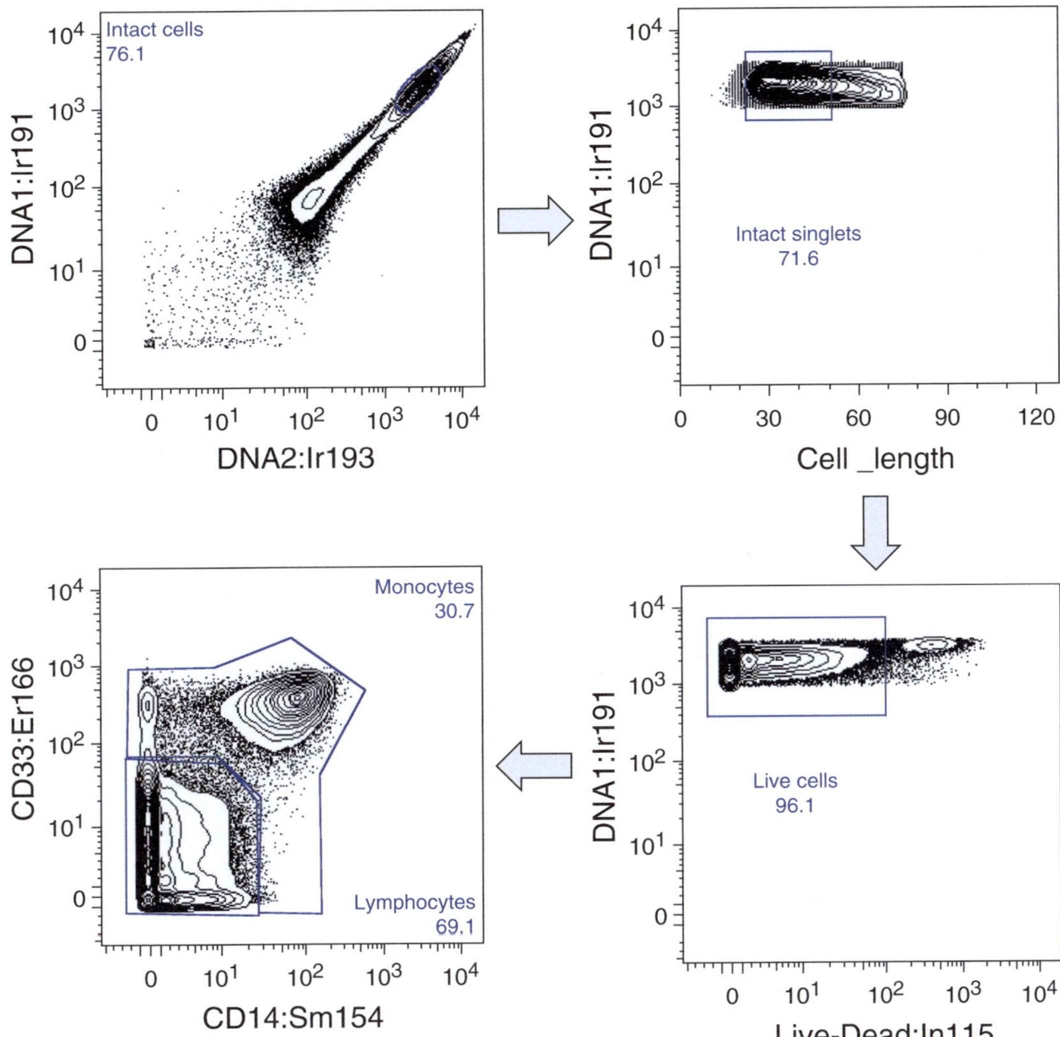

Fig. 1 Initial gating of a PBMC sample in CyTOF. *Top, left*: Gating on the dense cluster of events with strong staining for the two isotopes of Ir intercalator eliminates much of the debris, and events within the gate are referred to as "intact cells." *Top, right*: Further gating on the Cell_length parameter eliminates some presumed cell aggregates, and events within this gate are referred to as "intact singlets." *Bottom, right*: A thiol-reactive dye is taken up by cells with compromised membranes, so those with low staining are gated as "live cells." *Bottom, left*: Initial marker-based gating is done on CD14 vs. CD33, to separate monocytes from lymphocytes. Because clean discrimination of these populations is essential to further analysis, we routinely use both markers for this purpose. All data was collected using Data Dual (Dd) calibration. The mass cytometer can give data in three different outputs: Intensity, Pulses Count, or Dual (d) mode. Dual mode is the calibration curve relating Intensity and Pulses Count, and is least dependent upon a particular machine. This calibration can be done using a commercial tuning solution containing known amounts of specified elements spanning the instrumental mass window (instrument Dual: Di), and will be saved as the calibration file until the calibration is run again. Data Dual (Dd) uses the first milliseconds of ion events from that particular sample to create the calibration, then uses that calibration to determine the cell event data. Di calibration information is written into the header of all files, regardless of whether the user specifies Di or Dd acquisition. Therefore, the data can be processed from one format to the other post-acquisition

The CyTOF 2 mass cytometer is currently tuned for a mass window approximately AM 89-209. The high end and the low end of the mass window have somewhat lower signal intensities ("dim channel") compared to the middle of the mass range ("bright channel"). Maximum sensitivity is centered slightly higher than the middle of the range. The lanthanide metals are La139-Yb176, and vary in signal intensity by less than a factor of 4. Nonetheless, it is important to understand that the relative "brightness" of the channels is a function of their position within the measured mass window. Therefore, if the mass window is significantly expanded or shifted to higher or lower masses, the peak intensities will shift accordingly.

Design of Antibody Panels for Mass Cytometry. The factors to consider when pairing antibodies with metals are similar to pairing an antibody with a fluorochrome [9–11].

1. The expression level of the marker. Markers with higher expression can be used in "dimmer" channels. Conversely, markers with lower expression require "brighter" channels in order for the positive population to be resolved from the background. For markers induced with in vitro stimulation, those with small fold changes in expression after stimulation would require brighter metals to resolve the difference over the unstimulated sample.

2. The resolution needed for gating. It is often beneficial to use two markers in a bivariate plot to cleanly resolve a population of interest, rather than relying on histograms. In such cases, one bright channel and one dimmer channel are usually sufficient for resolution: for instance, B cells (CD19+ CD20+) can be cleanly gated from total CD3– cells using CD20-Dy164 (bright) vs. CD19-Nd142 (dim). In some instances, two channels of intermediate sensitivity may be needed, such as when both bivariate markers are of medium or low expression.

3. The type of expression. Some markers, such as CD27, exhibit bimodal expression: These can generally be labeled with dimmer metals, since they exhibit clearly resolved positive and negative populations, with no intermediate population.

   Alternatively, other markers such as CCR7 or CD45RA have a spectrum or "smear" of expression. These often require brighter metals to allow finer distinction between important cell populations, even in bivariate plots.

4. If you need to redesign a panel, shifting metals up or down by one or two mass units will generally not impact signal/resolution.

5. Tm169 is the brightest metal for the AM 89-209 mass window for current commercially available polymer reagents/lanthanides. If labeling with Tm169 yields no signal for cells of

known positivity, either: (1) the target molecule is not expressed in sufficient density for resolution by mass cytometry; or (2) the antibody is losing binding specificity upon labeling. Use of different labeling chemistry, or polymer-labeling a commercial fluorescent conjugate and checking it for binding by fluorescence analysis, can help resolve the second possibility.

6. Quantum dots (Qdots) and nanocrystals. Particles of hundreds to tens of thousands of metal atoms can efficiently be burned in the mass cytometry argon plasma, and the resulting ions can be quantified. Therefore, Qdots and similar nanocrystals labeled with antibodies can be one way to boost signal for a particular marker. As in fluorescence, non-specific binding needs to be carefully monitored.

Most commercial Qdots contain cadmium (usually CdSe), which lies within the mass cytometer mass window. Typically, only one Cd-Qdot can be used in a given panel: they contain natural-abundance Cd, which has eight naturally occurring isotopes (AM 106-116, 114 the most abundant). Cadmium is at the very low end of the sensitivity range and therefore would normally only be useful for markers of extremely high abundance. However, each Qdot contains thousands of Cd atoms, effectively increasing the signal of most markers to a reasonable level.

CdSe/CdTe Qdots contain tellurium (AM 120-130). However, since they also contain Cd, they cannot easily be used simultaneously with CdSe Qdots. Additionally, the xenon impurities (AM 124-136) present in the argon gas could potentially cause a noticeable background in the tellurium mass range.

Commercial InGaP Qdots contain primarily In115 (95.71% natural abundance). Cadmium lacks a 115 isotope, so these could be compatible with Cd Qdots, if Cd112 and In115 are monitored.

Potential Sources of Contaminating Signals. Due to the mass resolution of the time-of-flight separation, there is little or no spillover from one channel to the next due to the detector itself. In addition, most of the metals used in the AM 89-209 window, such as the lanthanides, Ir, Pt, In, Pd, or Cd, are seldom found in biological samples from healthy individuals. Therefore, there is no equivalent to "autofluorescence."

However, other sources of contaminating signals must be considered, including metal and environmental impurities, and oxidation products [12].

1. Metal impurities. These can be impurities either of different elements, or of alternative isotopes of the same element; most typically, the greatest amount of impurity is seen in the next higher mass channel ("M+1"), with sometimes significant impurity in "M−1" or "M+2" as well; this is due to the nature of the isolation procedure.

The metals that are sold as part of antibody labeling kits are of very high purity (98% and higher in most cases). As a practical matter, this means that "compensation" analogous to fluorescent antibodies is not needed, as most of the signal will be of the specified mass, with little to no signal at "M+1" or another contaminating mass. However, metal salts from other commercial sources may be of lesser purity. For example, the chemistries of the lanthanides (Ln) are sufficiently similar that undesired lanthanides (often La139) can be contaminants in purchased salts since they are difficult to purify using only chemical methods. There are currently no labeling kits containing Gd157 due to purity concerns about the available salts. If using these less-pure isotopes, some caveats to consider include the following:

(a) Consider using them for "dump" channels or exclusion markers. If only events that are negative for the label in question are subjected to further analysis, the impurities present should not cause any issues.

(b) Put a lower-abundance marker at a less-pure "M" so that the absolute spillover (usually up to 0.5–1% of "M" signal) is reduced. If "M" is a less pure isotope and is labeling a high-abundance marker, do not put a low-abundance marker at the M+1 position. Aim for at least medium-abundance so that positive and negative populations can still be clearly resolved if there is isotopic "spillover."

(c) For channels that have significant spillover, use combinations of markers that label mutually exclusive populations. For instance, put a T-cell-specific marker at M+1 when using a B-cell-specific marker labeled with a less-pure isotope M.

2. Impurities from the sample or environment. There are several sources of impurities to guard against. When in doubt, a highly diluted aliquot of the suspected stock can be injected into the mass cytometer in tuning/liquid mode and observed for contamination.

(a) Many laboratory dish soaps have high levels of barium (AM 130-138). Barium tends to persist even after multiple rinses. This is a problem even if these masses are not being used in the experiment, as it leads to detector aging, and can result in oxidation signals in M+16 channels (see point #3 below). It is therefore generally advised to store mass cytometry buffers in brand-new plastic or glass vessels that have never been through laboratory wash.

(b) Low levels of mercury, lead, or tin can sometimes be found in lab buffers, especially those made with "house" distilled water rather than reverse osmosis (e.g., MilliQ) water, or from commercial stock solutions that were not specified as metal-free. Even iodine (mass 127) is in the mass window of the mass cytometer.

(c) Unexpected sources of contamination include, for example, striker flints for Bunsen burners. These contain high levels of cerium (AM 136-142) and lanthanum, as well as traces of neodymium and other lanthanides.

3. Oxidation products. All metals exhibit some degree of oxidation in the argon plasma. This cannot be eliminated, but can be minimized with proper instrument warm-up and tuning of the current and make-up gas each day. This tuning should result in oxides <3% of maximum signal. Technically, oxide formation decreases signal at M, while increasing signal at M+16. However, it is easier to detect a small increase in oxide at M+16 than to detect a small decrease in signal at M.

Some lanthanides are more easily oxidized than others. La139 is the worst (oxide mass 155). Pr141 (oxide AM 157), Nd (oxide AM 158-166), and Gd (oxide AM 172-176) have notable levels of oxidation as well. Eu (oxide AM 167, 169) has very low oxide levels. When using a more-easily oxidized metal, it is useful to use it for markers that are relatively low-abundance compared to the marker at M+16, so that M+16 spillover ($\leq$0.5–1% of "M" signal) is minimized.

It is important to remember that the undesired signals listed above are all a function of the signal intensity of M. Even with a less pure isotope such as Gd157, the total interference may only add up to a few percent of M signal, distributed among all spillover channels (M+1, M–1, M+16, environmental contamination, Ln, etc.). Therefore, careful pairing of marker abundance and metal signal intensity, along with metal salt purity will minimize any potential spillover. Generally, a signal of $<10^1$ Dual counts can be considered as background. Therefore, if the signal at M is $<10^3$ Dual counts, any spillover contribution would be at or below background level in the affected channels.

Qualification of Antibody Conjugates. As with standard fluorescence flow cytometry, qualification of antibodies for assay purposes is critical. This is particularly relevant since comparatively few pre-conjugated metal–antibodies are currently commercially available. Therefore, many antibody–metal conjugates will have to be conjugated in-house by the end-user. In most cases, an antibody clone that works for fluorescence flow cytometry can be successfully conjugated for use in mass cytometry. In most of the remaining cases, another widely used clone can be substituted successfully. *See* Fig. 2 for some representative examples comparing various markers in fluorescence and mass cytometry. However, with the relatively young state of the field, there are occasionally markers for which no suitable antibody clone has yet been identified.

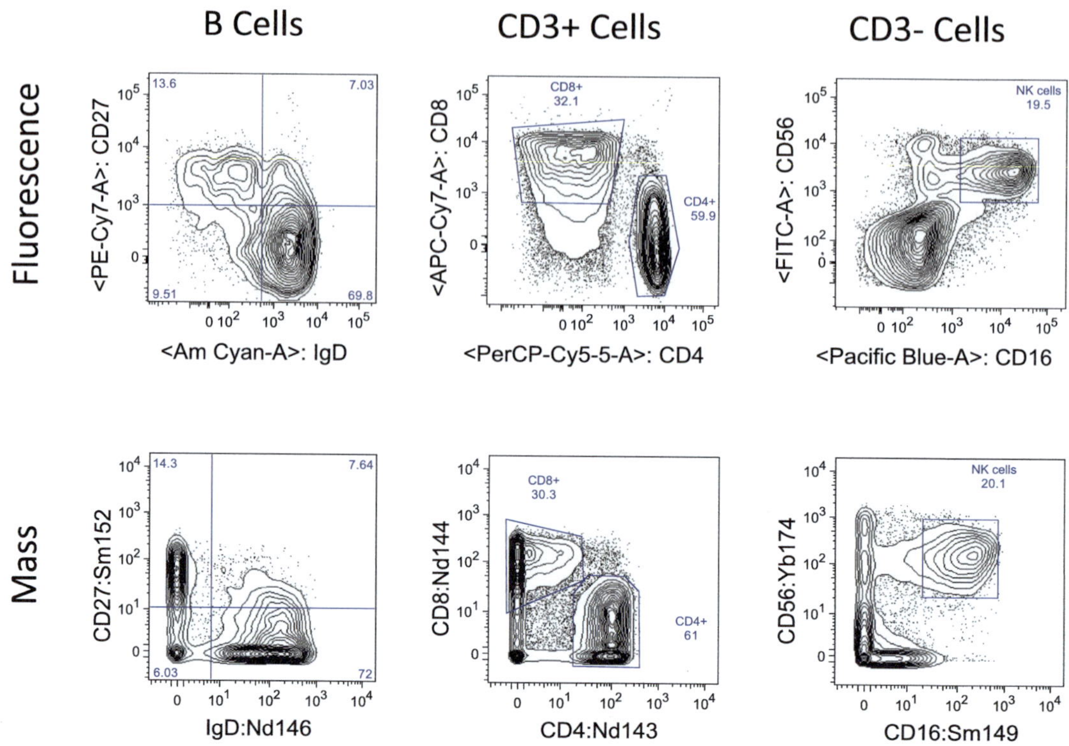

Fig. 2 Representative comparisons of fluorescence (*top row*) and mass cytometry (*bottom row*) for the same antibody combinations on cryopreserved PBMC from the same donor. Parent populations are shown at the *top of each column*. *Left to right*: naïve and memory B cell sub-populations, CD4+ and CD8+ T cells, and NK cells. In each case, the staining patterns differ somewhat, especially with regard to background staining of negative populations; but overall frequencies of each gated population are very similar. All data was collected using Data Dual (Dd) calibration

Furthermore, we recommend that even after a successful antibody clone–metal pairing is found, each new batch of conjugated antibodies should be checked for activity against a reference before use in assays with unknown samples.

There are several points to keep in mind when testing new antibody conjugates.

1. The expected expression pattern of the marker. This includes: cell type (monocytes, NK cells, T cells, B cells, etc.); location (peripheral circulation, bone marrow, lymph node, gut lumen, etc.); and effects of stimulation, differentiation, or cell cycle phase. For example, one might test an antibody on stimulated cells if antigen expression is not expected on unstimulated cells.

2. Effects of sample processing. Some markers (e.g., CD62L, PD-1) are reduced upon cryopreservation (though these can

be partially restored after resting of thawed cells). Some cell types are also lost or reduced after processing (e.g., granulocytes and dendritic cells after Ficoll gradient separation). Finally, staining after fixation and/or permeabilization can destroy epitopes. For example, many anti-CD16 antibodies lose binding after fixation. Conversely, there can be a large increase in nonspecific binding of many anti-CD56 antibodies after fixation.

3. Use of both positive and negative controls. Often, different cell types within the same sample can provide positive and negative controls for antibody staining. For example, B cells can serve as a negative control for T cell markers, etc. However, beware of limitations of this approach, as many markers are expressed by more than one type of cell, often at lower levels or in small subpopulations.

   If doing two-step staining with element-labeled secondary antibodies, one should include additional controls such as: secondary antibody in the absence of the primary antibody, and secondary antibody in the presence of a known primary antibody.

   Cell lines can be useful for antibody qualification (see proteinatlas.org for immunohistochemistry data for ~4300 proteins on 47 cell lines). Of course, the antigen expression on a cell line may be higher or lower than seen on primary cells. Also, data from proteinatlas.org are from samples fixed, paraffin-embedded, deparaffinized with xylene, rehydrated with ethanol, boiled in antigen-retrieval solution, stained, then read by a computer. Thus, the staining may not match that seen on fresh samples in flow cytometry.

4. Use of more than one donor during antibody-conjugate validation. Some donors have unusual patterns of expression or cell distribution. TCRγδ+ T cells are an example of a highly donor-dependent population. We have observed occasional donors with low or negative expression of CD33 on monocytes, or very skewed distributions of memory T-cell subsets (e.g., nearly all CD8+ T cells are CD28+ or CD28−). By use of more than one donor, false conclusions about the performance of the antibody are less likely.

Once a panel is designed and conjugates are tested and titrated, it is advisable to test performance and reproducibility of the panel on control samples such as healthy subject PBMC. *See* Fig. 3 for an example of the staining pattern of PMA+ionomycin-activated normal PBMC with a selection of markers from a 38-antibody intracellular cytokine panel.

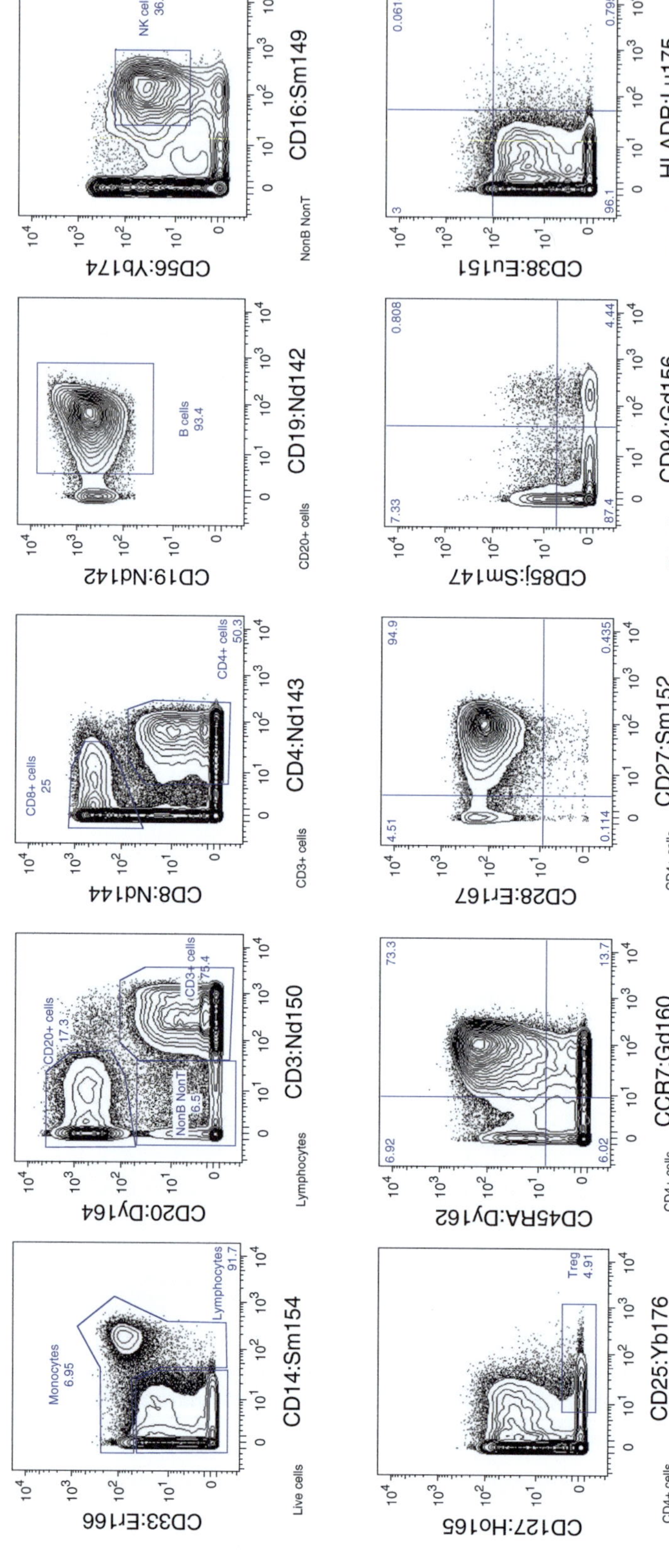

Fig. 3 Representative staining of various cell-surface (**a**) and intracellular (**b**) markers in a 38-antibody panel that includes eight intracellular cytokines. Plots show staining from a positive control, stimulated with PMA+ionomycin, but the panel has been successfully used with antigen-specific stimulations as well. Resolution of surface and intracellular markers is generally quite good. The parent population is shown at the bottom of each plot. All data was collected using Data Dual (Dd) calibration

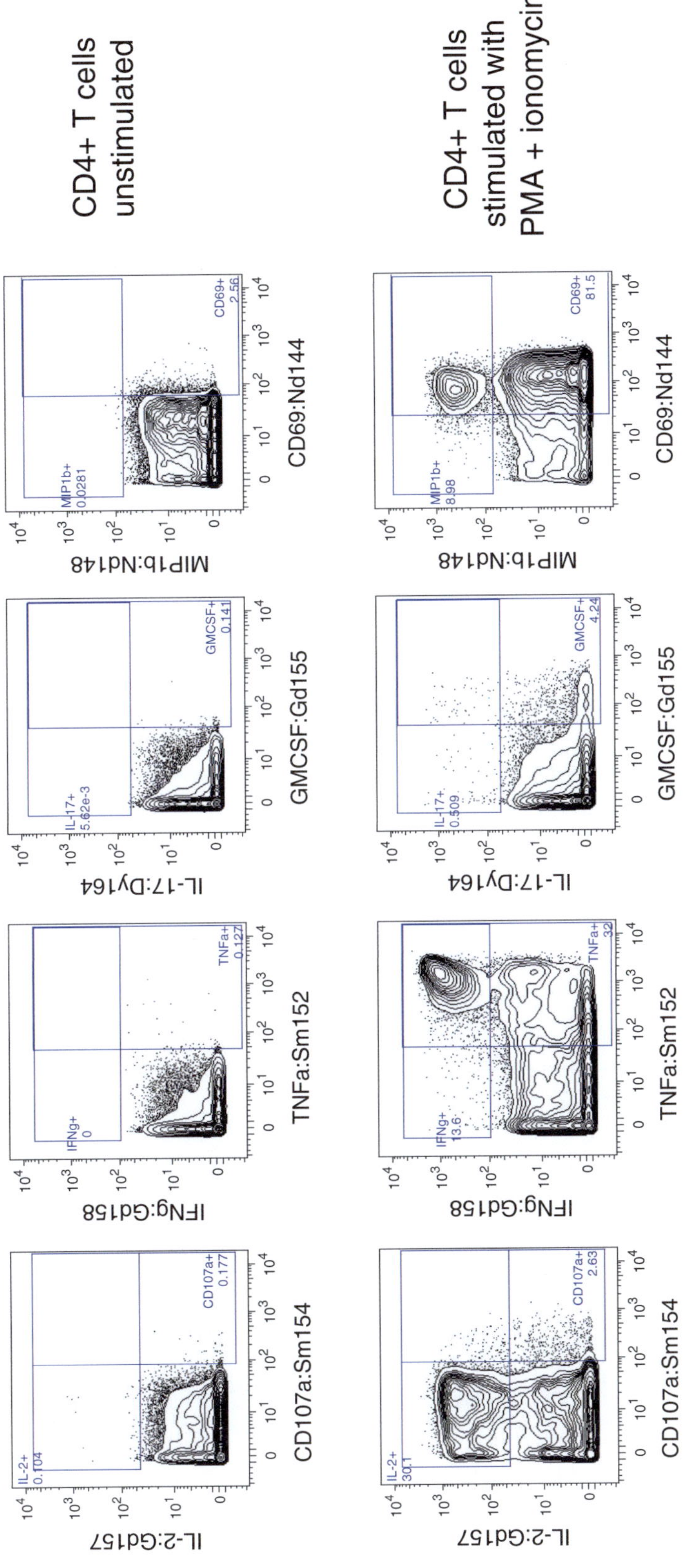

Fig. 3 (continued)

2 Materials

1. 96-well round bottom plates (*see* **Note 1**).

2. CyFACS buffer: 0.1% BSA+ 2 mM EDTA+ 0.1% NaAzide in PBS made with MilliQ water and no heavy metal contaminants (no glass or beakers washed with soap). Filter with a 0.2 μm filter; store at room temperature.

3. CyPBS: PBS without heavy metal contaminants (10× PBS from Rockland). No contact with beakers or bottles washed with soap. Filter with a 0.2 μm filter; store at room temperature.

4. MilliQ dH$_2$O: No contact with beakers or bottles washed with soap.

5. DOTA-maleimide: B-272 from Macrocyclics.
   - Use to make 5 mg/mL In115*-DOTA-maleimide, dissolved in MilliQ water. Add 100 μl 3% nitric acid per 10 mL solution to maintain low pH and store at 4 °C.
   - In115* is natural-abundance indium from a high-purity metal salt.

6. 0.1 μm spin filters: Millipore UFC30VV00.

7. 16% Paraformaldehyde: Electron Microscopy Sciences Cat. 15710.

8. DVS Sciences iridium intercalator solution: 2000× or 500× stock, use at final 1×.

9. Saponin-based permeabilization buffer (Ebioscience Cat. 00-8333-56).

10. Set of MAXPAR-labeled antibodies–labeled as per MAXPAR kit from DVS Sciences (*see* **Note 2**).

3 ICS Staining Protocol

3.1 Sample Collection

1. Two million viable cells per well (as measured by dye exclusion method such as Vicell; rested, if desired) (*see* **Note 3**).

3.2 Cell Activation

1. Perform as described in Lovelace and Maecker [13].

3.3 Sample Processing

1. Wash 1× in CyFACS buffer (flick plate or aspirate to remove supernatant).

2. Make Ab cocktail in CyFACS buffer (Filter with 0.1 μm spin filter).

3. Resupend cells in 50 μL filtered Ab cocktail.

4. Incubate for 30–60 min on ice.

5. Wash 2× in CyFACS buffer (*see* **Note 4**).

6. Resuspend cells in 100 μl of 1:3000 diluted In115-DOTA maleimide in CyPBS.

7. Incubate for 30 min on ice.

8. Wash 3× in CyFACS buffer.

9. Resuspend in 100 μl of 2 % PFA in CyPBS (*see* **Notes 5** and **6**).

10. Incubate at 4°C overnight.

11. Wash 2× in 1× eBioscience perm buffer (1× in MilliQ water).

12. Make intracellular staining cocktail in 1× perm. buffer and filter with 0.1 μm spin filter.

13. Incubate on ice for 45 min.

14. Wash 3× in CyFACS buffer.

15. Resuspend in 2 % PFA+ 1× Ir-Interchelator in CyPBS.

16. Incubate for 20 min at room temperature.

17. Wash 1× in CyFACS buffer.

18. Wash 3× in MilliQ water (*see* **Note 7**).

19. Resuspend in MilliQ water for running on mass cytometer (*see* **Note 8**). Filter through a 25 μM cell strainer prior to acquisition (*see* **Note 9**).

To perform only surface phenotyping: Subheading 3.1: 1 million live cells are usually sufficient. Omit stimulations in Subheading 3.2. In Subheading 3.3, omit **step 13**, and 2 % PFA in **step 16**.

3.4 Data Acquisition and Analysis

1. Start the machine. Warm up and tune as in Ref. [14].

2. Acquire data as in Ref. [14]. The length of the run will be dependent upon the volume of your sample: dilution with MilliQ water to ~1 million cells/mL is recommended for minimizing doublets as well as maximizing sample throughput (*see* **Note 10**).

3. Analyze data using third-party flow analysis software such as FlowJo (Treestar) or Cytobank (*see* **Note 11** and Fig. 1). Note that some display settings may need to be altered for proper viewing.

---

4 Notes

1. Plates vs. tubes: cells can be handled in 96-well microtiter plates or in 12 × 75 mm polystyrene tubes. Deepwell plates are useful for additional volume per wash (*see* **Note 4**).

2. Lanthanides cannot be photobleached. Therefore, there is no need to protect antibody stocks or samples from standard lab lighting.

3. The current cell transmission efficiency of the mass cytometer is 20–25%, compared to 95+% for a standard fluorescence flow cytometer. Therefore, coupled with cell loss due to the suggested number of wash steps (*see* **Note 4**) greater starting numbers of cells will be required for similar cell event counts.

4. Due to the sensitivity of the detector, mass cytometry samples require a large number of washes to minimize nonspecific background from staining steps. While this must be balanced against the loss of cells with each wash step, reducing the number of washes below what is listed here is not recommended.

5. All cells that are injected into the mass cytometer have been fixed and permeabilized. This is necessary to allow the iridium intercalator to effectively enter the cell.

6. MilliQ water can cause improperly fixed cells to lyse (*see* **Note 5**). Therefore, ensure that your PFA is fresh. While it is not always necessary to open a new bottle/ampule, PFA should be generally protected from light and exposed to atmosphere for less than a month to be completely active.

7. Ultrapure (e.g., MilliQ) water is required for washes and final resuspension at the end of the staining protocol. This helps ensure that there is little or no free metal or antibody upon injection into the mass cytometer. This also ensures that there are no buffer salts carried along with the sample. While most buffer salts will not make it through the quadrupole mass filter window (AM 89-209), they will accumulate on the metal cones at the entry to the machine. Over long run-times, buffer salts can accumulate and cause the tuning to drift, particularly the Current setting.

8. Stained samples can be kept at 4 °C for up to a week. However, fresher samples are optimal. If samples must be stored, it is preferable that they be stored in 2 % PFA/CyPBS, or at least in CyFACS. Regardless of the storage conditions, it will be necessary to do at least one MilliQ water wash prior to resuspension in MilliQ water and injection. Do not freeze stained samples.

9. All samples must be filtered through 25 μm cell strainers before injecting into the mass cytometer. This will minimize the likelihood that a clog will form in the nebulizer tubing or the nebulizer itself.

10. While the mass cytometer is capable of acquiring cells at up to 1000 cells/s, this usually causes an unacceptable number of doublets. Event rates of approximately 300–500 cells/s strike a better balance between optimizing the number of singlet events while still allowing sample acquisition in a reasonable timeframe. The event viewing window in the software shows ~1/350 snapshot of the data actually being acquiring per second. Therefore, an average of ~1 cell event/screen refresh would be in this 300–500 cells/s range.

11. The number of cell events counted by the mass cytometer during acquisition is an upper limit to the number of true cell events. The software registers a cell event as metal signal in any mass channel that is a number of standard deviations above background (default = 3 S.D.). Therefore, debris or other background signal from your sample could achieve this threshold and be counted. High signal in both iridium channels (Ir191 and Ir193) represents intact cells and is a useful first gate (Fig. 1). The number of Intact cells/Singlets/Live cells in a standard sample is often 50–60% of the total initially counted by the machine.

Acknowledgments

The authors thank Sean Bendall for helpful discussions, and Sheena Gupta and Meena Malipatlolla for contributing example data. Development of this protocol was funded in part by grant 2 U19 AI057229 S4 from the National Institutes of Health.

References

1. Kalisky T, Quake SR (2011) Single-cell genomics. Nat Methods 8:311–314

2. Ornatsky O, Bandura D, Baranov V, Nitz M, Winnik MA, Tanner S (2010) Highly multiparametric analysis by mass cytometry. J Immunol Methods 36:1–20

3. Bandura DR, Baranov VI, Ornatsky OI, Antonov A, Kinach R, Lou X, Pavlov S, Vorobiev S, Dick JE, Tanner SD (2009) Mass cytometry: technique for real time single cell multitarget immunoassay based on inductively coupled plasma time-of-flight mass spectrometry. Anal Chem 81:6813–6822

4. Newell EW, Sigal N, Bendall SC, Nolan GP, Davis MM (2012) Cytometry by time-of-flight shows combinatorial cytokine expression and virus-specific cell niches within a continuum of CD8(+) T cell phenotypes. Immunity 36:142–152

5. Bendall SC, Simonds EF, Qiu P, Amir el AD, Krutzik PO, Finck R, Bruggner RV, Melamed R, Trejo A, Ornatsky OI, Balderas RS, Plevritis SK, Sachs K, Pe'er D, Tanner SD, Nolan GP (2011) Single-cell mass cytometry of differential immune and drug responses across a human hematopoietic continuum. Science 332:687–696

6. Bodenmiller B, Zunder ER, Finck R, Chen TJ, Savig ES, Bruggner RV, Simonds EF, Bendall SC, Sachs K, Krutzik PO, Nolan GP (2012) Multiplexed mass cytometry profiling of cellular states perturbed by small-molecule regulators. Nat Biotechnol 30:858–867

7. Behbehani GK, Bendall SC, Clutter MR, Fantl WJ, Nolan GP (2012) Single-cell mass cytometry adapted to measurements of the cell cycle. Cytometry A 81:552–566

8. Fienberg HG, Simonds EF, Fantl WJ, Nolan GP, Bodenmiller B (2012) A platinum-based covalent viability reagent for single-cell mass cytometry. Cytometry A 81:467–475

9. Maecker HT (2009) Multiparameter flow cytometry monitoring of T cell responses. Methods Mol Biol 485:375–391

10. Maecker HT, Frey T, Nomura LE, Trotter J (2004) Selecting fluorochrome conjugates for maximum sensitivity. Cytometry A 62:169–173

11. Rundberg Nilsson A, Bryder D, Pronk CJ (2013) Frequency determination of rare populations by flow cytometry: a hematopoietic stem cell perspective. Cytometry A 83:721–727

12. Ornatsky OI, Kinach R, Bandura DR, Lou X, Tanner SD, Baranov VI, Nitz M, Winnik MA (2008) Development of analytical methods for multiplex bio-assay with inductively coupled plasma mass spectrometry. J Anal At Spectrom 23:463–469

13. Lovelace P, Maecker HT (2010) Multi-parameter intracellular cytokine staining. Methods Mol Biol 699:165–178

14. Leipold MD, Maecker HT (2012) Mass cytometry: protocol for daily tuning and running cell samples on a CyTOF mass cytometer. J Vis Exp. doi:10.3791/4398

Chapter 8

Imaging Immunosenescence

Feng Qian and Ruth R. Montgomery

Abstract

To demonstrate effects of aging visually requires a robust technique that can reproducibly detect small differences in efficiency or kinetics between groups. Investigators of aging will greatly appreciate the benefits of Amnis ImageStream technology (www.amnis.com/), which combines quantitative flow cytometry with simultaneous high-resolution digital imaging. Imagestream is quantitative, reproducible, feasible with limited samples, and it facilitates in-depth examination of cellular mechanisms between cohorts of samples.

Key words Flow cytometry, Microscopy, Image analysis, Immune response, Signal transduction, Aging, Monocyte, Dendritic cell, Neutrophil

1 Introduction

Advances in imaging techniques and analysis modalities present an unprecedented ability to view cellular events and trace intracellular signaling pathways and mechanisms [1]. Using transfected fluorescent proteins, it is now possible to resolve kinetics of cellular processes, organelle localization, and dynamic interactions in living cells by fluorescence recovery after photobleaching (FRAP). Fluorescence resonance energy transfer (FRET) can localize molecules interacting within 2–6 nm or resolve temporal interactions in living cells [1]. Super-resolution microscopy combines increased sensitivity of imaging hardware with novel image analysis to achieve nanometer resolution at the light level [2], and multiphoton imaging allows deep penetration (500 nm) into living tissue with minimal damage to surrounding tissue [3]. These dramatic advances in imaging are now feasible for many general uses in cell biology, but remain for the most part impractical for the study of aging, although multiphoton imaging may be valuable for investigation of differences in murine models of aging [3]. The use of imaging to demonstrate effects of aging requires a robust visualization technique that can detect small differences (10–30 %) in efficiency or kinetics between groups and can be repeated routinely so that

Albert C. Shaw (ed.), *Immunosenescence: Methods and Protocols*, Methods in Molecular Biology, vol. 1343,
DOI 10.1007/978-1-4939-2963-4_8, © Springer Science+Business Media New York 2015

samples from older or younger subjects may be directly compared. The technique should be able to be conducted with minimal manipulation of cells ex vivo and should not introduce new sources of variability. Both FRAP and FRET entail introducing fluorescently labeled components into cells—by transfection or injection—to detect their localization or interaction in the cells. The variability associated with adding these manipulations—potentially different in cells of different ages—may mask the ability to detect effects of aging.

For these reasons, the benefits of Amnis ImageStream technology (www.amnis.com/) will be greatly appreciated among investigators of aging. Imagestream combines quantitative flow cytometry, which can be employed without manipulation of cells and has sufficient sensitivity to assess differences from only a few thousand cells, and combines it with simultaneous high-resolution digital imaging. ImageStream allows gating of cell subsets and imaging of cell responses from gated, but unsorted cell populations. Imagestream has been employed to elucidate many cellular functions, e.g. to quantify nuclear translocation of transcription factors [4], bacterial phagocytosis and oxidative burst [5], as well as differences in signaling in studies of aging subjects and disease cohorts [6–8]. Imagestream's advantages include quantitation, reproducibility, feasibility with limited samples, and ability to promote in-depth examination of cellular mechanisms between cohorts of samples. Here, we provide a protocol to evaluate Toll-like Receptor (TLR) function in monocytes from human peripheral blood mononuclear cells.

2   Materials

All samples must be collected in accordance with appropriate IACUC, IRB, and biosafety regulations governing laboratory investigation. Comparison groups must be carefully selected to reduce any variations other than age such as manner of sample collection and handling. Sufficient samples must be collected to support robust statistical analysis such as mixed effects modeling [9] of factors such as gender, race, and co-morbid conditions.

1. AMNIS ImageStream X imaging cytometer (Amnis.com) equipped with ≥4 lasers (Excitation lasers: 488 nm blue laser, 561 nm green laser, 642 nm red laser, 405 nm violet laser and a Darkfield (SSC) laser 785 nm laser).

2. Computer: The Amnis IDEAS software currently requires a 32- or 64-bit Windows computer with recommended minimum specifications as follows: a quad core processor with 4GB of RAM and a PC bus speed of at least 1066 MHz. We have not found the Imagestream analysis program files to be compatible with MAC computers.

3. Fresh blood samples from younger and older human subjects collected in anticoagulated vacutainer tubes or BD Vacutainer® CPT™ Cell Preparation Tubes; or equivalent source of murine cells.

4. Cell culture media and sera: RPMI, MEM, pooled human serum or FBS for murine cells. We pre-screen aliquots of multiple test lots of serum from commercial sources (Lonza Group Ltd., Gemini Bio-Products, Valley Biomedical Products & Services, Inc.) to identify sera that optimize cell conditions. We culture monocytes from two to five donors in each sera and assess viability, morphology, and cytokine production in response to ligand stimulation.

5. Buffers for flow cytometry: We use phosphate-buffered saline (PBS) to wash cells, BD Staining Buffer and Perm/Wash buffer (BD Biosciences, NJ) for antibody labeling, we fix cells in 4 % paraformaldehyde (Electron Microscopy Sciences) in PBS (PFA/PBS), freezing buffer is 90 % FBS containing 10 % DMSO.

6. Fluorescently conjugated monoclonal antibodies: lineage markers Lin-1 (lineage-1 marker includes CD3, CD14, CD19, CD20, CD56), HLA-DR, CD45, CD11c, CD123. Functional markers: TLRs, signaling components (e.g., IRF1, IRF3, IRF5, IRF7, NF-κB). Commercial sources for these antibodies include BD Biosciences, BD Pharmingen, eBioscience, Invitrogen, CA, SantaCruz Biotechnology, CA (Table 1).

Table 1
Antibody panel for cell lineage staining of signaling pathways

Cell type	FITC	PE	Alexa 647	Pacific blue
Monocyte		Anti-CD14 (61D3; eBioscience)	NF-κB (anti-p65, C-20; Santa Cruz)	
Neutrophil		Anti-CD15 (HI98; BD Biosciences)		
mDC	Lin1	Anti-CD11c (S-HCl-3; BD Biosciences)	NF-κB (anti-p65, C-20; Santa Cruz)	Anti-CD4 (RPA-T4; BD Biosciences)
pDC	Lin1	Anti-CD123 (9-F5; BD Biosciences)	NF-κB (anti-p65, C-20; Santa Cruz)	Anti-CD4 (RPA-T4; BD Biosciences)

Monocyte: CD14+
Neutrophil CD15+
mDC: Lin1−, CD4dim, CD11c+
pDC: Lin1−, CD4dim, CD123+
Lin1 (lineage) marker includes CD3 (SK7), CD14 (MφP9), CD16 (3G8), CD19 (SJ25C1), CD20 (L27), CD56 (NCAM16.2)—the combination available from BD Biosciences

3 Methods

1. Procedures with human blood should be conducted in a laminar flow hood for Biosafety level 2 containment. Carry out procedures at room temperature unless otherwise specified. To minimize technical variability, samples can be collected and treated as available and frozen to be assessed together at one time.

2. Obtain 10–50 ml heparinized blood from study volunteers after written informed consent under the guidelines of the local Institutional Review Board (*see* **Note 1**).

3. Dilute blood 1:1 with PBS.

4. Prepare 50 ml tubes with 12.5 ml filtered Ficoll-Hypaque Plus gradient separation gradient gel (GE Healthcare, NJ, density 1.077 g/ml). Dispense approximately 35 ml diluted blood very slowly and gently down the side of tube so that it forms a layer of diluted blood over the Ficoll. Take care to minimize any blood entering into the Ficoll layer.

5. Centrifuge at $800 \times g$ for 20 min at RT with brake off; for CPT tubes, centrifuge at $1500–1800 \times g$ for 20 min at RT.

6. Peripheral blood mononuclear cells (PBMCs) will form a white band in the middle of the tube. Using a pipette, remove and discard the upper supernatant to within 0.5 cm of the cell layer. Collect cells from the white layer into a new 15 ml tube containing 5–7 ml RPMI.

7. Pellet cells at $500 \times g$ for 10 min at 4 °C, discard supernatant, and resuspend PBMC pellet in culture medium. For human cells we use RPMI with 20 % human serum. With murine cells, we use MEM with 10 % FBS.

8. Count cells and divide for treatment groups, $\sim 1 \times 10^6$ cells/condition. You may use wells of a 96-well plate or autoclaved 1.5 ml Eppendorf tubes.

9. To study kinetics of cell responses, add the stimulating agent to the series of samples. In the example shown in Figs. 1 and 2, we show mock treated cells and cells stimulated with flagellin (2.5 μg/ml), a TLR5 agonist (*see* **Note 2**).

10. Incubate cells at 37 °C in 5 % CO_2 incubator for the desired time(s). If cells are to be incubated in PBS rather than tissue culture medium, incubations should not be done in a 5 % CO_2 atmosphere as PBS will not have sufficient buffering capacity to maintain cultures at physiological pH. Instead when using PBS choose a warm room or incubator with room air at 37 °C.

11. We label surface markers on the day of isolation and then cells are fixed and stored in freezing buffer at −80 °C until all the samples are collected. Intracellular markers are labeled in batches of cells at one time to minimize assay variability.

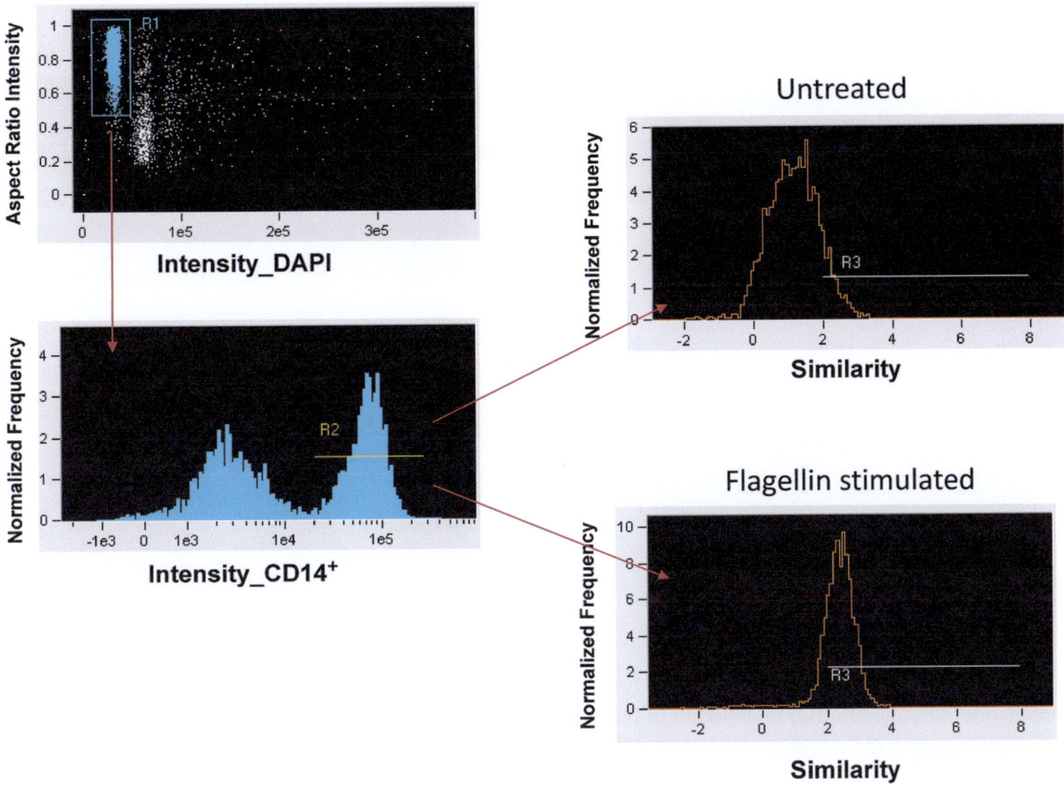

Fig. 1 Gating strategy for human monocytes from PBMCs. Monocytes are distinguished in gates with normal nuclear dye DAPI intensity and high DAPI aspect ratio (R1) which are labeled with lineage marker CD14 (R2). A high correlation of NF-κB with DAPI nuclear dye localization is reflected in a high similarity score and indicates the degree of activation in CD14+ monocytes (R3)

12. To label cell surface lineage markers, we first remove the stimulation medium by centrifuging samples at $300 \times g$ for 10 min at 4 °C, then remove the supernatant taking care to avoid disturbing the pellet.

13. Wash cells once by resuspending samples in 200 μl cold Staining Buffer, centrifuge at $300 \times g$ for 10 min at 4 °C, and discard the supernatant.

14. Label cells by resuspending samples in 50 μl Staining Buffer containing specific antibodies or isotype controls and incubate for 20 min at 4 °C protected from light. A sample staining panel is shown in Table 1 (*see* **Note 3**).

15. At the end of the staining period, wash cells by adding 200 μl cold Staining Buffer, and centrifuge at $300 \times g$ for 10 min at 4 °C. Remove the supernatant.

16. Fix cells by adding 0.1 ml 4 % paraformaldehyde in PBS for 10 min at RT protected from light.

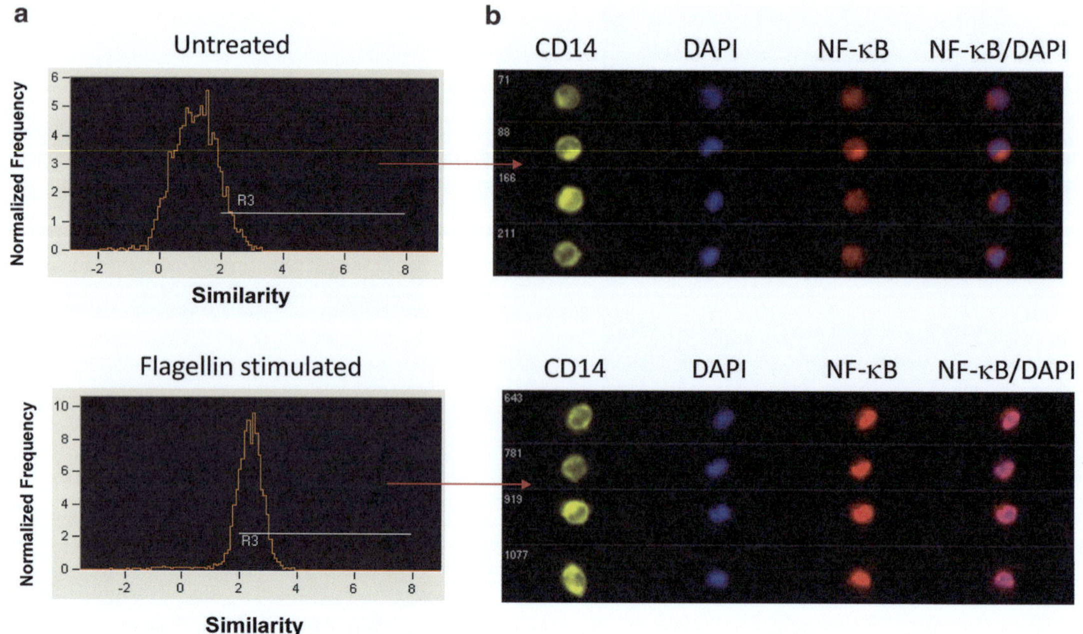

Fig. 2 Translocation of NF-κB in human monocytes after stimulation. The translocation of NF-κB (p65) into the nucleus after stimulation (R3) is depicted in populations of untreated and stimulated cells. The median value of similarity scores is 1.16 in untreated sample and 2.34 in stimulated sample (**a**). Digital images collected simultaneously of the untreated or flagellin-stimulated cell populations show representative cells and the intensity of NF-κB translocated into the cell nucleus (**b**)

17. At the end of the fixation period, centrifuge samples at $500 \times g$ for 10 min at 4 °C. Remove the supernatant and resuspend cells in 0.1 ml 90 % fetal calf serum/10 % DMSO for storing at −80 °C.

18. To minimize technical variability, batches of untreated and stimulated cells from a group of donors should be processed together. On the day of analysis, thaw cells quickly in a 37 °C water bath, and centrifuge at $500 \times g$ to remove freezing buffer.

19. Wash cells by adding 0.3 ml Staining Buffer (BD Biosciences), and centrifuge at $500 \times g$ for 10 min at 4 °C. Remove the supernatant.

20. Before intracellular staining, resuspend cells in 0.2 ml PermWash Buffer (BD Biosciences). Centrifuge at $500 \times g$ for 10 min at 4 °C. Remove the supernatant.

21. Resuspend cells in 0.1 ml PermWash Buffer and incubate for 15 min at 4 °C. Centrifuge at $500 \times g$ for 10 min at 4 °C. Remove the supernatant.

22. Label intracellular signaling components or organelle structures with specific antibodies and isotype controls in PermWash Buffer for 20 min at RT, e.g. rabbit anti-NF-κB (p65) antibody (10 μg/ml, SantaCruz Biotechnology, CA), detected using F(ab')$_2$ goat anti-rabbit IgG-Alexa647 (Invitrogen, CA). These incubations are conducted at RT according to the instrument manufacturer.

23. Immediately prior to imaging, counterstain nuclei with DAPI (final concentration 0.2 μg/ml, Invitrogen) or propidium iodide (PI; final concentration 20 ng/ml, Invitrogen). These concentrations should be optimized for new stocks of reagents and for different cell types.

24. Power up ImageStream, launch INSPIRE software and load default template as the setting. The calibration steps are automated by the instrument software. Initialize Fluidics and load the SpeedBead calibration reagent (Amnis) until the Flow Speed CV is consistently less than 0.2 %. To calibrate and test the instrument, use "Start All" command in the ASSIST tab.

25. After the ImageStream system is calibrated, define instrument settings using a sample that is bright in all the fluorescent channels employed for the study samples. Load the experiment's brightest sample and set the laser power for each fluorochrome to show maximum pixel values between 100 and 4000 counts, as measured in the dot plots. To normalize settings of batches of samples, primary cells may be used if in plentiful supply, or stored aliquots of frozen cells may be used. Compensation beads are not recommended by Amnis because speed control beads are used during the sample runs.

26. Set the "Cell Classification" criteria to eliminate collection of unwanted events, and set a number of events to acquire (a minimum of 5000 events for monocytes).

27. Click "FLL: Flush, Lock, Load." The sample pathway will be flushed first so wait until prompted before placing the sample on the left sample uptake line. To initiate readings, load labeled cells into sample chambers—either place a 96-well plate of labeled cells in the sample plate dock for autoplate reader instruments, or add tubes to the loading rack for instruments that use tubes.

28. Begin collecting sample data using the "Run Acquire" command to collect the data and save the file. Once acquisition finishes, click "FLL" to load the next sample. When finished collecting data on the last sample, click "FLL" and leave the system on. When the last user of the day is finished, choose Sterilize System from the instrument menu to prepare for shutting down.

29. Design a gating strategy template for the study and apply the gates equivalently across all study samples (*see* **Note 4**).

30. For data processing, identify monocytes using Amnis IDEAS software and follow gates as shown in Fig. 1. To distinguish in-focus single cells from debris, gate on events with a normal nuclear dye DAPI intensity and high aspect ratio (defined as the ratio of the width of a shape to its height) for DAPI (R1).

31. To identify monocytes, choose cells gated with high intensity labeling of the CD14 marker (R2).

32. To identify activated cells after stimulation, the similarity score of NF-κB and the nuclear dye DAPI will be calculated in CD14+ cells. Similarity measures the degree to which two images (NF-κB/DAPI) are correlated on a pixel-by-pixel basis. A high correlation of NF-κB with DAPI, indicating co-localization of the two markers, is reflected in a high "Similarity" score (R3). After stimulation, the treated cells were determined to have a significantly higher similarity score of NF-κB p65 with DAPI, indicating that NF-κB p65 translocated into the nucleus after stimulation. Representative images of cells are shown in Fig. 2.

33. The labeling and gating strategy described here works well for both monocytes and dendritic cells and should be effective for other cell types that show nuclear translocation of NF-κB after stimulation.

34. Differences between subject groups will be readily apparent through dot plots, histograms, and cell images. Data representative of the study cohort may be presented as populations in histogram format, and/or representative images (where they are particularly compelling). Data from within a defined gate—such as the "Similarity" score—can be tabulated for each study subject and/or group and is suitable for statistical determinations.

4 Notes

1. Design your experimental plan so that you can efficiently handle the number of samples sufficiently quickly. Examining samples from multiple study subjects at once reduces variability but only when the protocol can be managed smoothly. If many conditions per subject are required you may need to cap the maximum number of subjects you can assess per study day.

2. We have found it more efficient to add the stimulus at staggered intervals and then harvest all the samples together to facilitate staining at the final time point. We have found this is more efficient for labeling all samples together at the final time point.

In the example shown in Figs. 1 and 2, Flagellin was added at time 0, 30, and 45 min for harvest at 60 min. In this way, we determined changes evident after 60, 30, and 15 min of stimulation.

3. To design a labeling panel, markers should be tested singly and in combination to build a panel with specific signal after subtraction of isotype staining, consistent detection across the channels, and faithful quantitation of each marker [6]. For transcription factors that translocate into the nucleus, it is better to use a small molecular weight dye such as Alexa 647 or FITC; larger molecular weight dyes such as PE and PE-Texas Red may reduce efficiency of translocation. Choices for additional antibodies to include in the panel will be driven by the availability of the antibody of choice in a given fluorochrome. Custom conjugations may be necessary for less common or lab-specific markers. It may be necessary to design separate panels to detect markers that form a complex in the cells of interest. For example, we have found that we cannot detect authentic levels of TLR4 in cells labeled with CD14, and we have substituted CD4 dim or CD11c staining to define cell lineage for samples in which we measure TLR4.

4. While automated gating strategies are becoming more accurate and gaining popularity, we find at present that individual variation among human subjects is best addressed by manual gating.

Acknowledgement

The authors are grateful to the Yale Human Immunophenotyping Consortium and IMAGIN teams for insightful discussions.

Funding: This work was supported in part by the National Institutes of Health (HHS N272201100019C, U19AI089992).

Conflicts of Interest: The authors declare no commercial or other association that might pose a conflict of interest for this work.

References

1. Higashi T, Watanabe W, Matsunaga S (2012) Application of visualization techniques for cell and tissue engineering. J Biosci Bioeng 115: 122–126

2. Herbert S, Soares H, Zimmer C et al (2012) Single-molecule localization super-resolution microscopy: deeper and faster. Microsc Microanal 18:1419–1429

3. Masedunskas A, Milberg O, Porat-Shliom N et al (2012) Intravital microscopy: a practical guide on imaging intracellular structures in live animals. Bioarchitecture 2:143–157

4. George TC, Fanning SL, Fitzgerald-Bocarsly P et al (2006) Quantitative measurement of nuclear translocation events using similarity analysis of multispectral cellular images obtained in flow. J Immunol Methods 311:117–129

5. Ploppa A, George TC, Unertl KE et al (2011) ImageStream cytometry extends the analysis of phagocytosis and oxidative burst. Scand J Clin Lab Invest 71:362–369

6. Qian F, Montgomery RR (2012) Quantitative imaging of lineage specific Toll-like receptor mediated signaling in monocytes and dendritic

cells from small samples of human blood. J Vis Exp 62:e3741

7. Qian F, Wang X, Zhang L et al (2012) Age-associated elevation in TLR5 leads to increased inflammatory responses in the elderly. Aging Cell 11:104–110

8. Stone RC, Feng D, Deng J et al (2012) Interferon regulatory factor 5 activation in monocytes of systemic lupus erythematosus patients is triggered by circulating autoantigens independent of type I interferons. Arthritis Rheum 64:788–798

9. Schluchter MD, Elashoff JD (1990) Small-sample adjustments to tests with unbalanced repeated measures assuming several covariance structures. J Statist Comput Simul 37:69–87

Chapter 9

Activation-Induced Cytidine Deaminase and Switched Memory B Cells as Predictors of Effective In Vivo Responses to the Influenza Vaccine

Daniela Frasca, Alain Diaz, and Bonnie B. Blomberg

Abstract

Aging impairs humoral immune responses, leading to increased frequency and severity of infectious diseases and reduced protective effects of vaccination. We have identified B-cell biomarkers that are reduced by aging and that can be used as predictive markers of the response of an individual to vaccination. The identification of these biomarkers will have an impact on the development of effective vaccines to protect the elderly from infections and other debilitating diseases.

Key words Activation-induced cytidine deaminase, Class switch recombination, Antibody vaccine response

1 Introduction

The enzyme activation-induced cytidine deaminase (AID) is essential for DNA cleavage required for both class switch recombination (CSR) and somatic hypermutation (SHM) of Ig genes [1, 2]. These processes are crucial for the generation of high-affinity antibodies and robust humoral immunity. CSR and SHM occur in germinal center B cells in response to both T-dependent and T-independent stimuli [3, 4]. AID triggers CSR and SHM by deaminating cytosines in the variable and switch regions of the Ig locus and converting them to uracils; the resulting mismatches are recognized by specific enzymes and excised, leading to DNA double strand breaks [5, 6].

We [7, 8] and others [9] have shown that specific B-cell defects occur during aging. These include decreases in CSR [7, 8, 10] and in the ability to increase antibody affinity after antigenic challenge, a direct result of SHM [11]—both dependent on the decrease in expression of AID and the transcription factor E47 [8], whose

Albert C. Shaw (ed.), *Immunosenescence: Methods and Protocols*, Methods in Molecular Biology, vol. 1343,
DOI 10.1007/978-1-4939-2963-4_9, © Springer Science+Business Media New York 2015

activity is required for the efficient induction of AID transcription [12]. These defects are at least in part responsible for the reduced ability of elderly individuals to respond well to vaccination against tetanus, encephalitis viruses, *Salmonella*, *S. pneumoniae* and influenza [7, 10, 13–15].

We have recently identified B-cell-specific biomarkers which can be used to track the in vivo response to the influenza vaccine. These biomarkers are the in vitro vaccine-induced increase in AID gene expression after vaccination and the ex vivo vaccine-induced increase in the percentage of switched memory B cells (CD19+IgD-CD27+), which are both significantly decreased with age [7, 10]. Our results showing that switched memory B cells are increased by influenza vaccination are of great importance because these cells carry the immune memory of the individual in terms of specific immune responses [16].

Moreover, AID expression can be measured in CpG-stimulated B-cell (or PBMC) cultures before vaccination and can be used as a predictive marker of the response of an individual to the influenza vaccine. This AID response decreases with age and is positively correlated with the in vivo humoral response, as evaluated by the increase in antibody titers after vaccination. Also the percentage of switched memory B cells measured in blood before vaccination decreases with age and is correlated with the in vivo response to the vaccine and therefore can be another good predictive marker of the vaccine response. Here, we describe our protocol to measure these two predictive markers of the response: AID in CpG-stimulated B-cell cultures by quantitative (q)PCR and switched memory B cells in blood by flow cytometry and we show how these are correlated with the in vivo antibody response, measured by hemagglutination inhibition assay (HAI) or by ELISA.

2 Materials

2.1 B-Cell Isolation

We perform this procedure using the MACS Cell separation protocol from Miltenyi Biotec (Miltenyi), that is why we buy most of the materials and reagents from this company.

1. Suspension of human PBMC in complete medium (RPMI 1640, supplemented with 10 % FBS, 10 µg/ml Pen-Strep, 1 mM Sodium Pyruvate, and 2×10^{-5} M 2-Mercaptoethanol and 2 mM L-glutamine).

2. CD19 Microbeads (Miltenyi Biotec).

3. MACS buffer. A solution of 0.5 % fetal bovine serum (FBS) or 0.5 % Bovine Serum Albumin in 1× Phosphate-Buffered Saline (PBS).

4. MS columns with plungers (Miltenyi).

5. MACS separator (Miltenyi).

6. Trypan blue 0.2 %. Dilute stock solution of Trypan blue 0.4 % 1:1 with 1× phosphate-buffered saline (PBS). Store at room temperature.

2.2 B-Cell Culture

1. Complete medium.

2. CpG (Invivogen ODN 2006).

2.3 mRNA Extraction

1. μMACS mRNA isolation kit (Miltenyi), containing Oligo (dT) Microbeads, Lysis/Binding, Wash and Elution buffers.

2. Lysate clear columns and μMACS columns (Miltenyi).

3. μMACS separator (Miltenyi).

2.4 Quantitative (q) PCR

To reverse transcribe mRNA and obtain cDNA:

1. PCR buffer II and $MgCl_2$, Deoxynucleoside triphosphates [dNTPs: dATP, dCTP, dGTP, dTTP], Random hexamers, MuLV Reverse transcriptase, RNase inhibitor. All reagents are from Life Technologies.

To amplify cDNA:

1. Taqman gene assay master mix, primers + probe mix (Hs00221068, AID; Hs99999905, GAPDH) (Life Technologies).

2. qPCR microplates and plastic covers (Life Technologies).

2.5 Flow Cytometry

1. Human blood.

2. APC-conjugated anti-CD19 (clone HIB19), PE-conjugated anti-CD27 (clone M-T271), FITC-conjugated anti-IgD (clone IA6-2) antibodies (*see* **Note 1**).

3. RBC Lysing Solution BD PharmLyse (BD).

4. FACS buffer (Dissolve 9.8 g Hanks Balanced Salts, 0.35 g $NaHCO_3$, 1 g BSA, 0.2 g Sodium Azide in deionized water for 1 L of buffer).

5. Fixation buffer (BD Cytofix).

2.6 In Vivo Antibody Response

This can be measured by the hemagglutination inhibition assay (HAI), which is the most established correlate with vaccine protection [7, 10, 17, 18]. The technique is not described here but it will be used below for correlations with our B-cell-specific biomarkers (*see* Figs. 1 and 2).

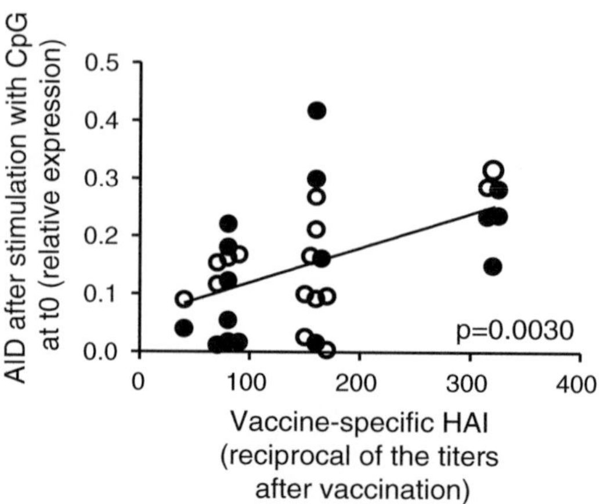

Fig. 1 The in vitro AID response of B cells to CpG at t0 is significantly correlated with the serum response. Thirty-two subjects (16 young and 16 elderly), enrolled during the 2011–2012 influenza vaccination season, were evaluated. Results are expressed as raw qPCR values of AID mRNA, calculated as $2^{-\Delta Ct}$. AID value is the fraction of the value of GAPDH, e.g. 0.25 means AID is ¼ of the amount of GAPDH. The serum response is measured by the reciprocal of the titers after vaccination as evaluated by the HAI assay. A titer of 1:40 indicates protection and a positive response. Pearson's $r = 0.5175$, $p = 0.0029$ (two-tailed). *Open symbols*: young; *filled symbols*: elderly

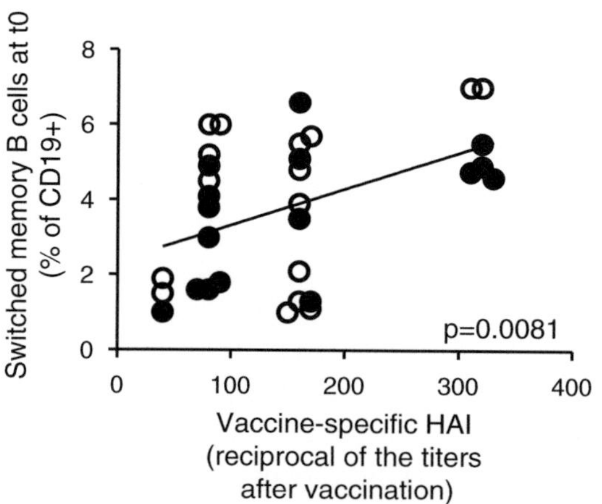

Fig. 2 The percentage of switched memory B cells at t0 significantly correlates with the in vivo serum response. The same subjects of Fig. 1 were evaluated. The percentages of switched memory B cells are evaluated by flow cytometry at t0. The serum response is measured by the reciprocal of the titers after vaccination as evaluated by the HAI assay. A titer of 1:40 indicates protection and a positive response. Pearson's $r = 0.4548$, $p = 0.0089$ (two-tailed). *Open symbols*: young; *filled symbols*: elderly

3   Methods

3.1   Isolation of Human B Cells by Positive Selection with CD19 Microbeads

This procedure should be performed under a laminar flow hood to preserve sterility and in a BSL-2 laboratory, implementing all the adequate safety measures for working with potentially infectious human samples. All personnel should be immunized with the Hepatitis B vaccine.

Positive selection of B cells is the best protocol to obtain highly purified B cells, without other contaminating cell types (T cells, NK cells, monocytes, macrophages). In long-term cultures (2–7 days), B cells isolated with this procedure, compared to B cells isolated with negative selection, give comparable results. Negative selection should be preferred only in studies on signal transduction performed in minutes from selection (5–30 min), in order to avoid effects of antibody cross-linking of cell surface proteins.

1. Resuspend PBMC in MACS buffer at a concentration of 10^7 cells/80 µl of buffer (*see* **Note 2**).

2. Add CD19 Microbeads (20 µl per 10^7 cells), mix well, and incubate for 15–20 min at 4 °C. Usually the B-cell yield is about 2–10 % of the total PBMC. A minimum of 10^5 B cells can be used for activation in culture and reliable detection of AID.

3. Wash cells with 5 ml of buffer, by centrifuging at $300 \times g$ for 10 min. Discard supernatant and resuspend in 500 µl of MACS buffer.

4. Place the MS columns (one per sample) in the MACS separator, rinse the columns with 500 µl of MACS buffer and apply cell suspension onto the column.

5. Wash the column twice with 500 µl of MACS buffer.

6. Remove column from the separator and place it in a centrifuge tube for collection of the adherent fraction.

7. Add 1 ml of complete RPMI onto the column, and collect CD19+ cells by pushing the plunger into the column. Count the cells by Trypan blue exclusion dye with a hemocytometer.

3.2   Culture and Stimulation of Human B Cells

1. Resuspend the B cells at a concentration of 10^6/ml of complete RPMI (*see* **Note 3**).

2. Add CpG to a final concentration of 1 µg/ml (*see* **Note 4**).

3. Incubate the cells at 37 °C, 5 % CO_2, for 5–7 days (*see* **Note 5**). In case cryopreserved PBMC are used, incubation time should be only 3 days.

3.3   mRNA Extraction from Activated Human B Cells

1. Extract mRNA from cultured cells using the µMACS mRNA isolation kit. Before starting, the Lysis/Binding buffer and the Wash buffer should be brought to room temperature, whereas the Elution buffer must be heated at 65 °C in a water bath.

2. Collect cultured cells by pipetting up and down several times (*see* **Note 6**).

3. Centrifuge at $300 \times g$ for 5 min and remove the supernatant.

4. Resuspend the cells in maximum of 0.7 ml of Lysis/Binding buffer.

5. Apply lysate on top of the LysateClear Column and centrifuge at $13,000 \times g$ for 3 min to remove any debris and reduce viscosity of the lysate.

6. Add 50 µl of Oligo (dT) Microbeads to the lysate and mix. Further incubation is not necessary for the hybridization of mRNA to Oligo (dT) Microbeads.

7. Place a µMACS Column in the magnetic field of the µMACS separator, rinse the column with 100 µl of Lysis/Binding buffer and let buffer run.

8. Apply cell lysate on top of the column matrix and let it run through. Magnetically labeled mRNA is retained in the column.

9. Rinse column twice with 200 µl of Lysis/Binding buffer to remove proteins and DNA and then four times with 100 µl of Wash buffer to remove rRNA and DNA. Wait until buffer runs through before each rinsing step.

10. To elute mRNA, apply 120 µl of 65 °C pre-heated Elution buffer to the column. mRNA is eluted by gravity. Collect the second, third, and fourth drops (*see* **Note 7**).

3.4 qPCR to Detect AID

1. To reverse transcribe mRNA and obtain cDNA, prepare a reaction RT mix by pipetting the following reagents: 1 µl DNase/RNase-free water, 4 µl $MgCl_2$, 2 µl PCR Buffer II, 2 µl of each dNTPs, 1 µl random hexamers, 1 µl MuLV Reverse transcriptase, 1 µl RNase inhibitor. This RT mix will be mixed in an Eppendorf (0.2 ml) tube with 18 µl (1:1; vol:vol) of the mRNA obtained as described above.

2. Place the Eppendorf tubes in the thermocycler and run the samples at the following conditions: 1 cycle of 40 min at 42 °C, followed by 1 cycle of 5 min at 65 °C.

3. To run qPCR and detect AID, prepare a reaction mix by pipetting the following reagents to the wells of a PCR microplate: 10 µl Taqman gene assay master mix, 1 µl primers + probe mix (for AID or GAPDH), 5 µl DNase/RNase-free water, 4 µl of the cDNA sample. Seal the microplate with an adhesive cover and quickly spin it for 20 s at $300 \times g$ to mix the reagents well.

4. Run the qPCR reaction in an ABI 7300 system machine. The settings are the following: 1 cycle of 2 min at 50 °C, then 1 cycle of 10 min at 95 °C, followed by 40 cycles of 15 s at 95 °C plus 1 min at 60 °C. The ABI 7300 software calculates

the number of amplification cycles at which transcripts reach a significant fluorescence threshold (Ct) for the sample gene (AID) and the housekeeping gene (GAPDH). Then Ct values for the housekeeping gene are subtracted from those of the target gene (ΔCt) and the following formula is calculated and used as qPCR value: $2^{-\Delta Ct}$, as reported previously [19]. CpG-induced AID expression before vaccination is positively correlated with the serum response and therefore can be used as a predictive marker of the response of an individual to the vaccine (Fig. 1).

3.5 Evaluation of Switched Memory B Cells by Flow Cytometry

1. To evaluate the switched memory B-cell subset, 100 μl of blood is stained with fluorescent-labeled antibodies to CD19, CD27, and IgD. Switched memory B cells are CD19+IgD–CD27+. With the same staining protocol, it is possible also to measure the other major B-cell subsets: naive (CD19+IgD+CD27–), IgM memory (CD19+IgD+CD27+), and late/exhausted memory (CD19+IgD–CD27–).

2. After 20 min incubation at room temperature, red blood cells are lysed using the RBC Lysing solution. Then samples are washed thoroughly with FACS buffer and fixed using Cytofix solution. Up to 10^5 events in the lymphocyte gate are acquired on an LSR-Fortessa (BD), equipped with five lasers, and analyzed using FACS Diva (BD) software. Any FACS equipment capable of measuring three colors simultaneously can be used. Single color controls are included in every experiment for compensation. Switched memory B-cell percentages before vaccination are positively correlated with the serum response and therefore can also be used as predictive markers of the response to the vaccine (Fig. 2).

4 Notes

1. We had previously used the IgG+/IgA+ stain instead of IgD to identify the memory subsets [7, 10, 20] which agree in general with these, but in order to measure B-cell subsets in cryopreserved cells the former is problematic because IgG and IgA markers are lost during the freezing/thawing procedure. Therefore, we switched to the protocol that includes IgD.

2. Cryopreserved PBMC can also be used, thawed and rested in complete medium in a 5 % CO_2 incubator at 37 °C, for at least 1 h (and up to 3 h).

3. For cultures of 5×10^5 cells or less, use a 48-well tissue culture plate, otherwise, seed the cells in a 24-well plate.

4. A stock solution of 1 mg/ml of CpG should be prepared and stored for use.

5. We have shown in kinetic experiments that the optimum expression of AID occurs after this time in culture.

6. At least 20 times are required to recover most of the cells from the wells.

7. The second to fourth drop will contain more than 90 % of the isolated mRNA in a volume of approximately 75 µl. Store mRNA at –80 °C until use.

References

1. Okazaki IM, Kinoshita K, Muramatsu M et al (2002) The AID enzyme induces class switch recombination in fibroblasts. Nature 416: 340–345

2. Yoshikawa K, Okazaki IM, Eto T et al (2002) AID enzyme-induced hypermutation in an actively transcribed gene in fibroblasts. Science 296:2033–2036

3. Pone EJ, Zan H, Zhang J et al (2010) Toll-like receptors and B-cell receptors synergize to induce immunoglobulin class-switch DNA recombination: relevance to microbial antibody responses. Crit Rev Immunol 30:1–29

4. Stavnezer J, Guikema JE, Schrader CE (2008) Mechanism and regulation of class switch recombination. Annu Rev Immunol 26:261–292

5. Muramatsu M, Nagaoka H, Shinkura R et al (2007) Discovery of activation-induced cytidine deaminase, the engraver of antibody memory. Adv Immunol 94:1–36

6. Rada C, Williams GT, Nilsen H et al (2002) Immunoglobulin isotype switching is inhibited and somatic hypermutation perturbed in UNG-deficient mice. Curr Biol 12: 1748–1755

7. Frasca D, Diaz A, Romero M et al (2010) Intrinsic defects in B cell response to seasonal influenza vaccination in elderly humans. Vaccine 28:8077–8084

8. Frasca D, Landin AM, Lechner SC et al (2008) Aging down-regulates the transcription factor E2A, activation-induced cytidine deaminase, and Ig class switch in human B cells. J Immunol 180:5283–5290

9. Gibson KL, Wu YC, Barnett Y et al (2009) B-cell diversity decreases in old age and is correlated with poor health status. Aging Cell 8:18–25

10. Frasca D, Diaz A, Romero M et al (2012) Unique biomarkers for B-cell function predict the serum response to pandemic H1N1 influenza vaccine. Int Immunol 24:175–182

11. Khurana S, Frasca D, Blomberg B et al (2012) AID activity in B cells strongly correlates with polyclonal antibody affinity maturation in-vivo following pandemic 2009-H1N1 vaccination in humans. PLoS Pathog 8:e1002920

12. Sayegh CE, Quong MW, Agata Y et al (2003) E-proteins directly regulate expression of activation-induced deaminase in mature B cells. Nat Immunol 4:586–593

13. Gardner EM, Bernstein ED, Dran S et al (2001) Characterization of antibody responses to annual influenza vaccination over four years in a healthy elderly population. Vaccine 19:4610–4617

14. LeMaoult J, Szabo P, Weksler ME (1997) Effect of age on humoral immunity, selection of the B-cell repertoire and B-cell development. Immunol Rev 160:115–126

15. McElhaney JE, Effros RB (2009) Immunosenescence: what does it mean to health outcomes in older adults? Curr Opin Immunol 21:418–424

16. Amanna IJ, Carlson NE, Slifka MK (2007) Duration of humoral immunity to common viral and vaccine antigens. N Engl J Med 357:1903–1915

17. Murasko DM, Bernstein ED, GardnerE M et al (2002) Role of humoral and cell-mediated immunity in protection from influenza disease after immunization of healthy elderly. Exp Gerontol 37:427–439

18. Skowronski DM, Tweed SA, De Serres G (2008) Rapid decline of influenza vaccine-induced antibody in the elderly: is it real, or is it relevant? J Infect Dis 197:490–502

19. Schmittgen TD, Livak KJ (2008) Analyzing real-time PCR data by the comparative C(T) method. Nat Protoc 3:1101–1108

20. Frasca D, Diaz A, Romero M et al (2011) Age effects on B cells and humoral immunity in humans. Ageing Res Rev 10:330–335

Chapter 10

Analyzing the Effect of Aging on CD8+ T-Cell Phenotype Using Flow Cytometry

Min Sun Shin and Insoo Kang

Abstract

One of the most noticeable changes in T-cell immunity with aging is the expansion of memory CD8+ T cells, with a decline in naïve phenotype T cells that reflects both diminished thymopoiesis and the effects of chronic antigenic stimulation with age. Flow cytometry is a useful tool in evaluating immune cells including the phenotype characteristics of different T-cell subsets. Here, we show flow cytometric methods measuring the different subsets of human CD8+ T cells that change with aging.

Key words Human, T cells, Flow cytometry

1   Introduction

T cells are a component of the adaptive immune system characterized by immunological memory. The progenitors for T cells that develop in the bone marrow migrate to the thymus where they become immature T cells or thymocytes [1, 2]. After undergoing positive and negative selection, a small number of immature T cells are exported into the circulation as mature but naïve T cells [2, 3]. Upon the recognition of appropriate antigen in the context of the major histocompatibility complex (MHC) and receiving co-stimulation from antigen-presenting cells (APCs) in secondary lymphoid tissues, naïve T cells become activated, proliferate, and differentiate into effector cells [2]. Once the source of antigen (e.g. viral infection) is removed, most effector T cells die but a few cells survive and become memory T cells providing long-term immune protection.

T cells can be classified into CD4+ and CD8+ T cells. The former cells recognize antigen presented in the context of MHC class II molecules while the latter cells recognize antigen presented in the restriction of MHC class I molecules. CD4+ and CD8+ T cells that are referred as T helper (Th) and cytotoxic T cells, respectively, have distinct functions although both cell populations can produce cytokines. The primary function of CD4+ T cells is to help other immune

Albert C. Shaw (ed.), *Immunosenescence: Methods and Protocols*, Methods in Molecular Biology, vol. 1343,
DOI 10.1007/978-1-4939-2963-4_10, © Springer Science+Business Media New York 2015

cells like B cells and monocytes become fully activated by producing cytokines and expressing co-stimulatory molecules [1, 4]. CD8+ T cells with the expression of cytotoxic molecules destroy infected host cells or tumor cells [5]. Th cells can be further divided into Th1, Th2, and Th17 cells based on the cytokines dominantly produced by these cells. Th1 and Th2 cells produce high levels of IFN-γ and IL-4, respectively, while Th17 cells produce IL-17 [2, 6]. Alterations in T-cell immunity occur with aging. Probably, the most noticeable change in T-cell immunity is the expansion of memory T cells, in particular CD8+ T cells [2, 7]. Such expanded memory CD8+ T cells have increased expression of natural killer (NK) cell-associated molecules, loss of CD28 expression as well as decreased expression of interleukin 7 receptor alpha chain (CD127) [2]. Of interest, reactivation of latent cytomegalovirus infection has been linked to the expansion of memory CD8+ T cells [8].

Human naïve and memory T cells are traditionally classified by the reciprocal expression of the T-cell receptor (TCR) co-receptors CD45RA and CD45RO. Memory T cells can be divided into central and effector memory cells (CM and EM, respectively) based on the expression of lymphoid tissue homing molecules such as CCR7 and CD62L [9]. CCR7 expressed on CM T cells allows them to migrate to secondary lymphoid tissues [9]. Based on the expression of CD45RA and CCR7, human CD4+ and CD8+ T cells are divided into naïve (CD45RA+CCR7+), central (CM, CD45RA-CCR7+), and effector (EM, CD45RA–CCR7–) memory cells (Fig. 1) [7, 9]. In CD8+ T cells, an additional subset of EM cells with the expression of CD45RA but not CCR7 is found. This subset can be referred to as CD45RA+ EM CD8+ T cells (Fig. 1). Aging also affects the expression of cell surface molecules such as IL-7Rα (CD127) on T cells [2, 10]. The expression of these molecules including CD45RA, CCR7, and IL-7Rα can be easily measured using flow cytometry.

Flow cytometry is a technology that is used to analyze the phenotype and function of cells that has become an essential tool in studying immune cells including T cells in humans and animals (reviewed in Ref. [11]). Over the past decade, hardware and software for flow cytometry have substantially advanced. Here, we show flow cytometric methods to identify subsets of human CD8+ T cells that change with aging.

2   Materials

1. Blood collection tubes with anticoagulants (heparin, EDTA, or acid citrate dextrose) (BD Bioscience).

2. Ficoll-Paque PLUS (GE Healthcare).

3. Antibodies to CD3, CD4, CD8, CD45RA, chemokine receptor (CCR7), and IL-7 receptor alpha chain (CD127) (*see* Table 1) (*see* **Note 1** for CD127 polyclonal goat antibodies).

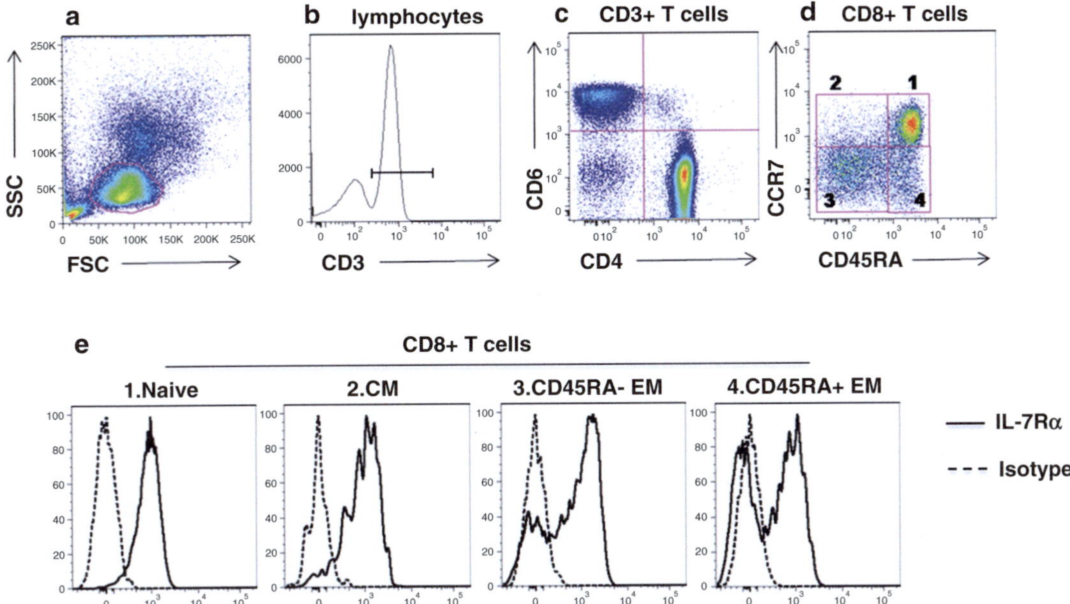

Fig. 1 Identification of different CD8+ T cell subsets with differential expression of IL-7Rα in human peripheral blood using flow cytometry. Peripheral blood was drawn into a heparinized tube from a healthy control after obtaining informed consent. Peripheral blood mononuclear cells (PBMCs) were purified by Ficoll-Paque centrifugation. PBMCs were stained with antibodies to CD3, CD4, CD8, CD45RA, CCR7 and IL-7Rα or isotype antibodies. Stained cells were analyzed on an LSRII® flow cytometer. (**a**) Lymphocytes were identified by forward and side light scatters. (**b–c**) CD4+ and CD8+ T cells were identified based on CD3, CD4 and CD8 expression. (**d**) Naïve (CD45RA+ CCR7+), central memory (CM, CD45RA– CCR7+), CD45RA– effector memory (EM, CD45RA– CCR7-) and CD45RA+ effector memory (CD45RA+ CCR7–) CD8+ T cells are identified. (**e**) IL-7Rα expression by different CD8+ T cell subsets is detected based on staining with antibodies to IL-7Rα (*open*) and isotype control

Table 1
Antibodies used in analyzing T-cell phenotype

Antibody	Clone (manufacturer)
APC-Cyc7 CD3	SK7 (BD Bioscience)
Alexa700 CD4	RPA T4 (BD Bioscience)
PB CD8	RPA-T8 (BD Bioscience)
PE Cy5 CD45RA	HI100 (BD Bioscience)
PE-Cy7 CCR7	3D12 (BD Bioscience)
IL-7Rα (CD127)	Clone 40131 (R&D Systems)

4. Donkey anti-goat IgG antibodies conjugated with FITC (Molecular Probes).

5. 1× Phosphate buffered saline (PBS) and FACS Buffer (PBS, 0.5–1 % bovine serum albumin (BSA, Sigma-Aldrich)).

6. 2 % paraformaldehyde (PFA) solution: Dilute 32 % PFA 1:32 in 1× PBS. Store at 4 °C.

3 Methods

1. Peripheral blood is collected into tubes containing heparin or EDTA (BD Vacutainer® or equivalent).

2. Mix blood with PBS at 1:1–3 ratio (V/V) (*see* **Note 2**).

3. Place 15 ml of Ficoll-Paque PLUS into a 50 ml conical tube.

4. Slowly layer the 20 ml of diluted blood onto the Ficoll, avoiding mixing the blood and Ficoll.

5. Spin sample at $400 \times g$ for 30 min at room temperature with no brake.

6. Carefully collect PBMC layer into a separate 50 ml tube using a Pasteur pipette and mix with PBS up to 40 ml.

7. Wash cells by spinning sample at $200 \times g$ for 5–10 min at room temperature. Repeat this step.

8. Count cells.

9. Resuspend cells with FACS buffer at $1 \times g$ 10^7 cells/ml (*see* **Note 3**).

10. Place 1×10^6 cells (0.1 ml) into a 12×75 mm, 5 ml polystyrene round bottom test tube (*see* **Note 4**).

11. Add the appropriate amounts of antibodies or isotype controls to each tube (*see* **Note 5**). Mix cells with antibodies by vortexing gently.

12. Incubate cells for 30 min at room temperature (*see* **Note 6**).

13. Wash cells with FACS buffer by spinning at $200–300 \times g$ for 5 min. This step can be repeated.

14. Add donkey anti-goat IgG antibodies conjugated with FITC and incubate for 30 min at room temperature.

15. Wash cells with FACS buffer by spinning at $200–300 \times g$ for 5 min. This step can be repeated.

16. Add 200 µl of 2 % PFA in FACS buffer and incubate at room temperature for 15–30 min.

17. Wash cells with FACS buffer by spinning at $200–300 \times g$ for 5 min.

18. Resuspend cells with 200 µl of FACS buffer.

19. Acquire data according to the flow cytometer instruction at individual institutions.

20. Analyze the acquired data using appropriate software (e.g. FlowJo). Identify lymphocyte population using forward and side scatter. Based on isotype control staining, populations positively and negatively stained for individual molecules can be identified.

4 Notes

1. Monoclonal and polyclonal antibodies are available for human IL-7Rα chain (CD127). We prefer goat polyclonal antibodies from R&D Systems since these antibodies provide the most optimal results in identifying EM CD8+ T cells with high and low levels of IL-7Rα.

2. Higher dilution with PBS may increase the yield of PBMC purification.

3. PBMCs can be resuspended at lower or higher concentrations.

4. A cocktail of multiple antibodies (e.g. anti-CD3, CD4, CD8, CD45RA, and CCR7) can be used to stain multiple samples.

5. The number of tubes to be set up depends on the number of antibodies to be used. Also, tubes for isotype, unstained, and single color controls should be included as appropriate.

6. Incubation temperature should be determined according to the manufacturer's instruction for individual antibodies.

References

1. Reiner SL (2007) Development in motion: helper T cells at work. Cell 129:33–36

2. Lee N, Shin MS, Kang I (2012) T-cell biology in aging, with a focus on lung disease. J Gerontol A Biol Sci Med Sci 67:254–263

3. Starr TK, Jameson SC, Hogquist KA (2003) Positive and negative selection of T cells. Annu Rev Immunol 21:139–176

4. Murphy KM, Stockinger B (2010) Effector T cell plasticity: flexibility in the face of changing circumstances. Nat Immunol 11:674–680

5. Cui W, Kaech SM (2010) Generation of effector CD8+ T cells and their conversion to memory T cells. Immunol Rev 236:151–166

6. Shin MS, Lee N, Kang I (2011) Effector T-cell subsets in systemic lupus erythematosus: update focusing on Th17 cells. Curr Opin Rheumatol 23:444–448

7. Hong MS, Dan JM, Choi JY et al (2004) Age-associated changes in the frequency of naive,

memory and effector CD8+ T cells. Mech Ageing Dev 125:615–618

8. Lee WW, Shin MS, Kang Y et al (2012) The relationship of cytomegalovirus (CMV) infection with circulatory IFN-alpha levels and IL-7 receptor alpha expression on CD8(+) T cells in human aging. Cytokine 58:332–335

9. Sallusto F, Lenig D, Forster R et al (1999) Two subsets of memory T lymphocytes with distinct homing potentials and effector functions. Nature 401:708–712

10. Kim HR, Hong MS, Dan JM et al (2006) Altered IL-7R{alpha} expression with aging and the potential implications of IL-7 therapy on CD8+ T-cell immune responses. Blood 107:2855–2862

11. Soloski MJ, Chrest FJ (2013) Multi-parameter flow cytometry for discovery of disease mechanisms in rheumatic diseases. Arthritis Rheum 65.1148–1156

Cell-Mediated Immune Response to Influenza Using Ex Vivo Stimulation and Assays of Cytokine and Granzyme B Responses

Janet E. McElhaney and Beth Gentleman

Abstract

The antibody response to vaccination has been the industry and regulatory standard for evaluating influenza vaccine efficacy. Although antibodies are an important defense mechanism providing sterilizing immunity, in older adults, the cellular immune response is also needed for clinical protection against the serious complications of influenza. Thus, the demonstration of enhanced antibody responses as a strategy for advancing new influenza vaccines through the standard clinical development pipeline may fail to translate to enhanced protection in the older population. In peripheral blood mononuclear cells (PBMC) challenged with live influenza virus, an increase in the interferon-γ:interleukin-10 (IFN-γ:IL-10) ratio and the level of the cytolytic mediator, granzyme B (GrzB), correlates with protection against influenza in vaccinated older adults. This chapter provides detailed methods for measuring these cell-mediated immune responses, which have been validated according to the International Conference on Harmonisation (ICH) guidelines. These immune correlates could be combined with antibody responses to improve the prediction of enhanced protection in vaccine trials in the older population.

Key words Influenza, Granzyme B, IL-10, IFN-gamma, Aging

1 Introduction

Largely supported by our work showing that antibody titers against influenza do not predict protection in older adults [1], there has been a paradigm shift in understanding the limitations of antibody titers as a sole measure of influenza efficacy [2]. Thus, antibody titers alone as a correlate of protection may fail to detect vaccine failures. This is not to say that antibodies are not an important defense mechanism, but suggests that the cellular immune response is also needed for clinical protection against influenza in older adults. In peripheral blood mononuclear cells (PBMC) challenged with live influenza virus, we have shown that risk for influenza illness in older adults correlates with a reduced interferon-γ:interleukin-10 (IFN-γ:IL-10) ratio in PBMC supernatants and a low level of the cytolytic mediator,

Albert C. Shaw (ed.), *Immunosenescence: Methods and Protocols*, Methods in Molecular Biology, vol. 1343,
DOI 10.1007/978-1-4939-2963-4_11, © Springer Science+Business Media New York 2015

granzyme B (GrzB), in PBMC lysates [1]. Assays of the ex vivo response (GrzB and IFNγ:IL-10) to influenza challenge have been developed, validated (according to the International Conference on Harmonisation guidelines) [3], and established as correlates of protection [1, 4] and as indicators of influenza disease severity [5] in older adults. The assay of GrzB activity capitalizes on the enzyme's unique substrate specificity for cleavage at the aspartate residue of the modified peptide IEPDpna, resulting in paranitroanalide (pna) release that correlates with cytolytic activity in influenza-stimulated peripheral blood mononuclear cells [6]. Assays of GrzB and the IFNγ:IL-10 ratio validated for precision and robustness in four international laboratories compare very favorably with humoral assays; a 25 % difference in the means can be detected with 95 % confidence in as few as 13 subjects/group for GrzB activity and 33 subjects/group for the IFNγ:IL-10 ratio [3]. To establish specificity with respect to the response to influenza virus, we have shown that in older adults with acute respiratory illness, GrzB levels increase following the illness only in those with laboratory-confirmed influenza illness (LCII). Prior to infection, a low level of GrzB and INFγ:IL-10 ratio was highly correlated ($r=0.99$, $p=0.03$) with the presence of febrile influenza illness (i.e., more severe illness) [5]. Thus, these assays of the cell-mediated immune response to influenza could complement serologic measures of vaccine efficacy in the selection of novel influenza vaccines to advance through the clinical development pipeline.

2   Materials

2.1   Abbreviations

PBMC Peripheral blood mononuclear cell.
TC   Tissue culture.
HAU   Hemagglutination units.
MOI   Multiplicity of infection.
VP   Virus particles.

2.2   Equipment/ Supplies for PBMC Stimulation with Influenza Virus and Culture Harvest

1. Biological safety cabinet (BSL2 facilities).
2. Microcentrifuge (Beckman, Eppendorf, or equivalent).
3. CO_2 Incubator (37 °C).
4. Refrigerator (2–8 °C) for storage of medium and reagents.
5. Freezer (–70/80 °C) for storage of supernatant and lysate samples.
6. Conical, PP 1.5 mL microcentrifuge tubes for collection of cell lysates (red color or equivalent).
7. Skirted, PP 2.0 mL cryogenic tube, siliconized/low retention, with screw caps, and O-rings for collection of culture supernatants.

8. Screw caps for 2.0 mL cryogenic tubes (yellow color or equivalent).

9. Sterile/autoclaved, conical polypropylene (PP) 5 mL centrifuge tubes.

10. Disposable, sterile, individually wrapped serological pipettes (10, 25, and 50 mL).

11. Pipette Aid for use with serological pipettes.

12. Rack, open, 42×1.5 mL microcentrifuge tubes.

13. Cardboard storage boxes, 81 place for supernatant and lysate tubes.

14. Tissue culture plates, 48 well, sterile, TC treated, individually wrapped (Corning or equivalent).

15. Micropipettes ranging from 10 to 1000 μL.

16. Sterile precision pipette tips (10–1000 μL) for micropipettes.

17. Equipment for counting cells: microscope, hemocytometer (Burker chamber, Kova chamber, or equivalent) or other counting instrument such as the Countess automated cell counter (Invitrogen) with counting chamber slides (Invitrogen).

18. Cryopreservation labels for identifying vials, 1.5–2 mL size vials.

19. Cryopreservation labels for identifying vials, circles for vial tops.

20. Tilting stand, adjustable for holding TC plates—optional Gloves (latex, vinyl, nitrile).

21. Laboratory Coat.

22. Appropriate biohazard waste bags and containers.

2.3 Equipment/ Supplies for Immunologic Assays

1. Plate reader.

2. Microcentrifuge with refrigeration (4 °C) capacity (Beckman, Eppendorf, or equivalent).

3. CO_2 Incubator (37 °C).

4. Refrigerator (2–8 °C) for storage of medium and reagents.

5. Freezer (–70/80 °C) for storage of lysate samples.

6. Vortex apparatus.

7. Humidified Chamber (*see* **Note 1**).

8. Water Bath (37 °C).

9. Conical, PP 1.5 mL microcentrifuge tubes for collection of cell lysates and for preparation of standards (red color or equivalent).

10. Microtiter plates, flat bottom, nontreated, 96 well (Nunc or Corning) (*see* **Note 2**).

11. Thermoplastic plate sealers.

12. Disposable, sterile, individually wrapped serological pipettes (10, 25, and 50 mL).

13. Pipette Aid for use with serological pipettes.

14. Rack, open, 42 × 1.5 mL microcentrifuge tubes.

15. Single channel micropipettes ranging from 10 to 1000 µL and multichannel pipettes with 200 µL dispense capacity.

16. Reagent reservoirs, to hold master mix when dispensing to plates.

17. Precision pipette tips (10–1000 µL) for micropipettes and multichannel pipettes.

18. Cryopreservation labels for identifying vials, 1.5–2 mL size vials.

19. Cryopreservation labels for identifying vials, circles for vial tops.

20. Laboratory Coat and Gloves (latex, vinyl, nitrile).

21. Appropriate biohazard waste bags and containers.

2.4 Reagents for Virus Stimulation

1. AIM V serum-free cell culture medium (Invitrogen, cat # 12055083 (Gibco)); store in refrigerator.

2. Trypan Blue (0.4 %) for staining cells during counting procedure; store at room temperature.

3. Influenza A/Puerto Rico/8/34 (H1N1), purified, live virus (Charles River, cat # 10100374); store at –80 °C.

4. Influenza A/Aichi/68 (H3N2), purified, live virus (Charles River, cat # 10100375); store at –80 °C.

5. Influenza A/Victoria/3/75 (H3N2), purified, live virus (Charles River, cat # 10100376); store at –80 °C.

6. Influenza B/Lee/40, purified, live virus (Charles River, cat # 10100379); store at –80 °C.

2.5 Reagent Preparation for Virus Stimulation

1. All the Influenza virus strains detailed are routinely used to stimulate PBMC samples but other virus strains or stimulants such as Concanavalin A can be used.

2. For each virus strain (stock tube and dilution tube), resuspend and mix well with micropipette before creating aliquots or stimulating cultures. Virus particles tend to settle to the bottom of the tube and may not reach full infectivity if insufficiently distributed.

3. Thaw each stock tube quickly by rolling in between hands and once thawed, create aliquots (to limit freeze/thaw cycles) of the appropriate size based on the number of stimulations to be performed per week, and then immediately refreeze and store at –80 °C. Do not create aliquots smaller than 100 µL. Also, if all of the aliquot is not used, do not refreeze as more

than a total of two freeze/thaw cycles will affect the viability of the virus.

4. Dilute the stock virus in Aim V medium to deliver a multiplicity of infection (MOI) of 2 in a 20 μL volume to each PBMC culture (*see* **Note 3**).

5. Make a fresh batch of diluted virus every week for PBMC culture stimulations, as it is only good for 5 days when stored at 4 °C.

6. Do not make up diluted virus at final volumes greater than 3 mL to effectively deliver the right amount of stimulation to each culture.

7. Concanavalin A (Con A) at a final concentration of 2 μg/mL is a good positive control for PBMC cultures.

2.6 Reagents for Immunologic Assays

1. Colorimetric Substrate—Isoleucine-Glutamate-Proline-Aspartate-paraNitroanalide (IEPDpNA) (EMD Chemicals, cat # 368067, 5 mg size); store at –20 °C for up to 2 years.

2. Triton X-100; store at room temperature.

3. Sodium Chloride (NaCl); store at room temperature.

4. CHAPS (Sigma Aldrich, cat # C5070, 5 g size); store at room temperature.

5. Dimethylsulfoxide (DMSO); store at room temperature.

6. HEPES; store at room temperature.

7. Tris-HCI store at room temperature.

8. Sucrose; store at room temperature.

9. Hydrochloric acid, 1 N (HCl); store at room temperature.

10. Sodium Hydroxide, 10 N (NaOH); store at room temperature.

11. Biomol Granzyme B, human recombinant (Enzo Life Sciences, cat # SE-238, 50 μL or 5000 U size); store at –80 °C (GrzB activity is quite stable across multiple years when stored at –80 °C).

12. BCA Protein Assay Kit (Pierce); store at room temperature.

13. Dithiothreitol, 99 % (DTT) (5 g size); store at 4 °C.

14. Bovine Serum Albumin (BSA) Fraction V, ≥96 % (Sigma Aldrich, cat # A9647, 10 g size); at 4 °C.

2.7 Reagent Preparation for Immunologic Assays

1. Cell Lysis Buffer—final concentrations:

   (a) 150 mM NaCl.

   (b) 15mM Tris-HCI.

   (c) 1 % Triton X-100.

For 200 mL volume Cell Lysis Buffer, combine:

Tris-HCl	3.63 g
Triton X-100	2 mL
Deionized H_2O	100 mL
NaCl	1.753 g

- Adjust pH to 8.0 using HCl (~15–20 mL of 1 N HCl) and adjust final volume to 200 mL. Store at 4 °C, expires after ~6 months (*see* **Note 4**).

2. Cell Lysis Buffer with BSA:

   (a) Cell Lysis Buffer with the addition of BSA is used specifically to prepare the GrzB standards (*ONLY* GrzB standards). Remove a portion of Cell Lysis Buffer from your stock bottle, add 2 µg/µL BSA (or 2 mg/mL), and transfer to new bottle and label appropriately. Store at 4 °C, expires after ~6 months.

3. 2× Reaction Buffer—final concentrations:

   (a) 20 % Sucrose.

   (b) 0.2 % CHAPS.

   (c) 100 mM HEPES, pH 7.5.

   For 500 mL volume 2× Reaction Buffer, combine:

Sucrose	100 g
CHAPS	1 g
HEPES	23.83 g
Deionized H_2O	400 mL

- Adjust pH to 7.5 using NaOH (~5 mL of 10 N NaOH) and adjust final volume to 500 mL. Store at 4 °C, expires after 6–9 months.

4. Biomol Granzyme B standard preparation:

   (a) Must be handled with particular care in order to retain maximum enzymatic activity.

   (b) Defrost quickly by rubbing between fingers, spin down briefly in mini-centrifuge (~5 s) to ensure all GrzB is collected in the base of the tube and then immediately place on ice.

   (c) To limit the number of freeze/thaw cycles, aliquot the GrzB into separate tubes (5 µL fractions). To create the aliquots, remove 1.5 mL precooled tubes from fridge and place on ice. Initially, resuspend the GrzB standard thoroughly and in between each 5 µL aliquot transfer also resuspend thoroughly to ensure delivery of the same amount of GrzB to each tube. Change pipette tips in between each transfer, and when dispensing 5 µL, place pipette tip right to bottom of the tube and ensure the entire contents in the tip are discharged.

(d) Immediately freeze the GrzB standard aliquots by placing the tubes in an open rack and snap freeze at −80 °C.

(e) The above steps should be performed as quickly as possible.

5. DTT Preparation:

(a) Combine 1.54 g of DTT (MW 154.25) with 10 mL deionized H_2O to make a 1 M solution. *Note*: When preparing DTT work in fume hood.

(b) Aliquot in to 1.5 mL tubes, store at −80 °C until ready for use, and limit to one freeze/thaw cycle. Once thawed, it should be stored at 4 °C and can be used for up to 1 week; the supply should be as fresh as possible.

6. Colorimetric Substrate Preparation:

(a) IEPDpNA, stored at −20 °C (5 mg of MW 634.6), is dissolved in 400 µL of DMSO to a concentration of 20 mM. When adding the DMSO, drip it along the sides of the vial to fully collect all the substrate, which may be adhering to the sides of the vial. After the addition of DMSO, roll the vial in between your hands to further encourage the substrate to dissolve and then vortex (medium speed for ~10 s). Resuspend well before addition to assay master mix. Undissolved substrate remnants may still persist in the bottom of the vial and appear almost gum-like; therefore, be diligent to ensure the entire vial contents are fully dissolved.

(b) Use fresh substrate preparations in the assay master mix and make up just before addition to the master mix. Leftover substrate preparations may be stored at −20 °C for later use but limit to one freeze/thaw cycle.

3 Methods

The purpose of this Standard Operating Procedure (SOP) is to describe the methodological steps necessary to: (1) stimulate PBMC with live influenza virus in order to obtain cell culture supernatants for cytokine assays and cell culture lysates for Granzyme B (GrzB) measurements; (2) determine Granzyme B (GrzB) levels from human peripheral blood mononuclear cell (PBMC) lysates using (a) assay of GrzB activity (Units) and (b) protein level to calculate GrzB levels as Units/mg protein. Cytokine assays on PBMC supernatants are completed using multiplex assays according to the manufacturer's directions.

3.1 Stimulation of PBMC with Live Influenza Virus

1. After isolation and counting of PBMC, the final cell concentration is to be adjusted to 3×10^6 *viable* PBMC/mL suspended in AIM V medium (*see* **Note 5**).

2. Distribute 0.6 mL of 3×10^6 cells/mL cell suspension to the appropriate number of wells in the tissue culture plate prepared for virus stimulation. Each culture well is stimulated with only one virus strain; therefore, when testing multiple strains of virus, set up the necessary number of cultures to test all the required strains/subject (final number of cells per well: 3×10^6 cells/mL $\times 0.6$ mL/well $= 1.8 \times 10^6$ cells/well).

3. Stimulate each well with virus (MOI $= 2$) by placing pipette tip directly into culture and injecting the contents. Place the TC plate in a 37 °C CO_2 incubator for 20 h and then harvest the culture supernatants and cell lysates (*see* **Note 6**).

3.2 Harvesting Cell Culture Supernatants and Cell Lysates

1. Remove cell culture plates from 37 °C CO_2 incubator, and inspect cultures under microscope to observe changes to PBMC. It is not necessary to centrifuge the plate as the cells will have all settled to the bottom of the culture wells within the 20 h incubation period.

2. Working in the biological safety cabinet, remove the supernatants and transfer to 2 mL cryogenic tubes. To avoid drawing up cells at the bottom of the well and remove as much supernatant as possible, tilt the plate towards you, at a *gentle/slight angle* so as to not draw the cells down, and get as close to the bottom of the well as possible without touching it. Then, draw up the supernatant from the front corner of the well very slowly. It's important that only approximately ≤20 μL of supernatant remains in the well to minimize dilution of the lysis buffer to be added.

3. During the collection process, tubes with cell supernatants should be placed on ice and then frozen at −80 °C for later use in assay for cytokines.

4. After removing the supernatant, add 200 μL Cell Lysis Buffer to the well containing 1.8×10^6 cells/culture. If the cell quantity/culture changes, adjust the amount of Cell Lysis Buffer added accordingly. Process at room temperature. To ensure no drying of the cells after you have removed the supernatant, immediately add the Cell Lysis Buffer and process each well individually before moving on to the next (*see* **Note 7**). To effectively lyse all the cells, scrape the bottom of the well *thoroughly* (approximately minimum of 1 min scrapping/well) with the pipette tip (use a motion as if coloring), being sure to scrape along the edges as well and then resuspend a couple times, from the front corner of the well, to fully collect all the lysate and transfer this suspension to 1.5 mL microcentrifuge tubes. During this step it is also important to avoid the formation of

bubbles, which will hinder the removal of all the lysate from the well. To avoid bubbles, use a fluid motion and avoid picking up the pipette tip, keeping it in constant contact with the well bottom. The well should appear clean after successful removal of cells (*see* **Note 8**).

5. Once the lysate has been transferred to a tube, let each lysate sit for approximately 5–10 min at room temperature to allow the Triton X-100 to fully permeate the cells. If processing larger batches of cultures, after 5–10 min at room temperature, transfer the lysate tubes to ice and then freeze within 30 min of collection to preserve GrzB activity. Freeze the lysates in open racks at −80 °C to ensure quick freezing and then once frozen transfer to freezer storage boxes. Do not store at −20 °C under any conditions.

6. When ready, continue to GrzB/Protein and Multiplex Cytokine assays.

3.3 Lysate Preparation

1. Prepare the cell lysates by completing three freeze/thaw cycles, vortexing after each thaw cycle:

   (a) Place tubes in −80 °C freezer until the lysates are frozen (~5 min in open racks to allow faster freeze cycles).

   (b) Immediately place the tubes into a 37 °C water bath for ~2 min or until the frozen lysates have thawed. Do not leave unattended in water bath.

   (c) Vortex the samples vigorously (high speed for 30 s).

   (d) Immediately repeat the freeze/thaw cycle two more times.

2. Using a refrigerated microcentrifuge, centrifuge samples at top speed (~16,000 × g) for 5 min to 4 °C to keep the lysates cold and to pellet cell debris, nuclei, and DNA.

3. Remove most of the lysate while safely avoiding contact with the pellet (~150 μL of lysate is removed if the original volume of Cell Lysis Buffer used to lyse the cells was 200 μL as leaving behind 50 μL is best to fully avoid the pellet—contact with the pellet introduces contaminants which introduces background activity to the GrzB assay) and transfer to two fresh-labeled tubes (100 μL dispensed into one tube and 50 μL in other tube). When splitting lysate between tubes, resuspend well in between to dispense the same concentration of protein into the tubes. One aliquot can be used for initial GrzB/Protein assays (need minimum of ~70 μL for both assays) and the other for later repeats if necessary. For this entire step all original sample tubes and transfer tubes (precool) need to be on ice (*see* **Note 9**).

4. Continue to keep samples on ice, to preserve GrzB activity, and proceed directly to GrzB/Protein assays or freeze at −80 °C until later use (limit to one freeze/thaw cycle) (*see* **Note 10**).

3.4 Determination of Granzyme B Activity (Part A: Granzyme Assay)

Assay Principle: Lysates are transferred to microtiter plates following three freeze/thaw cycles and incubated with the substrate IEPDpNA (Isoleucine-Glutamate-Proline-Aspartate-paraNitroanalide). GrzB (a serine protease) levels are measured by cleavage of the substrate, IEPDpNA at the aspartate (D) residue. The released paranitroanalide (pNA) forms a yellow colored end product within 20 h at 37 °C in a humidified container.

1. Biomol Standard Preparation:

   (a) Standards are prepared from Biomol GrzB units; initial stock is supplied as 100 U/μL in 50 μL total starting volume. Begin with a 1:67 dilution for the top (A) standard by adding 328.3 μL cell lysis buffer containing 2 μg/μL BSA (BSA preserves the GrzB enzyme activity) to a 5 μL stock aliquot of Biomol GrzB. This will result in a new concentration of 1.5 GrzB units/μL (*see* **Note 11**).

   (b) Prepare an additional seven standard tubes; label "B to H" (*see* recipe below).

Volume of biomol GrzB	Volume of diluent[a] (μL)	Final volume (μL)	Final biomol units
5 μL stock	328.3	166.7	30 units (A)
166.7 μL of (A)	166.7	166.7	15 units (B)
166.7 μL of (B)	166.7	166.7	7.5 units (C)
166.7 μL of (C)	166.7	166.7	3.75 units (D)
166.7 μL of (D)	166.7	166.7	1.875 units (E)
166.7 μL of (E)	166.7	166.7	0.938 units (F)
166.7 μL of (F)	166.7	166.7	0.469 units (G)
0 μL	166.7	166.7	0 units (only Cell Lysis Buffer with 2 μg/μL BSA) = blank (H)

[a]Cell lysis buffer w/BSA

   (c) When performing the standard serial dilutions, be sure to vortex each tube (medium speed for ~5 s), resuspend well, transfer appropriate volume, and change pipette tip after every volume transfer. Also, minimize bubble formation. After final volume transfer to standard G, draw up and discard 166.7 μL which will result in the same volume of standard in all tubes (*see* **Note 12**).

2. Pipette 20 μL in duplicate of each standard (A–H) to the appropriate wells of microtiter plate using a micropipette (*see* plate template below). Before use, vortex the tube (medium speed for ~5 s), resuspend and directly dispense the appropriate

volume to the plate. Resuspend standards between replicates (*see* **Note 13**).

3. Pipette 20 μL in duplicate of each lysate sample after standards to the appropriate wells. Before use, vortex the tube (medium speed for ~5 s), resuspend well, and directly dispense the appropriate volume to the plate. Also resuspend sample between replicates (*see* **Notes 13** and **14**).

	1	2	3	4	5	6	7	8	9	10	11	12
A	30 units		Unknown samples 1–40 in duplicate									
B	15 units											
C	7.5 units											
D	3.75 units											
E	1.875 units											
F	0.938 units											
G	0.469 units											
H	0 units											

4. Master Mix Preparation:

   (a)

Individual well	Final concentration
50 μL (2×) Reaction Buffer	1×
1 μL (1 M) DTT	10 mM
2 μL (20 mM) Colorimetric Substrate, IEPDpNA 27 μL Deionized H$_2$O 80 μL total/well	400 μM

   (b) Be sure to make up enough master mix daily to run all plates (# of samples + # standards + minimum 20 % extra).

   (c) Directly after a batch of master mix is prepared and just before addition to the plates, thoroughly mix by very gentle inversion of tube to avoid formation of bubbles.

5. Pipette 80 μL of previously prepared master mix to all wells with a multichannel pipette (*see* **Note 15**).

6. Cover each plate with a thermoplastic seal and seal very well to prevent moisture from entering wells.

7. Incubate for 20 h in a dark humidified chamber at 37 °C (*see* **Notes 1** and **16**).

8. Once the plates have been placed in the incubator, immediately proceed to the protein assay (Part B).

9. After 20 h incubation, read the plates using a single wavelength on the plate reader. Measure the absorbency of GrzB at 405 nm (*see* **Note 17**).

10. Determine the concentration of GrzB in Biomol units/20 μL lysate using a quadratic curve with a log (concentration)-linear (absorbance) plot (*see* **Note 18**).

3.5 Determination of Granzyme B Activity (Part B: Protein Assay)

Assay Principle: The BCA Protein Assay is a detergent-compatible formulation based on bicinchoninic acid (BCA) for the colorimetric detection and quantitation of total protein. This method combines the well-known reduction of Cu^{2+} to Cu^{1+} by protein in an alkaline medium (the Biuret reaction) with the highly sensitive and selective colorimetric detection of the cuprous cation (Cu^{1+}) using a unique reagent containing bicinchoninic acid. The purple-colored reaction product of this assay is formed by the chelation of two molecules of BCA with one cuprous ion. This water-soluble complex exhibits a strong absorbance at 562 nm.

1. Initial BCA Standard Preparation:

   (a) Prepare 9×1.5 mL tubes; label one tube "Stock" and the remaining eight "A–H".

   (b) Transfer contents of BSA standard vial to "Stock" tube. Vortex vial vigorously (between medium to high speed for ~10 s), resuspend thoroughly, and then transfer to the tube.

   (c) Add the appropriate volume of Cell Lysis Buffer to the remaining tubes (see recipe below).

   (d) At this point, keep the Stock tube and standard tubes containing Cell Lysis Buffer at *room temperature*. The final preparation of the standards, with the addition of BSA, will be completed after the lysate samples are plated (*see* **Note 19**).

Volume of BSA	Volume of diluent[a] (μL)	Final volume (μL)	Final BSA concentration (standard letter)
50 μL Stock	50	50	1000 μg/mL (A)
50 μL of (A)	50	50	500 μg/mL (B)
50 μL of (B)	50	50	250 μg/mL (C)
50 μL of (C)	50	50	125 μg/mL (D)
50 μL of (D)	75	75	50 μg/mL (E)
50 μL of (E)	50	90	25 μg/mL (F)
10 μL of (F)	40	50	5 μg/mL (G)
0 μL	50	50	0 μg/mL (only Cell Lysis Buffer) = blank (H)

[a]ONLY pure Cell Lysis Buffer used as standard diluent for BCA Assay

2. Pipette 10 μL in triplicate of each lysate sample to the appropriate wells of microtiter plate (leave columns 1–3 of the plate

free for standards and begin plating the samples at column 4). Before use, vortex the tube (medium speed for ~5 s), resuspend well, and directly dispense the appropriate volume to the plate. Also, resuspend between replicates (*see* **Note 13**). Keep samples and microtiter plate cold at all times during the plating process in same manner as the GrzB assay.

3. Final BCA Standard Preparation:

   (a) While the plates, loaded with samples, remain in the fridge, complete preparation of the standards by adding the appropriate volume of BSA to tubes as per the recipe.

   (b) When performing the standard dilutions be sure to vortex each tube (between medium to high speed for ~5 s), resuspend well, transfer appropriate volume, and change pipette tip after every volume transfer. Also, minimize bubble formation.

4. Unused BSA stock should be stored at 4 °C and is good for 1 week. Pipette 10 μL in triplicate of each standard (A–H) to the appropriate wells of microtiter plate (columns 1–3). Before use, vortex the tube (between medium to high speed for ~5 s), resuspend well, and directly dispense the appropriate volume to the plate. Also, resuspend between replicates (*see* **Notes 13** and **20**).

5. Determine quantity of A + B reagent needed at 200 μL per well, then dilute A:B at 50:1, and mix by inversion/swirling until the solution becomes clear green (for a single plate: 22.540 mL reagent A + 460 μL reagent B → provides 20 % extra).

6. Add 200 μL of the A + B mixture to all wells with a multichannel pipette (*see* **Note 21**).

7. Cover each plate with a thermoplastic seal and incubate in CO_2 incubator at 37 °C for 30 min (*see* **Note 22**).

8. Wipe bottom of microtiter plate before inserting in plate reader.

9. Read plate immediately at 560 nm.

10. Determine the concentration of protein in μg/mL using linear curve fit.

3.6 Calculation of Granzyme B Activity (Units/mg Protein)

1. Limits of the assay:

   (a) Check the uniformity of the standard curves intra-assay and inter-assay and check that the r^2 value of the standard curve is greater than 0.990 prior to accepting the results. Any plate that does not meet these criteria is rejected.

   (b) Check that each standard dilution point has a Coefficient of Variance (CV) ≤ 20 %. Any standard curve not meeting these criteria is rejected.

(c) Check that each sample concentration (after subtraction of the blanks) is ≥blank concentration. If the concentration of an unknown is less than the concentration of the blank, then the sample concentration is rejected and must be re-assayed.

(d) Check that each sample concentration has a %CV ≤ 20 % for GrzB assay and %CV ≤ 10 % for protein assay. If the result gives a %CV ≥ 20 % or %CV ≥ 10 % or if only one of the replicate wells is calculated, do not accept the result. The unknown must be re-assayed (*see* **Note 23**).

2. Obtain GrzB concentration in Biomol units/20 μL lysate and protein concentration in μg/mL from the plate reader software reports.

   (a) Divide the Biomol units/20 μL of GrzB by the μg protein/mL.

   (b) To determine the protein values in mg protein/mL, divide the μg/mL protein by 1000.

   (c) Multiply your answer by 1000 μL (same as 1 mL) to correct for the 1 mL unit in the protein concentration (mg/mL) and cancel the μL unit from 20 μL lysate. Express the final answer as Biomol units/mg protein (*see* **Note 24**).

3.7 Determination of INFγ and IL-10 Cytokine Levels

We use the Bio-Ples Pro color-coded, bead-based multplex assays that are designed to measure multiple cytokines in diverse solutions including serum, plasma, and tissue culture supernatants. IFNg and IL-10 levels are measured in harvested PBMC supernatant samples.

4 Notes

1. For the humidified chamber, any plastic container with a lid will be sufficient, line the bottom with a layer of wet paper towels and an additional top layer to cover the assay plate.

2. Plates which provide optical clarity are necessary and newer plates are preferred, old stock may not be optimal due to the sensitivity of the assay; therefore, only purchase the plates as specified.

3. The following are the calculations for preparation of the virus strains:

   (a) To set up 3.0×10^6 PBMC/mL at 0.6 mL volume cultures = $3.0 \times 10^6 \times 0.6$ mL = 1.8×10^6 cells/culture. PBMC are stimulated at a MOI of 2, which means there should be twice as many virus particles (VP) as PBMC; therefore 1.8×10^6 cells $\times 2 = 3.6 \times 10^6$ VP/culture is needed.

(b) An effective volume of diluted virus to add to each culture has been determined to be 20 µL; therefore the 20 µL aliquot contains 3.6×10^6 VP $= 3.6 \times 10^6$ VP$/20$ µL $= 1.8 \times 10^5$ VP$/$µL *OR* 1.8×10^8 VP$/$mL. 20 µL is the optimized volume to reproducibly deliver the same amount of virus without appreciably changing the overall culture volume.

(c) Convert the titer of the stock virus to the concentration VP$/$mL, using the approximated conversion factor for influenza virus, that 1 Hemagglutination Unit (HAU)$= 1 \times 10^4$ VP. Alternatively, the antilog of the median tissue culture infective dose (TCID$_{50}$) or the number of plaque forming units (pfu) is equivalent to the number of VP in your calculations.

(d) To prepare the final virus dilution, use the following calculation:

- C1V1 $=$ C2V2.

- C1 $=$ Virus concentration of original stock virus.

- V1 $= X$ (the volume of virus to be prepared).

- C2 $=$ Final concentration of diluted virus to effectively deliver a MOI of 2 to each culture.

- V2 $=$ Final volume of diluted virus you will use for stimulations, i.e.: *20 cultures to stimulate per day* $\times 5$ *days (1 week)* $\times 20$ *µL per culture* $\times 1.20$ *(20 % extra)* $= 2.400$ *mL.*

(e) *Example calculations:*

- *Charles River Influenza Strain: A/Victoria/3/75 (H3N2)*
    Original total volume: 1 mL.
    Stock $\rightarrow$ 32,768 HAU$/50$ µL.
    $= 655.36$ HAU$/$µL.
    $= 655,360$ HAU$/$mL.
    Conversion: 1 HAU $= 1 \times 104$ VP.
    655,360 HAU$/$mL $\times 1 \times 10^4$ VP$/$HAU $= 6.5536 \times 10^9$ VP$/$mL.
    Using C1V1 $=$ C2V2:
    $(6.5536 \times 109$ VP$/$mL$)$ $(V1) = (1.8 \times 108$ VP$/$mL$)$ $(2.400$ mL$)$.
    V1 $= 0.066$ mL virus stock $+ 2.334$ mL Aim V Media

- *Charles River Influenza Strain: B/Lee/40*
    Original total volume: 1 mL
    Stock $\rightarrow$ 262,144 HAU$/50$ µL
    $= 5242.88$ HAU$/$µL
    $= 5.24288 \times 106$ HAU$/$mL
    Conversion: 1 HAU $= 1 \times 104$ VP

$$5.24288 \times 106 \ \ HAU/mL \times 1 \times 104 \ \ VP/HAU = 5.24288 \times 1010 \ VP/mL$$

Using C1V1 = C2V2:

$$(5.24288 \times 1010 \ \ VP/mL) \ \ (V1) = (1.8 \times 108 \ VP/mL) \ (2.400 \ mL)$$

V1 = 0.008 mL virus stock + 2.392 mL Aim V

If dealing with a highly concentrated stock virus as specified for B/Lee above, a 2-step dilution is alternatively recommended as follows:

- *Dilution 1*:

  If prepared 100 µL aliquots of stock virus, you would use almost the entire aliquot:

  $$(5.24288 \times 1010 \ \ VP/mL) \ \ (0.085 \ \ mL) = (C2) \ (2.400 \ mL) \rightarrow add \ 0.085 \ mL \ virus \ stock + 2.315 \ mL \ Aim \ V$$

  C2 = 1.85685 × 109 VP/mL

- *Dilution 2*:

  $$(1.85685 \times 109 \ VP/mL) \ (V1) = (1.8 \times 108 \ VP/mL) \ (2.400 \ mL)$$

  V1 = 0.233 mL virus from Dilution 1 + 2.167 mL Aim V

4. The Cell Lysis Buffer is used to prepare the standards for both the GrzB and protein assays, so the same batch of Cell Lysis Buffer should ideally be used to prepare the standards and the subject samples to be tested. To ensure the same batch of Cell Lysis Buffer is used, the buffer can be used up to 9 months if necessary. This can be an important consideration if subject lysates samples are being collected over a longer period of time prior to being tested. As microbial growth in the Cell Lysis Buffer will affect the blank sample reading for the protein assay, to a greater degree with time, it is advisable to further minimize microbial growth by removing desired quantities under a biosafety cabinet with sterile serological pipettes.

5. To set up a smaller number of culture quantities per subject, such as five or less, it may be best to make up the desired final cell concentration in a new tube (i.e., 5 mL tube), which can help minimize the amount of culture media used, particularly when starting with concentrated cell suspensions.

(a) Example: if original cell concentration is 8×10^6 cells/mL and only three cultures required.

(b) Use C1V1 = C2V2:

- $(8 \times 10^6 \ cells/mL) \ (V1) = (3 \times 10^6 \ cells/mL) \ (2.0 \ mL) \rightarrow 3 \ cultures \times 0.6 \ mL \times 0.200 \ extra = 2.0 \ mL$

- Solve for V1, V1 = 0.750 mL; therefore, transfer 0.750 mL of your original cell suspension to a new tube and add 1.250 mL Aim V (2.0 mL – 0.750 mL = 1.250 mL) to make up your desired final cell concentration.

(c) If you notice what may appear to be any remaining platelet clusters in your original cell suspension, avoid drawing them up in your pipette tip when transferring to make up your final cell concentration as it can affect culture purity and thus cell performance during the incubation with the virus (platelets can deplenish culture media nutrients).

6. If time constraints do not permit harvesting the cultures at exactly 20 h, the incubation period can range from a minimum of 20 h to an absolute maximum of 24 h.

7. The maximum amount of time allowed between removing the supernatant and adding the Cell Lysis Buffer, to prevent any drying of the cells, is 5 min.

8. To remove the supernatant without touching the cell pellet and to effectively collect all of the cell lysate from the culture well, it can be helpful to use an adjustable tilting stand to hold the TC plate, at the appropriate angle, during the above process. The tilting stand can help you acquire the right angle to be able to observe the bottom of the culture well and positioning of your pipette tip while removing the supernatant but also avoid tilting the plate too much as to draw the cells down. The stand can also help you find the right angle to make sure the Cell Lysis Buffer covers the entire well surface, during the lysing process, and ensures the best tilt for resuspension and collection.

9. The pellet may look more like mucous at the bottom of the tube rather than a dense pellet; therefore take note of this to further aid in pellet avoidance.

10. Both the GrzB and Protein assays should be performed on the same day to leave one lysate aliquot banked for any future repeat assays (order: first GrzB assay and second Protein assay). In the case of preparing lysates and proceeding directly to performing the assays on the same day, limiting the number of plates to be run per day (i.e., ~5 plates total = 2 GrzB + ~3 Protein) is suggested. If all your lysates are first prepared and frozen, then more plates/day can be run (i.e., 8 plates total = 3 GrzB + 5 Protein). This will better preserve GrzB activity in the sample and limit the gap in time between when the samples were first plated and the master mix added.

11. Standard Dilution Explanation:

(a) Using C1V1 = C2V2.

- C1 = 100 U/μL; V1 = 5 μL; C2 = if plate 20 μL/well and desire 30 U/well top standard, what are the final units/μL = 30 U/20 μL = 1.5 U/μL; V2 = the volume of standard to be prepared $\rightarrow$ (100 unit/μL) (5 μL) = (1.5 unit/μL) (V2).

- V2 = 333.3 μL.

- Add 328.3 μL Cell Lysis Buffer w/BSA to 5 μL Biomol GrzB to create top standard (A).

12. To ensure everything is kept cold, precool the standard tubes, only add cold Cell Lysis Buffer w/BSA, and place all tubes on ice the entire time.

13. Due to the nature of the Cell Lysis Buffer as media, if the micropipette leaves an insignificant residual sample in the tip at the first dispensing stop point, it is not necessary to go to the second stop of the pipette to dispense the correct amount of GrzB units to each well and no tip change is required between replicates. If the pipette leaves a significant residual sample in the tip at the first stop, it is best to go to the second stop of the pipette and tip change is recommended between replicates, as the Cell Lysis Buffer (detergent base) will create a bubble in the tip after a full blowout. When undertaking a full blow out, make sure to do so gently to minimize the development of any bubbles in the plate well.

14. Keep standards, samples, and microtiter plate cold at all times during the plating process. Precool the plates in the fridge and when loading, place the plate ideally upon a cold pack which was stored at 4 °C (not frozen) and then return the plate to the fridge immediately afterwards. If the plate is placed directly on ice, any residual moisture should be wiped off the bottom of the plate when loading is finished. Replenish the cold packs often (ideal is a fresh cold pack for every plate) and ensure that the plates are covered when in the fridge, which can be accomplished by stacking the plates and placing an empty plate on top of the stack. Standards may be prepared and plated up to a maximum of 3 h in advance of sample plating completion. If the standards are plated ahead of time, keep the plates in the fridge and covered.

15. Avoid bubbles and do not vortex. When loading wells, do not dispense to second stop point to further avoid bubble formation and no change in pipette tips are required between additions. Simply dispense high enough against well wall to ensure no contamination with samples. In addition, when drawing the master mix into the pipette tip, do so in a steady and controlled manner for vigorous uptake can cause bubbles to form in the tips. Dispense in similar fashion. After every third dispense, re-mix the master mix gently once again by moving the reservoir dish back and forth, to ensure equal distribution of master mix to sample wells. The master mix may be prepared

up to a maximum of 3 h in advance of addition to the plates and should be stored in the fridge until time of use.

16. Do not stack the plates in the container to limit edge effects. Simply place them side by side; this may require use of more containers based on plate quantity. Place container(s) in 37 °C incubator.

17. Before reading, with plate sealers still on, thoroughly wipe off the plates to remove all moisture. When slowly removing the plate sealer, bubbles may form at the top of the plate wells, briefly allow the bubbles to settle, and then directly read the plate.

18. The GrzB results can be affected to a significant degree by plate-to-plate standard curve variability. To limit this effect the following should be undertaken:

    (a) *Biomol GrzB Standard Lot Variation*:
    There can be lot differences for the GrzB standard obtained from the manufacturer. Therefore, it is advisable to test all samples using the same lot. If comparing data between sites, ensure each site is using the same lot of GrzB standard. If comparing data between years of a study, ordering enough vials for the duration of the study is recommended. To further aid in curve reproducibility, use the same lot of colorimetric substrate as well.

    (b) *Distribution of Biomol GrzB Standard in Aliquot Tubes*:
    When creating aliquots of the GrzB standard, unequal distribution of GrzB between tubes can also contribute to curve variability. Generally, within the same lot, the top standard between plates should not differ by more than 0.1 OD. If there is greater variability than this, more diligence may be needed when creating the stock aliquots.

    (c) *Sample Organization on Plate*:
    Before sample plating, decide how the data will be analyzed and presented, then plate the samples accordingly. That is, if examining the response to vaccination across four visits based on certain culture conditions, it would be best to plate all four visit samples, inclusive of all the conditions, for one subject on the same plate; including any background and control samples.

    (d) Overall, if OD readings are as low as 0.300 s OD for the highest concentration of the standard, which is too low for 30 units of expected GrzB activity, it may be due to the following contributing factors:

    - Loss of activity within Biomol GrzB standard due to prolonged thaw cycle when creating stock aliquots.

    - Colorimetric substrate not fully dissolved in DMSO before addition to master mix.

- Using diluted standards which are not freshly prepared (use within 3 h of preparation).

- Expired solutions/reagents (follow all suggested expiration dates).

19. The standard preparation recipe provides sufficient quantities for one plate; therefore, if running multiple protein plates/day, increase recipe quantities by the appropriate factor.

20. When you begin plating the standards, remove all plates from the fridge to ensure samples and plates come to room temperature before addition of the final reagent A + B mixture. Keep plates covered.

21. When loading wells, do not dispense to second stop point and no change in pipette tips is required between additions. As the 200 μL volume size will come close to the top of the well, be extra careful when dispensing to ensure no contamination with samples. After every few dispenses mix the A + B reagent before draw up, by moving the reservoir dish back and forth, to ensure equal distribution of the mixture to sample wells. The standards and master mix should be as freshly prepared as possible and plated right after final preparation to ensure good standard curves.

22. Do not stack the plates on the incubator shelf; place them side by side, to limit edge effects.

23. Overall, in general the protein levels can be more variable, between replicates, due to utilizing a smaller volume of lysate sample (10 μL) and create the need for samples to be run in triplicate. Also, the %CV requirement, between replicates, is lower for the protein assay due to the fact that the protein value is in the denominator of the calculation and can more greatly affect the overall result; therefore, it is quite important to ensure the most precise value is represented.

24. *Grz B Activity Calculations:*

    (a) (GrzB assay concentration ÷ Protein assay concentration).

    - (Biomol units/20 μL) ÷ (μg protein/mL).

    - μg protein/mL × 0.02 = μg protein/20 μL then calculate.

    - Biomol units/20 μL ÷ μg protein/20 μL = Biomol units/μg protein.

    (b) Biomol units/μg protein × 1000 = Biomol units/mg protein.

    (c) Excel Formula: 1000 × (Cell A/20)/(Cell B/1000).

    - Cell A = Biomol U/20 μL and Cell B = protein μg/mL.

References

1. McElhaney JE, Xie D, Hager WD et al (2006) T cell responses are better correlates of vaccine protection in the elderly. J Immunol 176:6333–6339

2. Effros RB (2007) Role of T lymphocyte replicative senescence in vaccine efficacy. Vaccine 25:599–604

3. Gijzen K, Liu WM, Visontai I et al (2010) Standardization and validation of assays determining cellular immune responses against influenza. Vaccine 28:3416–3422

4. McElhaney JE, Ewen C, Zhou X et al (2009) Granzyme B: correlates with protection and enhanced CTL response to influenza vaccination in older adults. Vaccine 27:2418–2425

5. Shahid Z, Kleppinger A, Gentleman B, Falsey AR et al (2010) Clinical and immunologic predictors of influenza illness among vaccinated older adults. Vaccine 28:6145–6151

6. Ewen CL, Rong J, Kokaji AI et al (2006) Evaluating antigen-specific cytotoxic T lymphocyte responses by a novel mouse granzyme B ELISPOT assay. J Immunol Methods 308: 156–166

Chapter 12

Assays for Monitoring Macroautophagy Activity in T cells

Yair Botbol and Fernando Macian

Abstract

Autophagy is an essential catabolic process that regulates a diverse array of functions by targeting cellular components for degradation by lysosomes. Studies in mammalian cells have shown that the regulation of autophagy is highly complex and optimization of experimental approaches to analyze this process needs to be developed for each model studied. This chapter provides an overview of two of the most commonly used ways to monitor autophagy activity in T cell. It involves description of common techniques, namely Western blot and cell immunostaining, giving specific recommendations for working with T cells and monitoring macroautophagy. We also discuss the analysis required for correct interpretation of the results and quantification of macroautophagy activity.

Key words: Macroautophagy, T cell, Lysosome, LC3

1 Introduction

Autophagy is an essential catabolic process that regulates cellular homeostasis through the lysosomal degradation of damaged or altered cellular components. Other than this crucial role, autophagy has also been shown to participate in the response to different environmental cues and the regulation of a wide array of cellular processes, ranging from the control of tissue remodeling or the regulation of the cell energetic balance to the development of adaptation responses to different types of cellular stress or aging [1–3]. In the immune system, autophagy has been reported to have specific functions in different cell types. For instance, in phagocytic cells such as macrophages, autophagy plays an important role during pathogen killing, either in cooperation with the phagocytic system or as an alternative system that can control pathogens that have developed virulence mechanisms to allow them escaping destruction following phagocytosis [4]. Autophagy also allows antigen presenting cells to process peptides derived from intracellular proteins in MHC class II molecules, by providing the class II loading compartment with additional input [5]. Three main

Albert C. Shaw (ed.), *Immunosenescence: Methods and Protocols*, Methods in Molecular Biology, vol. 1343, DOI 10.1007/978-1-4939-2963-4_12, © Springer Science+Business Media New York 2015

different forms of autophagy have been described in mammalian cells: macroautophagy, microautophagy, and chaperone-mediated autophagy. Each of these forms of autophagy has different mechanisms of regulation and distinct functions; therefore, specific assays have been developed to measure their activity. This manuscript will focus on macroautophagy, a process through which in-bulk or targeted cargo (which can include, among others, soluble cytosolic proteins, lipid droplets, whole organelles, or pathogens) is engulfed in a de novo formed double membrane vesicle, the autophagosome, which will deliver the cargo to lysosomes for degradation.

As with other tissues and systems, the immune system is affected by aging. The age-associated decline in immune responses has been termed immunosenescence. The T cell compartment is specially affected by age, and defective T cell function underlies inefficient responses to pathogens and diminished efficacy of vaccinations, which are commonly found in aging organisms [6]. Decline of different forms of autophagy has been reported in many cell types and tissues [1] including T cells [7]. In T lymphocytes, macroautophagy can be induced in response to TCR engagement and contributes to the control of cell homeostasis and survival, activation-induced responses, and energy metabolism [8–11]. Accurately measuring autophagic activity in aged T cells could therefore constitute an indicator of age-associated decline in T cell function. Although the protocols we will describe are tailored for the analysis of the regulation of macroautophagy in T cells, they can be easily applied to other cells of the immune system to measure basal or induced macroautophagy in response to specific signals (e.g., TLR engagement in macrophages, or BCR activation in B cells) that may activate or inhibit this process in a given cell type.

Several methods to monitor macroautophagy have been developed, including image-based procedures such as electron microscopy (which is commonly used for morphology analysis and quantification of autophagosomes), direct fluorescence through the use of fluorescent reporter proteins and immunostaining, as well as biochemical procedures such as immunoblot to measure steady-state levels of related proteins and macroautophagy flux [12]. In this chapter, we describe two of the most widely employed methods to measure macroautophagy activity, which we routinely use in our laboratory to monitor macroautophagy in T cells. First, we will address how to measure endogenous microtubule-associated protein 1 light chain 3 (LC3) conjugation and degradation by immunoblot, and then we will describe how to quantify autophagosome generation and turnover in cells using LC3 immunostaining.

LC3 protein is one of the most common and reliable markers for macroautophagy quantification. LC3 coexists in the cell in two forms: LC3-I (cytosolic form) and LC3-II (membrane-bound lipidated form). During autophagosome formation, LC3 is converted to LC3-II through a process that involves proteolytic processing by Atg4 to form LC3-I, and subsequent Atg7/Atg3-mediated conjugation to phosphatidylethanolamine of the newly exposed C-terminal glycine residue. The lipidated LC3-II can now associate to the membrane of the forming autophagosome [13]. Hence, LC3-II can be used to quantify autophagosome formation in the cell by comparing levels and subcellular localization of this protein under different experimental conditions. However, since macroautophagy is a dynamic process, the simple static quantification of LC3-I or LC3-II levels does not provide an accurate measure of macroautophagy activity. Therefore, specific experimental approaches have been developed to monitor the dynamic macroautophagy flux combining different static measurements [12, 14]. The macroautophagy flux represents the fraction of autophagosomes undergoing a full cycle of macroautophagy, from autophagosome formation to degradation in the lysosome. Static quantifications of autophagosomes by electron microscopy, immunofluorescence, or LC3 conversion by immunoblot do not represent macroautophagy flux, and changes in their steady-state levels could be the result of very different conditions. For example, an increased number of autophagosome structures seen in a snapshot of a cell could be the consequence of either increased autophagosome formation or inhibition of autophagosome degradation. However, the rate of macroautophagy flux would be completely different for these two possibilities. The best way to assess macroautophagy flux is to block the last step of the process (degradation of autophagosomes) and analyze the effect of this treatment on levels of autophagosome markers. We use the combination of ammonium chloride (increases lysosomal pH) and leupeptin (a protease inhibitor) to inhibit lysosomal degradation (other lysosomal inhibitors such as bafilomycin are also widely utilized). This treatment must be as short as possible to minimize effects on the cells studied but long enough to ensure quantifiable accumulation. The level of accumulation of LC3-II and/or autophagosomes caused by this treatment in a given experimental condition compared to the same condition without any inhibitors allows measurement of the flux of macroautophagy (i.e., LC3-II turnover) [15]. In our case, we use basal level of autophagy on resting cells as a reference to measure enhanced macroautophagy following T cell activation.

In the following paragraphs, we will describe protocols we have improved to obtain reliable and reproducible conditions to study macroautophagy induction in activated mouse CD4+ T cells (*see* Figs. 1 and 2). As stated above, this method may be easily adapted to measure macroautophagy in other cell types or other conditions.

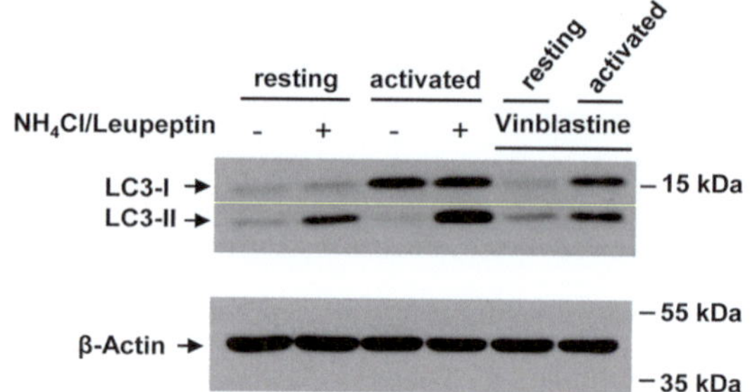

Fig. 1 Macroautophagy flux monitored by LC3-II turnover on immunoblot. Freshly isolated mouse CD4+ T cells were incubated in TCM for 24 h in resting or activated conditions. Cells were treated with or without the indicated autophagy inhibitors for the last 3 h (NH_4Cl and leupeptin are respectively at 20 mM and 100 μM, and vinblastine at 100 μM). Twelve micrograms of protein extract was loaded per well

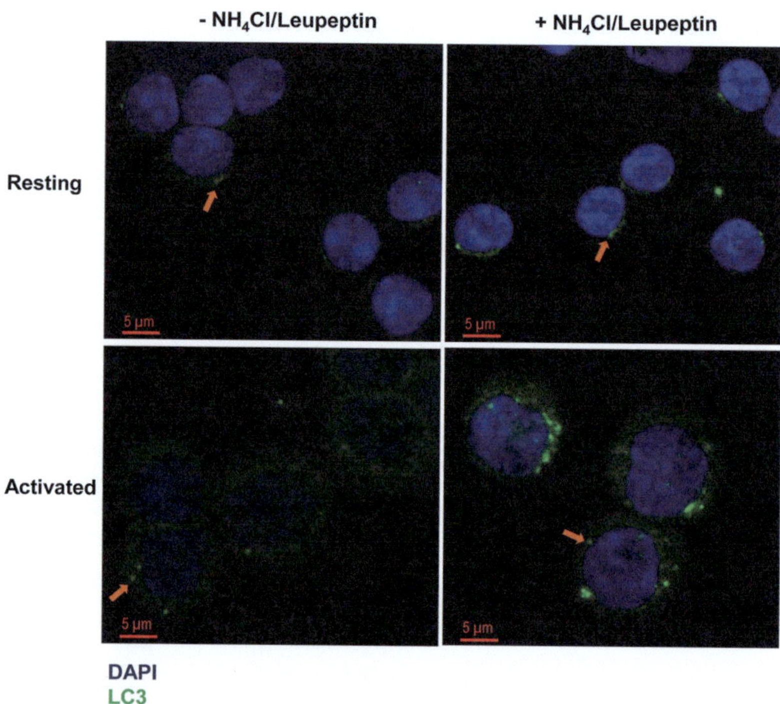

Fig. 2 Macroautophagy flux monitored by LC3-II turnover by immunofluorescence. Freshly isolated mouse CD4+ T cells were incubated in TCM for 24 h in resting or activated condition. Cells were treated with or without the indicated autophagy inhibitors for the last 3 h. Macroautophagy flux was monitored by measuring LC3 puncta accumulation using immunostaining. *Orange arrows* indicate the LC3-II puncta (autophagosome) in each condition (magnification ×630)

2 Materials

2.1 Common Reagents, Solutions, and Equipment

1. Phosphate-buffered solution, PBS 1×.
2. Protein SDS-PAGE and Blotting buffers and equipment.
3. CO_2 tissue culture incubator.
4. Image J software (National Institutes of Health, http://imagej. nih.gov/ij/).

2.2 CD4+ T Cell Culture

1. C57BL/6 mice, 6–10 week old.
2. T cell media (TCM): DMEM/high glucose (Hyclone), supplemented with, 10 % (v/v) FBS, 5 IU/mL Penicillin, 5 μg/mL streptomycin, 4 mM glutamine, 1× Non-Essential Amino acids (Lonza), 1× MEM Eagle Vitamin Mixture (Lonza), 50 μM β-Mercaptoethanol, 660 μM L-Arginine, 270 μM L-Aspartic acid, 6 μM Folic Acid, 10 mM HEPES, 1 mM Sodium Pyruvate in the composition of media.
3. Dynabeads® Mouse CD4 (L3T4) (Invitrogen), DETACHa-BEAD® Mouse CD4 (Invitrogen), and magnet.
4. Activator antibodies (Ab): anti-mouse CD3ε (clone 145-2C11), anti-mouse CD28 (clone 37–51).
5. 24-well tissue culture plate.
6. 2 M Ammonium chloride freshly prepared and filtered sterilized.
7. 100 mM leupeptin in sterile H_2O. Aliquots can be stored at –20 °C.

2.3 Cell Lysis and Western Blot

1. RIPA buffer 1×: 50 mM Tris–HCl pH 7.7, 150 mM NaCl, 1 % (v/v) NP40, 0.5 % Sodium deoxycholate, 0.1 % SDS. Add fresh Complete Protease Inhibitor cocktail 1× (Roche), 2 mM PMSF, 1 mM DTT.
2. 15 % Tris-Glycine SDS-PAGE buffers and solutions and nitro-cellulose membrane.
3. Blocking buffer: 1× PBS, 0.1 % (v/v) Tween-20, 5 % Non-fat dry milk.
4. Antibody Incubation Buffer (AIB): 1× PBS, 0.1 % Tween-20, 4 % BSA.
5. Wash buffer (WB): 1× PBS, 0.1 % (v/v) Tween-20.
6. Anti-mouse LC3 (MBL PM036), anti-mouse β-Actin (clone AC-15 from Abcam).
7. HRP-conjugated secondary antibodies (rabbit and mouse).

2.4 Immunostaining: Tools and Reagents

1. Cytology Funnel and cytospin centrifuge.
2. Cell Fixation Buffer: 4 % Paraformaldehyde (PFA) solution in 1× PBS, pH adjusted to 7.5.

3. Cell Permeabilization Buffer: 1× PBS, 0.015 % (v/v) Digitonin.

4. Cell Blocking Buffer (CBB): 1× PBS, 10 % (v/v) FBS.

5. Wash buffer (WB): 1× PBS.

6. DAPI-Fluoromount-G (Southern Biotech).

7. Anti-mouse LC3 (MBL PM036).

8. Secondary fluorophore-conjugated antibody.

3   Methods

3.1   CD4+ T Cell Isolation and Activation

1. Prepare plate with bound anti-mouse CD3ε using a 10 μg/mL Ab solution in sterile 1× PBS. Add 250 μL per well in 24-well plate and incubate for 3.5 h at 37 °C in a tissue culture incubator under 10 % CO_2. Wash the wells twice with 1× PBS just before adding the cells on **step 2** (*see* **Note 1**).

2. Isolate Lymph nodes and/or spleen from the mouse and perform CD4+ isolation using Dynabeads® Mouse CD4 (L3T4) and following the manufacturer's protocol (*see* **Note 2**). Bring cells to a final density of 1.25×10^6 cells/mL of TCM. Add 0.5 μg/mL of anti-mouse CD28 and seed the cells in the plate with bound antiCD3e prepared in **step 1** of Subheading 3.1 (1 mL per well). Incubate at 37 °C in 10 %-CO_2 incubator (*see* **Note 3**).

3. After 21 h of culture add ammonium chloride/Leupeptin solution (NL) to a final concentration of 20 mM and 100 μM, respectively, for 3 h to half of the wells used for each condition analyzed (*see* **Note 4**).

3.2   Cell Lysate and Western Blot

1. From this step on keep everything on ice. Harvest T cells after the 3 h treatment with NL, centrifuge 5 min at $300 \times g$ at 4 °C, and discard the supernatant.

2. Wash cell pellet with 1 mL of ice-cold 1× PBS (for immunostaining take an aliquot of these cells and go to Subheading 3.3), pellet the cells as in **step 1**, and gently aspirate the supernatant.

3. Flick the tube to break up the cell pellet and resuspend it in RIPA buffer. Homogenize by pipetting up and down 5–10 times (*see* **Note 5**). Leave the tubes on ice for 30 min to complete lysis. Flick the tubes a couple of times during the lysis. Freeze at −80 °C for storage or proceed directly to **step 4**.

4. Centrifuge the crude extract at 4 °C, for 30 min at $20,000 \times g$. Transfer the supernatant to a new tube and perform an additional run of centrifugation. Collect the supernatant.

5. Measure the protein concentration (*see* **Note 6**).

6. Add Laemmli sample buffer and load 10 μg of your samples per lane on a Tris-glycine SDS-PAGE (4 % stacking and 15 % resolving) and run it at constant current (*see* **Note 7**).

7. Electrotransfer the protein from the gel to a nitrocellulose membrane and probe the membrane with the appropriate antibodies (*see* **Note 8**).

   All following blot steps are performed at room temperature with agitation.

8. Block the membrane for 45 min in western blot blocking buffer.

9. Remove blocking buffer and add LC3 antibody solution (1/1500 in AIB). Incubate for 45 min (*see* **Note 9**).

10. Wash the membrane three times (10 min each) in WB.

11. Add anti-rabbit HRP-conjugated secondary antibody diluted in AIB and incubate for 45 min.

12. Wash as in **step 10**, and perform an additional final wash in 1× PBS.

13. Develop the blot.

14. Blot the membrane with anti β-Actin antibody (1/100000 in AIB) repeating **step 9–13** (use anti-mouse secondary Ab).

3.3 LC3 Immuno-staining in T Cells

1. From **step 2** of Subheading 3.2, take an aliquot of cells, pellet down (5 min at 300 g) and resuspend in ice-cold 1× PBS at 10^6 cells/ml.

From here on all steps are performed at room temperature.

2. Load cells into a cytology funnel (~10^5 cells in 100 μL) attached to a glass slide.

3. Centrifuge in cytospin for 5 min at $220 \times g$.

4. Immediately draw a ring in the slide around the cells using a hydrophobic-ink pen and add fixation buffer. Incubate for 10 min.

5. Wash once with 1× PBS.

6. Add permeabilization buffer and incubate for 12 min.

7. Wash cells with 1× PBS, twice for 10 min each time.

8. Incubate cells with CBB for 45 min to block unspecific binding of the antibodies.

9. Incubate cells with LC3 antibody dilution (1/750) in CBB for 30 min.

10. Wash the cells in WB, three times for 10 min.

11. Incubate with secondary Ab fluorophore conjugated in CBB for 45 min.

12. Wash as in **step 10**.

13. Wash once with 1× PBS for 10 min.

14. Briefly wash with water to remove salts, and add a drop of mounting solution DAPI-Fluoromount-G and mount your slide immediately.

15. Let slide dry for 20 min in the dark before microscope visualization and acquisition of images.

3.4 Data Acquisition and Macroautophagy Flux Quantification

As described previously, macroautophagy is a dynamic process and quantification of the flux is required to assess macroautophagy activity.

On Immunoblot, the protocol gives a clear separation between LC3-I and LC3-II, and allows quantification of LC3-II turnover in every condition.

1. Quantify bands for LC3-II and β-actin using ImageJ analyze/measure/gel function (*see* **Note 10**).

2. Normalized LC3-II value to its corresponding β-actin (*see* **Note 11**).

3. Subtract the normalized LC3-II densitometric value in the sample without lysosomal inhibitors from the one with inhibitors. This value corresponds to the amount of LC3-I converted to LC3-II and degraded during the time of the lysosome inhibition treatment (flux) (*see* **Note 12**).

4. Divide each flux value to your reference condition to represent fold change in the tested conditions.

On the immunofluorescence images the number of LC3 puncta in cells has to be quantified.

1. Count LC3-II(+) puncta and number of cells in all conditions (*see* **Note 13**).

2. Calculate the number of puncta per cell.

3. Subtract the puncta per cell value in the sample without lysosomal inhibitors from the value measure in the sample treated with inhibitors. This value corresponds to the accumulation of autophagosome during the time of the lysosome inhibition treatment (flux).

4. Finally, calculate the fold of this accumulation normalizing to your reference condition.

4   Notes

1. Coat only half of the wells in a plate to keep the other half for resting condition. For other plate sizes, use the same CD3ε Ab dilution adjusting the volume in proportion to the surface area (1 well of 24-well plate is 1.9 cm^2).

2. We observe the same results using T cells isolated with MACS and also with primed Th1 and Th2 cells restimulated after 5 or 6 days of culture. However, experimental conditions on primed cells require few modifications of the described protocol.

3. We recommend starting with 24-well plates and using at least three wells per condition to get enough protein. For each condition tested you will need double the number of wells: for untreated cells and cells treated with the lysosomal inhibitors, to get the value of the macroautophagy flux.

4. Several inhibitors of autophagy acting at different stages of the process have been used in the literature. For instance we have also used 100 µM Vinblastine for 3 h instead of NL to measure macroautophagy flux in T cells (*see* Fig. 1). But, since vinblastine inhibits macroautophagy before autophagolysosome formation (by preventing autophagosome and lysosome fusion), the absolute quantity of LC3-II accumulated might be slightly lower than the one observed with NL and corresponds to autophagic structures before autophagosome-lysosome fusion. Bafilomycin and chloroquine can also be used to alter the lysosome acidification and prevent LC3 degradation, although chloroquine is less recommended because it can alter protein synthesis in some cells. The use in parallel of more than one method to inhibit LC3 turnover and measure macroautophagy flux is recommended.

5. Use 20 µL of RIPA per ~3×10^6 cells to obtain enough protein concentration to get reliable quantification.

6. Quantification of protein extract can become tricky especially when using high percentage of detergents in the lysis buffer. We optimized the Bradford protocol using 2 µL of lysate in 18 µL of water added to 1 mL of 1× Bradford solution. Do not use more than 2 µL of sample, which corresponds to a 1/500 dilution of the RIPA buffer, since the detergent concentration can start to significantly disturb measurements above that dilution. A standard curve using BSA must be linear between 1 and 8 µg of BSA per mL of 1× Bradford in the same RIPA dilution as the samples. Following the recommendation in this protocol, one should get all samples' OD in the linear part of this standard curve, and enough proteins to run 2–3 gels.

7. Since LC3 is a small protein (~16 kDa apparent size of LC3-I) and LC3-II shift to a lower size (~14 kDa), we recommend starting with a 15 % polyacrylamide gel. Then, after becoming familiar with the pattern of LC3 on the blot, the polyacrylamide concentration may be reduced to 13 % without losing LC3-I/LC3-II resolution but allowing a better separation of higher MW protein in case other proteins in addition to LC3 and β-Actin need to be analyzed in the same blot. Running conditions for Mini-Protean size:Setup the current at 20 mA

per gel and fixed Voltage max at 125 V. The voltage at the beginning of the run should be around 70 V and then will increase up to the max setup.

8. Transfer at no more than 150 mA per transfer cell (mini size of Protean Biorad) for at least 3 h, rather than using higher current and shorter times. This will avoid excessive heating of the transfer buffer, producing a cleaner membrane and a more reproducible blot.

9. Increasing LC3-Ab binding time does not usually improve specific signal, but will increase the appearance of nonspecific bands.

10. Follow ImageJ commands for gel densitometry. Select both LC3-I and LC3-II bands. Even if macroautophagy flux quantification considers only LC3-II accumulation, this allows to precisely quantifying background around LC3 bands by measuring pixel intensity between the two peaks. We have observed that the level of LC3-II protein in the absence of lysosome inhibitors is very low in both resting and activated T cells, which suggest a very fast rate of macroautophagy activity in T cells. However, with lysosome inhibitors the bands become very intense, especially in activated cells, where macroautophagy is highly induced. In any case, if the signal is still low, increase the quantity of protein loaded on gel to 12–15 μg per lane (no more than 15 μg is recommended to avoid saturation of LC3-II signal in activated cells).

11. We have checked protein level as well as mRNA level of β-Actin and we did not observe any differences in any of the conditions used to study macroautophagy in T cells so far, making this protein a good housekeeping gene.

12. The ratio of the LC3-II levels between samples treated with or without inhibitors has also been used and it provides a measurement of the "speed of the process"; however subtraction will quantify the real net change in total levels of LC3-II. Although initially ratio of LC3-II to LC3-I was widely used, it has become clear that the amount of LC3 primed for conjugation (LC3-I) is very cell type dependent and this ratio is not indicative of macroautophagy activity. Furthermore, differences in the affinity of different anti-LC3 antibodies for LC3-I and LC3-II may lead to inaccurate estimations of the real rate of conversion of LC3-I into LC3-II.

13. This process can be done manually or using an image analysis software such as ImageJ. The particle-counting's functions of ImageJ must be used very carefully and always with a shrewd eye since many parameters still need to be defined manually (threshold, particles size, etc.). We found that ImageJ MaxEntropy auto-threshold method appeared to be a good

tools in order to keep same threshold calculation in all pictures and to give a reliable estimation of LC3 punctates. Also, to avoid any user bias, it is important to count a high number of cells and if possible to perform an additional analysis by another experimenter, both in blind conditions. In any case, clear and clean images are strictly required to make this analysis reliable. If the experimental conditions used lead to a high density of LC3 positive structures that prevents their resolution as individual puncta, area positive for LC3 (also calculated when using the measure particles option in Image J) can be used instead.

Acknowledgments

This work was supported by NIH grant AG021904.

References

1. Cuervo AM (2008) Autophagy and aging: keeping that old broom working. Trends Genet 24:604–612

2. Mizushima N (2009) Physiological functions of autophagy. Curr Top Microbiol Immunol 335:71–84

3. Sridhar S, Botbol Y, Macian F, Cuervo AM (2012) Autophagy and disease: always two sides to a problem. J Pathol 226:255–273

4. Deretic V (2012) Autophagy as an innate immunity paradigm: expanding the scope and repertoire of pattern recognition receptors. Curr Opin Immunol 24:21–31

5. Gannage M, Munz C (2009) Autophagy in MHC class II presentation of endogenous antigens. Curr Top Microbiol Immunol 335:123–140

6. Maue AC, Yager EJ, Swain SL, Woodland DL, Blackman MA, Haynes L (2009) T-cell immunosenescence: lessons learned from mouse models of aging. Trends Immunol 30:301–305

7. Phadwal K, Alegre-Abarrategui J, Watson AS, Pike L, Anbalagan S, Hammond EM et al (2012) A novel method for autophagy detection in primary cells: impaired levels of macroautophagy in immunosenescent T cells. Autophagy 8:677–689

8. Hubbard VM, Valdor R, Patel B, Singh R, Cuervo AM, Macian F (2010) Macroautophagy regulates energy metabolism during effector T cell activation. J Immunol 185:7349–7357

9. Bell BD, Leverrier S, Weist BM, Newton RH, Arechiga AF, Luhrs KA et al (2008) FADD and caspase-8 control the outcome of autophagic signaling in proliferating T cells. Proc Natl Acad Sci U S A 105:16677–16682

10. Pua HH, Dzhagalov I, Chuck M, Mizushima N, He YW (2007) A critical role for the autophagy gene Atg5 in T cell survival and proliferation. J Exp Med 204:25–31

11. Li C, Capan E, Zhao Y, Zhao J, Stolz D, Watkins SC et al (2006) Autophagy is induced in CD4+ T cells and important for the growth factor-withdrawal cell death. J Immunol 177:5163–5168

12. Klionsky DJ, Abdalla FC, Abeliovich H, Abraham RT, Acevedo-Arozena A, Adeli K et al (2012) Guidelines for the use and interpretation of assays for monitoring autophagy. Autophagy 8:445–544

13. Mizushima N, Yoshimori T, Ohsumi Y (2011) The role of Atg proteins in autophagosome formation. Annu Rev Cell Dev Biol 27:107–132

14. Mizushima N, Yoshimori T, Levine B (2010) Methods in mammalian autophagy research. Cell 140:313–326

15. Tanida I, Minematsu-Ikeguchi N, Ueno T, Kominami E (2005) Lysosomal turnover, but not a cellular level, of endogenous LC3 is a marker for autophagy. Autophagy 1:84–91

Chapter 13

Fluorescence-Based Approaches for Quantitative Assessment of Protein Carbonylation, Protein Disulfides, and Protein Conformation in Biological Tissues

Asish R. Chaudhuri, Rochelle Wei, Arunabh Bhattacharya, and Ryan Hamilton

Abstract

Protein oxidation and misfolding have been considered as key players for progression of aging and etiology of various pathological conditions. However, few attempts have been made to develop sensitive and reproducible assays to quantify the changes in protein oxidation and alteration in structure. Here we describe three distinct fluorescence-based assays to quantify changes in protein oxidation, namely carbonylation and disulfides and alteration in protein surface hydrophobicity as a reporter for protein conformation. These techniques will provide investigators the opportunity to address important biological questions in their experimental models.

Key words Protein oxidation, Carbonylation, Disulfide, Oxidative stress

1 Introduction

Substantial evidence in the literature has elegantly shown that protein oxidation has deleterious effects in aging and in the etiology of several age-related diseases, including diabetes, cardiovascular disease, and neurodegenerative diseases [1–8]. Most of the amino acids in proteins are sensitive to oxidation; for instance, side chains on amino acids such as lysine, arginine, proline, and cysteine are susceptible to carbonylation [9–11]. In addition, the thiol group in cysteine is particularly important because it is often found at the catalytic and regulatory sites of proteins and enzymes and is highly sensitive to oxidation. It undergoes various reversible (disulfide, S-thiolated, S-nitrosylated, and sulfenic acid) as well as irreversible (sulfinic and sulfonic acids) oxidations depending on the status of intracellular glutathione [12–15]. Oxidation of critical amino acid residues often leads to protein misfolding/conformational changes that lead to the formation of deleterious oligomers or aggregates

Albert C. Shaw (ed.), *Immunosenescence: Methods and Protocols*, Methods in Molecular Biology, vol. 1343, DOI 10.1007/978-1-4939-2963-4_13, © Springer Science+Business Media New York 2015

which could be damaging to normal cellular homeostasis and contribute to the pathophysiology of several diseases. Therefore, it is essential to utilize sensitive and reliable assays for quantitative assessments of the oxidation and conformational states of proteins. In this chapter, we provide detail on three distinct and sensitive fluorescence-based assays developed by our group to monitor specific types of protein modifications [8, 16–23], which include (1) protein carbonylation, (2) protein disulfides, and (3) alteration of protein surface hydrophobicity as a reporter of protein conformation. Protein carbonyls are one of the most commonly measured modifications over the past 20 years. However, the sensitivity and precision of the spectrometric and immunological based assays are compromised by interference from the free probe, dinitrophenyl hydrazine (DNPH), and by nonspecific interactions of anti-DNPH with proteins. In contrast, our gel-based fluorescent technique using a fluorescein thiocarbazide probe detects only bound protein carbonyls; the free probe does not interfere in the quantification as it is removed during sample preparation. Importantly, all the protein carbonyl data reported in the literature have been performed with the soluble cellular fractions, while our fluorescence-based assay can quantify both soluble and detergent-soluble states of protein carbonyls [8, 17, 18]. The thiol group in cysteine is sensitive to oxidation and undergoes several oxidation states including the disulfide bond which often initiates the formation of both intramolecular and intermolecular bonds usually observed in higher-order protein aggregates. Our fluorescence-based assay [16, 19] using the probe, 6-iodoacetamidofluorescein, specifically recognizes the disulfide linkage on proteins. Our third assay utilizes an apolar fluorescent probe, 4, 4′-dianilino-1,1′-binaphthyl-5,5′-disulfonic acid, to monitor the alteration of the surface hydrophobic domains globally or in specific proteins [20, 21, 23]. UV crosslinking of the probe with surface exposed hydrophobic domain in proteins can distinguish these changes in protein conformation.

These gel-based assays can be used in both in vitro and in vivo studies to determine the effect of oxidative stress on protein oxidation and misfolding. One of the common and unique aspects of all these technologies is the use of fluorescent molecules as probes. This is important as fluorescent probes in general give high quantum yields (the number of fluorescent photons emitted per excitation photon absorbed) which helps quantify low levels of oxidation and conformational changes in potential target proteins during aging and in age-related diseases. Development of these techniques is an important part of basic and clinical research, particularly since the oxidative stress theory remains one of the most widely accepted theories in explaining biochemical changes in various pathophysiological conditions. Thus, these techniques will give investigators necessary tools to delve into the molecular mechanisms involved in various oxidative stress-related disease conditions. Using mouse models that are either deficient in the superoxide radical detoxifying enzyme, copper-zinc superoxide dismutase (SOD), or overexpress the human mutant SOD protein (familial Amyotrophic Lateral Sclerosis model), we demonstrate here that the techniques are not restricted to studies on aging and age-related diseases but may also be applicable in any disease state that is associated with an increase in oxidative stress. Most importantly, all three techniques can also be used as proteomic tools to identify the potential target proteins that are carbonylated, undergo aberrant disulfide formation or alteration in protein conformation [17, 19, 20].

2 Materials

Prepare all solutions using sterile filtered deionized water with a resistance of 18 MΩ/cm unless indicated otherwise. Prepare and store all reagents as indicated.

2.1 SDS Polyacrylamide Gel Components

1. Resolving gel buffer: Prepare a 1 L stock of 2 M Tris–HCl, pH 8.8. Weigh 242.28 g Tris–HCl and transfer to a 1 L graduated cylinder. Add water to graduated cylinder up to a volume of 900 mL. Mix until Tris is dissolved in the water, then adjust for pH with HCl (*see* **Note 1**). When pH is adjusted, add water to graduated cylinder up to a volume of 1 L and mix. Store at 4 °C.

2. Stacking gel buffer: Prepare a 350 mL stock of 1.25 M Tris–HCl, pH 6.8. Weigh 53.0 g Tris–HCl and transfer to a 500 mL graduated cylinder. Mix, adjust pH, and store as described in **step 1**.

3. 30 % Acrylamide/Bis solution 37.5:1.

4. Ammonium persulfate (APS): 10 % solution dissolved in water (*see* **Note 2**).

5. Sodium dodecyl sulfate (SDS): Prepare a 10 mL stock of 10 % SDS dissolved in water. Add 1 g SDS, add water up to a volume of 10 mL, and mix (*see* **Note 3**).

6. *N*,*N*,*N*,*N'*-tetramethyl-ethylenediamine (TEMED). Store at room temperature in fume hood (*see* **Note 4**).

7. Prepare 10× Tris/glycine running buffer by adding 30.3 g of Tris, and 144 g of glycine into 1000 mL of water or use (Bio-Rad catalog number 161-0772): Prepare 1 L 1× working solution by mixing 100 mL 10× buffer with 900 mL water with 4 g of SDS. Store at room temperature (*see* **Note 5**).

8. 10× loading dye: 0.2 M Tris–HCl (pH 6.8), 10 % SDS, 40 % glycerol, 10 % β-mercaptoethanol (β-ME), 0.2 % bromophenol blue.

The mixture is dissolved in water and separated into 1 mL aliquots. Store at –20 °C (*see* **Note 6**).

9. Precision Plus Kaleidoscope protein standards (Bio-Rad catalog number 161-0375) (*see* **Note 7**).

10. Gel loading tips.

11. 1.0 mm thick Criterion Empty Cassettes (Bio-Rad catalog number 345-9903) (*see* **Note 8**).

12. Criterion Cell and PowerPac Basic Power Supply.

2.2 BisANS, Disulfide, and Carbonyl Assay Shared Equipment and Components

1. Homogenizer (Glas-Col catalog number 099C K54).

2. Tissue Grind Tube (Kimble Chase catalog number 885452-0021) (*see* **Note 9**).

3. Tissue Grind Pestle SZ 21 (Kimble Chase catalog number 885451-0021) (*see* **Note 9**).

4. Sonic Dismembrator F60 (Fisher Scientific) (*see* **Note 10**).

5. Sorvall Discovery M120 SE or equivalent centrifuge.

6. 1.0 mL PC thick-walled tubes (Thermo Scientific catalog number 45237).

7. 0.2 mL PC thick-walled tubes (Thermo Scientific catalog number 45233).

8. S120-AT2 rotor (Thermo Scientific catalog number 45583) (*see* **Note 11**).

9. S100-AT3 rotor (Thermo Scientific catalog number 45595) (*see* **Note 11**).

10. Protease inhibitor cocktail set III (pi) (Calbiochem catalog number 539134) (*see* **Note 12**).

11. Pierce BCA protein assay kit (Thermo Scientific catalog number 23227).

12. Water bath or incubator set to 37 °C.

13. Aluminum foil.

14. Plastic wrap.

15. Bio-safe Coomassie stain (Bio-Rad catalog number 161-0772) (*see* **Note 13**).

16. AlphaImager 3400 (Alpha Innotech) or equivalent imaging system.

2.3 BisANS Assay Components

17. 1× BisANS labeling buffer: 50 mM Tris–HCl and 1 mM Magnesium Sulfate ($MgSO_4$), pH 7.4 with pi. Prepare a 50 mL stock by adding 0.303 g Tris and 0.006 g Magnesium Sulfate (*see* **Note 14**). Add up to 50 mL water, mix, and adjust for pH. Store at room temperature if pi has not yet been added (*see* **Note 12**).

18. 4,4′-Dianilino-1,1′-Binaphthyl-5,5′-Disulfonic Acid, Dipotassium Salt (BisANS) (Invitrogen catalog number B-153) fluorescent probe: Prepare 10 mM aliquots by adding 1.486 mL dimethyl sulfoxide (DMSO) to 10 mg of BisANS and mix. Cover aliquots with foil and store at −20 °C (*see* **Note 14**).

19. Flat-bottomed 96-well plate (*see* **Note 16**).

20. Handheld long wave UV light (UVP Model UVL-56) (*see* **Note 17**).

2.4 Disulfide Assay Components

1. 10× KP buffer, pH 8.0: 200 mM potassium phosphate (KP), 5 mM magnesium chloride ($MgCl_2$), and 10 mM ethylenediamine-tetraacetic acid (EDTA), pH 8.0. First, prepare 50 mL stocks of 200 mM KP monobasic and dibasic. Add 1.36 g of KP monobasic, add up to 50 mL water, and mix. Add 1.74 g of KP dibasic, add up to 50 mL water, and mix. Next, prepare a 50 mL stock of 10× KP buffer, pH 8.0. Add 0.24 g of $MgCl_2$, 0.146 g of EDTA, 47 mL of KP dibasic, and 3 mL KP of monobasic (*see* **Note 18**). Add up to 50 mL water and mix (the 10× KP buffer should be pH 8.0). Store at room temperature.

2. 1× KP buffer, pH 8.0: 20 mM KP, 0.5 mM $MgCl_2$, and 1 mM EDTA, pH 8.0 with pi. To make 50 mL stock, mix 5 mL of 10× KP buffer, pH 8.0 and 45 mL water. Store at room temperature if protease inhibitors have not yet been added (*see* **Note 12**).

3. 1× KP buffer, pH 8.0 with 200 mM iodoacetamide (IAM) and pi: 20 mM KP, 0.5 mM $MgCl_2$, and 1 mM EDTA, pH 8.0 with pi. Add IAM, dilute 10× KP buffer, pH 8.0 to 1× with water, and mix. Store at room temperature if IAM and pi have not yet been added (*see* **Notes 12** and **19**).

4. 1× P3 buffer, pH 8.0: 1× KP buffer, pH 8.0 with 2 % SDS, 0.5 % IGEPAL CA-630, 0.5 % Sodium Deoxycholate, and pi (*see* **Note 12**). Prepare a 50 mL stock by adding 1 g of SDS, 750 µL of IGEPAL CA-630, 0.75 g of Sodium Deoxycholate, and 5 mL of 10× KP buffer, pH 8.0. Add up to 50 mL of water and mix. Store at room temperature if pi has not yet been added (*see* **Note 12**).

5. 1× P3 buffer, pH 8.0 with 200 mM IAM and pi (*see* **Notes 12** and **19**).

6. 6 and 8 M Urea dissolved in water (*see* **Note 20**).

7. 20 % trichloroacetic acid (TCA) dissolved in water.

8. 1:1 ethanol/ethyl acetate: Prepare 50 mL of 1:1 ethanol/ethyl acetate mixture by adding 25 mL of 200 proof ethanol and 25 mL ethyl acetate.

9. Dithiothreitol (DTT): Prepare a 1 mL stock of 200 mM DTT. Dissolve 0.031 g of DTT, add up to 1 mL of water, and mix. Store at 4 °C.

10. 6-iodoacetamidofluorescein (6-IAF) fluorescent probe (Invitrogen catalog number I-30452): Prepare 100 mM aliquots by adding 485.19 µL DMSO to the bottle (25 mg) and mix. Cover aliquots with foil and store at –20 °C (*see* **Note 15**).

11. Typhoon 9400 Variable Mode Imager (GE Healthcare Life Sciences).

2.5 Carbonyl Assay Components

1. 10× KP buffer, pH 6.0: 200 mM potassium phosphate (KP), 5 mM magnesium chloride (MgCl$_2$), and 10 mM ethylenediamine-tetraacetic acid (EDTA), pH 8.0. First, prepare 50 mL stocks of 200 mM KP monobasic and dibasic. Add 1.36 g of KP monobasic, add up to 50 mL water, and mix. Add 1.74 g of KP dibasic, add up to 50 mL water, and mix. Next, prepare a 50 mL stock of 10× KP buffer, pH 6.0. Add 0.24 g of MgCl$_2$, 0.146 g of EDTA, 6.6 mL of KP dibasic, and 43.4 mL KP of monobasic (*see* **Note 18**). Add up to 50 mL water and mix (the 10× KP buffer should be pH 6.0). Store at room temperature.

2. 1× KP buffer, pH 6.0: 20 mM KP, 0.5 mM MgCl$_2$, and 1 mM EDTA, pH 6.0 with pi. To make 50 mL stock, mix 5 mL of 10× KP buffer, pH 6.0 and 45 mL water. Store at room temperature if pi has not yet been added (*see* **Note 12**).

3. 1× P3 buffer, pH 6.0: 1× KP buffer, pH 6.0 with 2 % SDS, 0.5 % IGEPAL CA-630, 0.5 % Sodium Deoxycholate, and pi (*see* **Note 12**). Prepare a 50 mL stock by adding 1 g of SDS, 750 µL of IGEPAL CA-630, 0.75 g of Sodium Deoxycholate, and 5 mL of 10× KP buffer, pH 6.0. Add up to 50 mL of water and mix. Store at room temperature if pi has not yet been added (*see* **Note 12**).

4. Dithiothreitol (DTT): Prepare a 1 mL stock of 200 mM DTT. Dissolve 0.031 g of DTT, add up to 1 mL of water, and mix. Store at 4 °C.

5. Fluorescein-5-thiosemicarbazide (FTC) fluorescent probe (Invitrogen catalog number F-121): Prepare 100 mM aliquots by adding 2.37 mL DMSO to the bottle and mix. Cover aliquots with foil and store at –20 °C (*see* **Note 15**).

6. Guanidine hydrochloride: Prepare 1 mL stock of 3 M guanidine hydrochloride. Add 0.287 g of guanidine hydrochloride, add up to 1 mL with water, then mix.

7. 20 % trichloroacetic acid (TCA) dissolved in water.

8. 1:1 ethanol/ethyl acetate: Prepare 50 mL of 1:1 ethanol/ethyl acetate mixture by adding 25 mL of 200 proof ethanol and 25 mL ethyl acetate.

9. 8 M Urea dissolved in water (*see* **Note 20**).

10. Typhoon 9400 Variable Mode Imager (GE Healthcare Life Sciences).

---

3 Methods

3.1 12 % Sodium Dodecyl Sulfate Polyacrylamide Gel Electrophoresis (SDS-PAGE)

All steps are performed at room temperature unless indicated otherwise.

1. Remove well comb from empty criterion cassette, and place cassette on a rack to keep it vertical.

2. Prepare the 12 % running gel by mixing 2.5 mL of resolving gel buffer, 5 mL of 30 % acrylamide/Bis solution, 125 μL of 10 % SDS, and 4.8 mL of water. Add 6 μL of TEMED and 63 μL of 10 % APS, then mix again (*see* **Note 21**).

3. Quickly fill empty criterion cassette with running gel mixture up to 2–3 mm below the bottom of the well insert.

4. Gently layer with 2 mL isopropanol (*see* **Note 22**).

5. Let set for 1 h to allow for full gel polymerization.

6. Rinse isopropanol out of the cassette with water, and briefly dry (*see* **Note 23**).

7. Prepare the 4 % stacking gel by mixing 833 μL of stacking gel buffer, 444 μL of 30 % acrylamide/Bis solution, 33 μL of 10 % SDS, and 2 mL of water. Add 3 μL of TEMED and 33 μL of 10 % APS, then mix again (*see* **Note 21**).

8. Quickly fill criterion cassette with stacking gel mixture to the top (*see* **Note 24**).

9. Carefully place well comb into the criterion cassette (*see* **Note 25**).

10. Let set for 40 min to allow for full gel polymerization.

11. Prepare samples to run in SDS-PAGE by adding appropriate volume of 10× loading dye and mix (*see* **Note 6**).

12. Warm samples to 37 °C for 5 min.

13. Spin down samples at $1000 \times g$ for 30 s to bring down any condensate or sample stuck on the walls.

14. Remove sticker strip from the bottom of the criterion cassette (*see* **Note 26**).

15. Place criterion cassette into criterion cell.

16. Fill criterion cell with 1× Tris/glycine/SDS running buffer up to marked fill line.

17. Fill top buffer reservoir of criterion cassette with 1× Tris/glycine/SDS running buffer (*see* **Note 27**).

18. Carefully remove well comb without disrupting polymerized stacking gel (*see* **Note 28**).

19. Load 5 μL of protein standard into the first well.

20. Carefully start loading samples into the gel (*see* **Note 29**).

21. After all samples are loaded, load 5 μL of protein standard into the next well.

22. Electrophorese at constant 130 V for 1 h 40 min or until the dye front has reached the bottom of the gel (*see* **Note 30**).

3.2 ***BisANS Assay***

1. Homogenize tissue/sonicate harvested cells in 1× BisANS labeling buffer, pH 7.4 with pi (*see* **Notes 9** and **10**).

    (a) Use 150–200 μL for ~100 mg of tissue.

    (b) Use 50–100 μL for cells harvested from 100 mm Petri dish (*see* **Note 31**).

2. Transfer to thick wall ultracentrifuge tubes.

3. Spin down at $100,000 \times g$ for 1 h at 4 °C.

4. Transfer supernatant to fresh tubes and keep on ice.

5. Measure protein concentration as instructed by BCA kit.

6. Turn lights off for as long as BisANS is being worked with.

7. Remove an aliquot of 10 mM BisANS and allow it to thaw before use.

8. In a clear flat-bottomed 96-well plate, prepare reaction mixtures at 1 mg protein/mL with 0.1 mM BisANS in 1×50 mM Tris–HCl, pH 7.4 (*see* **Note 32**).

9. Place the 96-well plate securely on ice and rest a handheld longwave UV light directly on the plate. Make sure the light will cover all of the wells uniformly.

10. Turn on the UV light and allow samples to crosslink with BisANS for 1 h in the dark (*see* **Note 33**).

11. Turn off the UV light, then add appropriate volume of 10× loading dye and buffer to prepare samples for SDS-PAGE (*see* **Note 6**).

12. Load 5–15 μg of BisANS-labeled protein per gel well and subject to SDS-PAGE (*see* **Note 29**).

13. After electrophoresis, place gel in a plastic container with wash consisting of 30 % methanol, 10 % 1× Tris/glycine/SDS running buffer, and 60 % water.

14. Leave plastic container gently rocking for 5 min.

15. Capture BisANS fluorescence image under 365 nm UV light.

16. Wash gel 3× in water for 5 min (at this point, the lights can be turned back on).

17. Add enough Bio-safe Coomassie stain to cover gel (*see* **Note 17**). This will correct for protein loading.

18. Wrap plastic container with plastic wrap and let gel stain overnight with gentle rocking.

19. Wash gel 3× in water for 5 min. There should be noticeable blue bands visible in the gel.

20. Capture Coomassie image under visible light.

21. Analyze all images using Unscanit software (*see* **Note 34**).

22. Figure 1 represents the use of the BisANS assay in two distinct mouse models of oxidative stress; (A) *Sod1*$^{-/-}$ and (B) f-ALS.

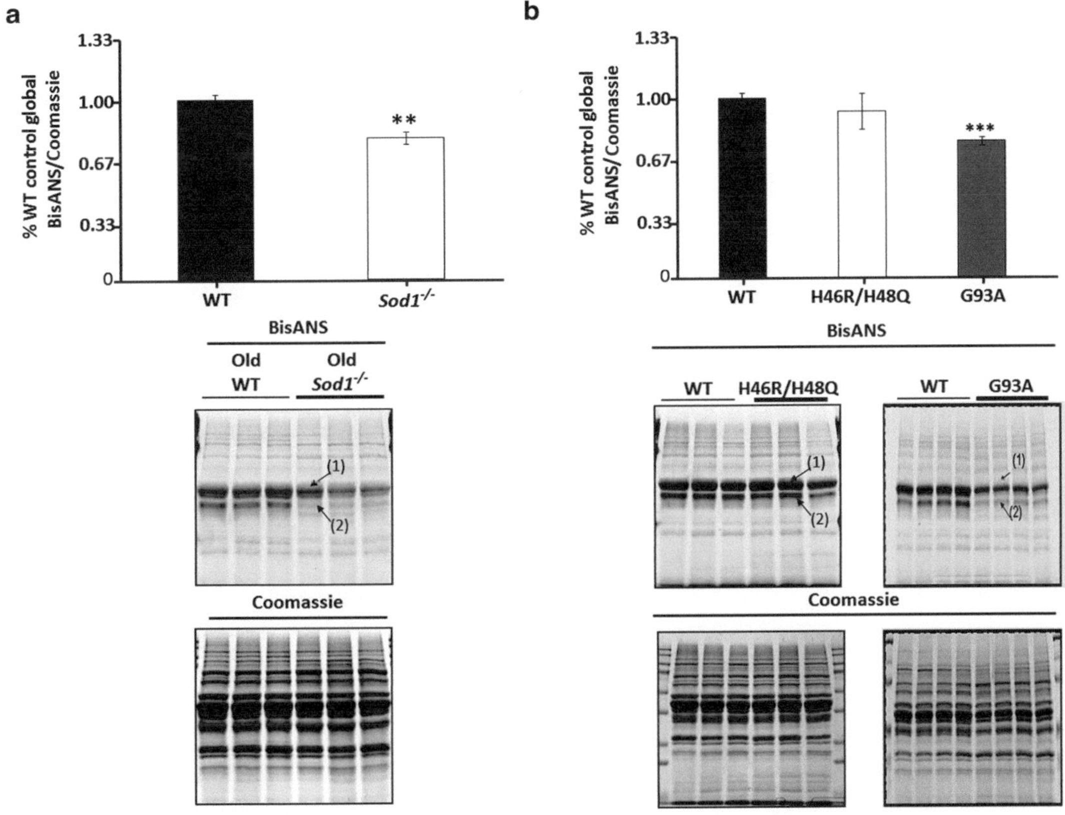

Fig. 1 Alteration in global protein conformation in mouse models of in vivo oxidative stress and f-ALS. BisANS UV crosslinked skeletal muscle proteins were analyzed by SDS-PAGE in (**a**) 20-mo-old wild-type (WT) and *Sod1*$^{-/-}$ mice and (**b**) SOD1^{G93A} and SOD1$^{H46R/H48Q}$ mouse models of human f-ALS. Results are expressed as mean ± standard error of the mean of 4–5 mice/group and analyzed by two-tailed *t*-test (*******p*<0.01, ********p*<0.001). *Panel* (**a**) demonstrates a 22 ± 3 % reduction in BisANS labeling in old *Sod1*$^{-/-}$ mice compared with old WT controls. *Panel* (**b**) demonstrates a 24 ± 2 % reduction in BisANS labeling in SOD1^{G93A} mice compared to the longer-lived SOD1$^{H46R/H48Q}$ mice. Previously, we reported that creatinine kinase (43 kDa) and glyceraldehyde 3-phosphate dehydrogenase (37 kDa) are affected conformationally in response to oxidative stress [20–22] and these proteins were also affected in the f-ALS and *Sod1*$^{-/-}$ mouse models as depicted in (**a**) and (**b**) by (1) and (2), respectively

3.3 Disulfide Assay

1. Homogenize tissue/sonicate harvested cells in 1× KP buffer, pH 8.0 with 200 mM IAM and pi (*see* **Notes 9** and **10**).

    (a) Use 150–200 μL for ~100 mg of tissue.

    (b) Use 50–100 μL for cells harvested from 100 mm Petri dish (*see* **Note 31**).

2. Transfer to thick-walled ultracentrifuge tubes.

3. Spin down at 100,000×*g* for 1 h at 4 °C.

4. Transfer supernatant to fresh tubes and keep on ice.

5. Add 1× P3 buffer, pH 8.0 with 200 mM IAM and pi to the remaining pellets.

    (a) Use 100–150 μL for pellet obtained from tissue.

    (b) Use 50–75 μL for pellet obtained from cells (*see* **Note 31**).

6. Sonicate samples to dissolve insoluble pellet (*see* **Note 10**).

7. Spin down at 100,000×*g* for 10 min at room temperature (*see* **Note 35**).

8. Transfer new supernatant to fresh tubes and keep at room temperature.

9. Measure protein concentration as instructed by BCA kit.

10. Prepare reaction mixtures at 1 mg protein/mL in 6 M Urea (*see* **Note 36**). Use 1× KP buffer, pH 8.0 with 200 mM IAM and pi for initial soluble supernatant; use 1× P3 buffer, pH 8.0 with 200 mM IAM and pi for insoluble pellet supernatant. This step will block all free sulfhydryl groups.

11. Incubate reaction mixtures for 1 h at 37 °C.

12. After incubation, add an equal volume of 20 % TCA to the samples in order to precipitate the protein (*see* **Note 37**).

13. Incubate for 15 min on ice (supernatant) or room temperature (pellet) (*see* **Note 38**).

14. Spin down at 16,000×*g* for 15 min at 4 °C (supernatant) or room temperature (pellet).

15. Carefully remove TCA and add 300 μL of 1:1 ethanol/ethyl acetate.

16. Break up the protein pellet using flattened pipette tip or sonicator (*see* **Note 10**).

17. Spin down at 16,000×*g* for 15 min at 4 °C (supernatant) or room temperature (pellet).

18. Carefully remove first 1:1 ethanol/ethyl acetate wash.

19. Add another 300 μL 1:1 ethanol/ethyl acetate.

20. Break up the protein pellet again using flattened pipette tip or sonicator (*see* **Note 10**).

21. Carefully remove second 1:1 ethanol/ethyl acetate wash.

22. Dissolve protein with 300 μL of 8 M Urea (sonicate if necessary) (*see* **Note 10**).

23. Add DTT to 1 mM final concentration and mix.

24. Incubate for 30 min at 37 °C. This step will break the disulfide bridges.

25. Turn lights off for as long as 6-IAF is being worked with.

26. Remove an aliquot of 6-IAF and allow it to thaw before use.

27. Add 6-IAF to samples to 1 mM final concentration and mix.

28. Incubate for 30 min at 37 °C in the dark. This step will label the reduced sulfhydryl groups that were previously oxidized in the disulfide bridges.

29. After incubation, add an equal volume of 20 % TCA to the samples in order to precipitate the protein (*see* **Note 37**).

30. Incubate for 10 min on ice (supernatant) or room temperature (pellet) (*see* **Note 38**).

31. Spin down at $16,000 \times g$ for 5 min at 4 °C (supernatant) or room temperature (pellet).

32. Carefully remove TCA and add 1 mL of 1:1 ethanol/ethyl acetate.

33. Continue with breaking the pellet, spinning down, removing wash, and adding a new wash until three washes have been completed (*see* **Note 39**).

34. After last wash, remove all excess 1:1 ethanol/ethyl acetate.

35. Dissolve supernatant protein with 8 M Urea with pi and pellet protein with 1× P3 buffer, pH 8.0 with pi.

36. Sonicate all samples (*see* **Note 10**).

37. If necessary, incubate samples for up to 30 min at 37 °C to help dissolve protein.

38. Spin down all samples at $16,000 \times g$ for 2 min at room temperature to pellet any insoluble protein.

39. Transfer supernatant to fresh tubes.

40. Measure protein concentration as instructed by BCA kit.

41. Add appropriate volume of 10× loading dye and buffer to prepare samples for SDS-PAGE (*see* **Note 6**).

42. Load 5–15 μg of labeled protein per well and subject to SDS-PAGE (*see* **Note 29**).

43. Place gel in a plastic container with water.

44. Leave plastic container gently rocking for 5 min.

45. Capture disulfide fluorescence image on Typhoon 9400 Variable Mode Imager under the settings 526 SP filter, 350 PMT sensitivity, 532 nm excitation (*see* **Note 40**).

46. Wash gel 3× in water for 5 min (at this point, the lights can be turned back on).

47. Add enough Bio-safe Coomassie stain to cover gel (*see* **Note 17**). This will correct for protein loading.

48. Wrap plastic container with plastic wrap and let gel stain overnight while gently rocking.

49. Wash gel 3× in water for 5 min. There should be noticeable blue bands visible in the gel.

50. Capture Coomassie image under visible light.

51. Analyze all images using Unscanit software (*see* **Note 33**).

52. Figure 2 represents the use of the disulfide assay in f-ALS mouse model.

53. Quantification for disulfides was performed utilizing Unscanit software as described previously for BisANS (*see* **Note 33**).

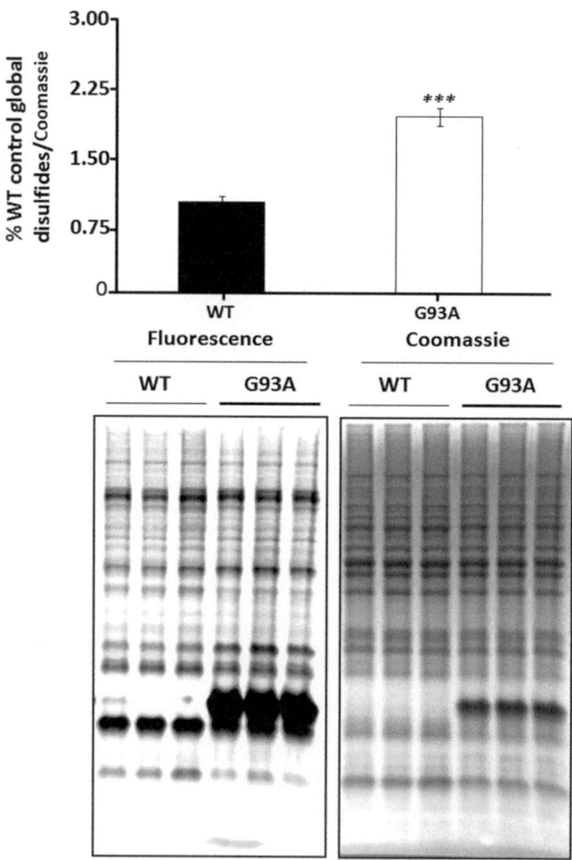

Fig. 2 Global change in protein disulfides in a mouse model of f-ALS. 6-IAF labeled spinal cord protein homogenates were run on 12 % SDS-PAGE and analyzed by fluorescence spectroscopy in postsymptomatic (140 days) SOD1^{G93A} mice and aged-matched wild-type (WT) mice. Results are expressed as mean±standard error of the mean of 3 mice/group and analyzed by two-tailed *t*-test (***$p<0.001$). Figure 2 shows a ~2-fold increase in protein disulfides in the postsymptomatic SOD1^{G93A} mice compared to WT littermate controls

3.4 Carbonyl Assay

1. Homogenize tissue/sonicate harvested cells in 1× KP buffer, pH 6.0 with pi (*see* **Notes 9** and **10**).

   (a) Use 150–200 μL for ~100 mg of tissue.

   (b) Use 50–100 μL for cells harvested from 100 mm Petri dish (*see* **Note 31**).

2. Transfer to thick wall ultracentrifuge tubes.

3. Spin down at 100,000×*g* for 1 h at 4 °C.

4. Transfer supernatant to fresh tubes and keep on ice.

5. Add 1× P3 buffer, pH 6.0 with pi to the remaining pellets.

   (a) Use 100–150 μL for pellet obtained from tissue.

   (b) Use 50–75 μL for pellet obtained from cells (*see* **Note 31**).

6. Sonicate samples to dissolve insoluble pellet (*see* **Note 10**).

7. Spin down at 100,000×*g* for 10 min at room temperature (*see* **Note 35**).

8. Transfer new supernatant to fresh tubes and keep at room temperature.

9. Measure protein concentration as instructed by BCA kit.

10. Prepare reaction mixtures at 1 mg protein/mL (*see* **Note 36**). Use 1× KP buffer, pH 6.0 with pi for initial soluble supernatant; use 1× P3 buffer, pH 6.0 with pi for insoluble pellet supernatant.

11. Add DTT to 1 mM final concentration to pellet samples only. This will help with dissolving the protein in subsequent steps.

12. Turn lights off for as long as FTC is being worked with.

13. Remove an aliquot of FTC and allow it to thaw before use.

14. Add FTC to 1 mM final concentration and mix.

15. Add guanidine hydrochloride to 0.3 M final concentration to all samples and mix (*see* **Note 37**).

16. Incubate for 2 h at 37 °C in the dark.

17. After incubation, add an equal volume of 20 % TCA to the samples in order to precipitate the protein (*see* **Note 38**).

18. Incubate for 15 min on ice (supernatant) or room temperature (pellet) (*see* **Note 39**).

19. Spin down at 16,000×*g* for 15 min at 4 °C (supernatant) or room temperature (pellet).

20. Carefully remove TCA and add 1 mL of 1:1 ethanol/ethyl acetate.

21. Break up the protein pellet using flattened pipette tip or sonicator (*see* **Note 10**).

22. Spin down at 16,000×*g* for 15 min at 4 °C (supernatant) or room temperature (pellet).

23. Carefully remove first 1:1 ethanol/ethyl acetate wash.

24. Continue with breaking the pellet, spinning down, removing wash, and adding a new wash until four washes have been completed (*see* **Note 40**).

25. After last wash, remove all excess 1:1 ethanol/ethyl acetate.

26. Dissolve supernatant protein with 8 M Urea with pi and pellet protein with 1× P3 buffer, pH 8.0 with 1 mM DTT and pi.

27. Sonicate all samples (*see* **Note 10**).

28. If necessary, incubate samples for up to 30 min at 37 °C to help dissolve protein.

29. Spin down all samples at 16,000×*g* for 2 min at room temperature to pellet any insoluble protein.

30. Transfer supernatant to fresh tubes.

31. Measure protein concentration as instructed by BCA kit.

32. Add appropriate volume of 10× loading dye and buffer to prepare samples for SDS-PAGE (*see* **Note 6**).

33. Load 5–15 µg of labeled protein per well and subject to SDS-PAGE (*see* **Note 29**).

34. Place gel in a plastic container with water.

35. Leave plastic container gently rocking for 5 min.

36. Capture carbonyl fluorescence image on Typhoon 9400 Variable Mode Imager under the settings 526 SP filter, 600 PMT sensitivity, 532 nm excitation (*see* **Note 41**).

37. Wash gel 3× in water for 5 min (at this point, the lights can be turned back on).

38. Add enough Bio-safe Coomassie stain to cover gel (*see* **Note 17**). This will correct for protein loading.

39. Wrap plastic container with plastic wrap and let gel stain overnight while gently rocking.

40. Wash gel 3× in water for 5 min. There should be noticeable blue bands visible in the gel.

41. Capture Coomassie image under visible light.

42. Analyze all images using Unscanit software (*see* **Note 33**).

43. Figure 3 represents the use of carbonyl assay in f-ALS mouse model.

44. Quantification of global carbonyls was performed utilizing Unscanit software as described previously for BisANS (*see* **Note 33**).

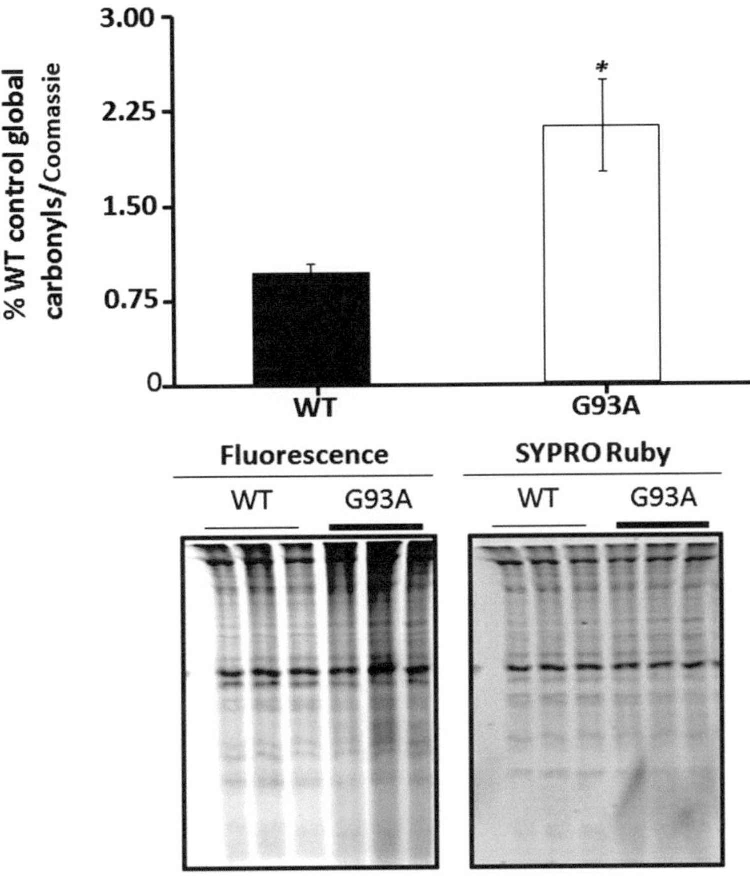

Fig. 3 Global change in protein carbonyls in a mouse model of f-ALS. Skeletal muscle protein carbonyls in post. Symptomatic ALS mice (140 days) and aged-matched wild-type (WT) mice were measured by FTC fluorescence. Results are expressed as mean ± standard error of the mean of 3 mice/group and analyzed by two-tailed t-test ($*p < 0.05$). Figure 3 demonstrates a ~2.3-fold increase in protein carbonyls in post. Symptomatic SOD1[G93A] mice compared to WT litter-mate controls

4 Notes

1. The 100 mL gap is to allow for the addition of concentrated HCl, as a considerable volume is used to adjust for pH in this solution.

2. 10 % APS solution is always prepared fresh.

3. Wear gloves and mask when handling powder; SDS is an irritant and harmful by inhalation, ingestion, skin or eye contact.

4. TEMED is stored and used in the fume hood to reduce odor.

5. 1× buffer: 25 mM Tris–HCl, 192 mM glycine, 0.1 % SDS, pH 8.3. 1× buffer may be used 4–5 times before discarding as waste.

6. SDS precipitates at 4 °C. Make sure loading dye is warmed to room temperature prior to use. β-ME is hazardous, avoid skin contact, eye contact, and inhalation.

7. Any gel protein standards will work. Make sure to take note of the molecular weight bands for that particular product.

8. We primarily use 26-well combs, but the company has a variety of other well comb sizes available.

9. Be very careful to only apply pressure vertically while homogenizing tissue, as the tissue grind pestle is made of glass and can easily break.

10. Wear sound mufflers to protect your hearing while sonicating. To avoid loss of precious sample, try to keep sonicator tip closer to the bottom of tube and carefully move tip up and down. Always keep sonicator tip away from the surface of sample as this will spray sample out of the tube.

11. Always double check for proper placement of rubber O-ring on the inner side of rotor cover. This will prevent loss of sample.

12. Hydrated magnesium sulfate ($MgSO_4$-xH_2O) can also be used in this case. Keep in mind that the amount weighed for the stock solution will be different in order to correct for higher molecular weight.

13. Stocks are prepared without pi and stored at room temperature. Pi is treated as 1000× (e.g., 5 μL of pi in 5 mL of buffer) and is added right before using buffer.

14. Fluorescent probe is light sensitive. Keep the lights off anytime fluorescent probe is being worked with.

15. Any flat-bottomed 96-well plate will work. It can be clear or black.

16. UV light wavelength 365 nm. UV light is harmful to bare skin and eyes, avoid exposure to those areas. Never look at the UV light while it is illuminated.

17. Coomassie is a total protein stain. Avoid using bare fingers when moving gel around, as this can leave fingerprints directly on the gel.

18. Combining certain percentages of KP monobasic and dibasic will result in a set pH. To obtain pH 8.0 for the disulfide assay, we combined 94 % KP dibasic with 6 % KP monobasic. To obtain pH 6.0 for the carbonyl assay, we combine 13.2 % KP dibasic with 86.8 % KP monobasic.

19. IAM is always prepared fresh.

20. 6 and 8 M Urea is always prepared fresh. It is normal for the solution to get colder while dissolving in water, let it warm to room temperature before use.

21. Always add TEMED and APS last to the mixture, as this will start the gel polymerization process.

22. It is normal to observe a slight rolling effect at the border of the running gel mixture and isopropanol.

23. To dry, invert the cassette onto paper towels and lightly tap to remove excess water.

24. Try to add stacking gel mixture carefully and avoid bubbles.

25. We try to push any bubbles to the side as we slide the well comb in. If bubbles remain in the stacking gel mixture, samples will not run properly.

26. Failure to remove sticker strip will prevent current flow and samples will not run down gel.

27. We completely fill the top buffer reservoir. It is crucial to have the wells covered in 1× Tris/glycine/SDS buffer. Failure to do so will prevent current flow and samples will not run down gel.

28. Stacking gel is fragile and can break off or bend if well comb removal is not careful.

29. We pipette samples starting from the bottom of the well and slowly raising pipette tip as well is filled with sample.

30. The dye front generally runs faster than the smallest molecular weight band of the precision plus kaleidoscope protein standards, so is easy to spot when to stop electrophoresis.

31. We generally try to prepare reaction mixtures of 100 μg protein in 100 μL total volume in 1× BisANS buffer plus protease inhibitors. A lower total volume will be difficult to uniformly cover the entire well surface of the 96-well plate.

32. It is very important to keep the plate on ice to avoid sample evaporation, as the plate will heat up over time while the UV light is on.

33. Unscanit software utilizes the area under the curve for given bands and allows you to calculate the areas under the curve for each band which can be summed after analysis for all bands on the gel. For all analysis, the total BisANS, disulfides, or carbonyls were measured as an area under the curve in arbitrary units for all bands and normalized to the area under the curve for the total protein loaded on the gels as measured by coomassie. Values were converted to fold change relative to the wild-type animals. Arrows located in Fig. 1 indicate two proteins that we observed in our 2006 manuscript which confirmed the proteins that were misfolded by mass spectrometry analysis [20]. Any alternative image analysis software will work for the analysis.

34. For sonicating volumes of 50–100 μL, we suggest using 0.2 mL thick wall ultracentrifuge tubes.

35. SDS precipitates at 4 °C; make sure that all samples containing P3 buffer are worked with at room temperature.

36. We generally try to prepare reaction mixtures of at least 200 μg protein in 200 μL total volume if limited on sample. Ethanol/ethyl acetate wash steps lose a lot of protein; use at maximum 500 μg protein in 500 μL total volume.

37. Add an equal volume of 20 % TCA as the total volume of reaction mixture (e.g., 200 μL TCA to 200 μL total volume reaction mixture).

38. Reaction mixture becoming cloudy or speckled is a good indication of protein precipitation. If working with very low amounts of protein, TCA precipitation time can be increased.

39. Several washes are required to get rid of excess TCA and free fluorescent probe. Failure to do so will cause the gel fluorescence to look streaky and lack distinguished band patterning.

40. Fluorescence imaging will also work with other imagers with similar excitation/emission/filter capabilities.

41. The addition of guanidine hydrochloride will make pellet samples difficult to work with, so make sure to add it last to the reaction mixture.

References

1. Christians ES, Benjamin IJ (2012) Proteostasis and REDOX state in the heart. Am J Physiol Heart Circ Physiol 302:H24–H37

2. Bokov A, Chaudhuri A, Richardson A (2004) The role of oxidative damage and stress in aging. Mech Ageing Dev 125:811–826

3. Butterfield DA, Kanski J (2001) Brain protein oxidation in age-related neurodegenerative disorders that are associated with aggregated proteins. Mech Ageing Dev 122:945–962

4. Olivares-Corichi IM, Ceballos G, Medina-Santillan R, Medina-Navarro R, Guzman-Grenfell AM, Hicks JJ (2005) Oxidation by reactive oxygen species (ROS) alters the structure of human insulin and decreases the insulin-dependent D-glucose-C14 utilization by human adipose tissue. Front Biosci 10:3127–3131

5. Uchida K, Toyokuni S, Nishikawa K, Kawakishi S, Oda H, Hiai H, Stadtman ER (1994) Michael addition-type 4-hydroxy-2-nonenal adducts in modified low-density lipoproteins: markers for atherosclerosis. Biochemistry 33:12487–12494

6. Nakamura A, Kawakami K, Kametani F, Nakamoto H, Goto S (2010) Biological significance of protein modifications in aging and calorie restriction. Ann N Y Acad Sci 1197:33–39

7. Curtis JM, Hahn WS, Long EK, Burrill JS, Arriaga EA, Bernlohr DA (2012) Protein carbonylation and metabolic control systems. Trends Endocrinol Metab 23:399–406

8. Bhattacharya A, Leonard S, Tardif S, Buffenstein R, Fischer KE, Richardson A, Austad SN, Chaudhuri AR (2011) Attenuation of liver insoluble protein carbonyls: indicator of a longevity determinant? Aging Cell 10:720–723

9. Uchida K (2003) Histidine and lysine as targets of oxidative modification. Amino Acids 25:249–257

10. Amici A, Levine RL, Tsai L, Stadtman ER (1989) Conversion of amino acid residues in proteins and amino acid homopolymers to carbonyl derivatives by metal-catalyzed oxidation reactions. J Biol Chem 264:3341–3346

11. Doorn JA, Petersen DR (2002) Covalent modification of amino acid nucleophiles by the lipid peroxidation products 4-hydroxy-2-nonenal and 4-oxo-2-nonenal. Chem Res Toxicol 15:1445–1450

12. Berlett BS, Stadtman ER (1997) Protein oxidation in aging, disease, and oxidative stress. J Biol Chem 272:20313–20316

13. Huggins TG, Wells-Knecht MC, Detorie NA, Baynes JW, Thorpe SR (1993) Formation of o-tyrosine and dityrosine in proteins during

radiolytic and metal-catalyzed oxidation. J Biol Chem 268:12341–12347

14. Thomas JA, Mallis RJ (2001) Aging and oxidation of reactive protein sulfhydryls. Exp Gerontol 36:1519–1526

15. Zhou JQ, Gafni A (1991) Exposure of rat muscle phosphoglycerate kinase to a nonenzymatic MFO system generates the old form of the enzyme. J Gerontol 46:B217–B221

16. Chaudhuri AR, Khan IA, Luduena RF (2001) Detection of disulfide bonds in bovine brain tubulin and their role in protein folding and microtubule assembly in vitro: a novel disulfide detection approach. Biochemistry 40: 8834–8841

17. Chaudhuri AR, de Waal EM, Pierce A, Van Remmen H, Ward WF, Richardson A (2006) Detection of protein carbonyls in aging liver tissue: a fluorescence-based proteomic approach. Mech Ageing Dev 127:849–861

18. Salmon AB, Leonard S, Masamsetti V, Pierce A, Podlutsky AJ, Podlutskaya N, Richardson A, Austad SN, Chaudhuri AR (2009) The long lifespan of two bat species is correlated with resistance to protein oxidation and enhanced protein homeostasis. FASEB J 23:2317–2326

19. Perez VI, Pierce A, de Waal EM, Ward WF, Bokov A, Chaudhuri A, Richardson A (2010) Detection and quantification of protein disulfides in biological tissues a fluorescence-based proteomic approach. Methods Enzymol 473: 161–177

20. Pierce A, deWaal E, Van Remmen H, Richardson A, Chaudhuri A (2006) A novel approach for screening the proteome for changes in protein conformation. Biochemistry 45:3077–3085

21. Pierce A, Mirzaei H, Muller F, De Waal E, Taylor AB, Leonard S, Van Remmen H, Regnier F, Richardson A, Chaudhuri A (2008) GAPDH is conformationally and functionally altered in association with oxidative stress in mouse models of amyotrophic lateral sclerosis. J Mol Biol 382:1195–1210

22. Pierce AP, de Waal E, McManus LM, Shireman PK, Chaudhuri AR (2007) Oxidation and structural perturbation of redox-sensitive enzymes in injured skeletal muscle. Free Radic Biol Med 43:1584–1593

23. Wei R, Bhattacharya A, Chintalaramulu N, Jernigan AL, Liu Y, Van Remmen H, Chaudhuri AR (2012) Protein misfolding, mitochondrial dysfunction and muscle loss are not directly dependent on soluble and aggregation state of mSOD1 protein in skeletal muscle of ALS. Biochem Biophys Res Commun 417:1275–1279

Chapter 14

Monitoring the DNA Damage Response at Dysfunctional Telomeres

Rekha Rai and Sandy Chang

Abstract

Telomeres are repetitive DNA repeats that cap the ends of all eukaryotic chromosomes. Their proper maintenance is essential for genomic stability and cellular viability. Dysfunctional telomeres could arise through natural attrition of telomeric DNA or due to the removal of shelterin components. These uncapped chromosomal ends are recognized as DSBs by the DDR pathway, leading to the accumulation of DNA damage sensors at telomeres. The association of these DDR proteins with dysfunctional telomeres forms telomere dysfunction induced DNA damage foci (TIFs). Detection of TIFs at telomeres provides an opportunity to quantify the extent of telomere dysfunction and monitor downstream DNA damage signaling pathways. Here we describe a method for the detection of TIFs using a fluorescent in situ hybridization (FISH) approach.

Key words DNA damage, Telomere dysfunction, Telomere induced foci, Telomere FISH

---

1 Introduction

DNA double-strand (ds) breaks are highly genotoxic lesions which must be repaired by the DNA damage response (DDR). Failure to properly repair these lesions results in genomic instability and could promote the onset of cancer. The DDR functions to delay cell cycle progression until the damaged DNA is repaired by either the non-homologous end joining or homologous recombination repair pathways, or if the damage is too severe for repair, the initiation of apoptosis. Persistent DNA damage promotes the onset of a permanent arrested state—termed senescence. Activation of a potent tumor suppressive senescence program is associated in vivo through the activation of the DDR by dysfunctional telomeres [1]. Telomeres are ribonucleoprotein complexes at the chromosome ends and consist of TTAGGG repetitive sequences. Telomeres terminate with a 3′ single-stranded G-overhang, and the enzyme telomerase utilizes this structure to add de novo telomere sequences to chromosome ends. In mammals, telomeres are bound by six

Albert C. Shaw (ed.), *Immunosenescence: Methods and Protocols*, Methods in Molecular Biology, vol. 1343,
DOI 10.1007/978-1-4939-2963-4_14, © Springer Science+Business Media New York 2015

telomeric core proteins: telomeric-repeat-binding factor 1 (TRF1) and 2 (TRF2), TRF1-interacting protein 2 (TIN2), transcriptional repressor/activator protein RAP1, protection of telomeres 1 (POT1), and POT1- and TIN2-organizing protein (TPP1) [2]. This so-called shelterin complex contributes to the formation of protective telomere loop (t-loop) structures in which the single-stranded 3′-overhang invades the telomeric duplex in order to prevent chromosome ends from being recognized as DSBs by the DDR pathway. Failure of the protective features of telomeres due to natural telomere attrition or to alterations in the shelterin complex leads to the formation of "dysfunctional" telomeres incapable of maintaining normal protective functions [3]. Dysfunctional telomeres are sensed by the MRN (Mre11/Rad50/Nbs1) complex, which activates an ATM/ATR dependent DNA damage signaling cascade leading to the recruitment of DNA damage response factors such as 53BP1, γ-H2AX, and MDC1 to initiate inappropriate non-homologous end joining (NHEJ) or homologous recombination (HR) DNA repair pathways at chromosome ends [4, 5]. The recruitment of DNA damage response factors to dysfunctional telomeres can be efficiently visualized in interphase nuclei using telomere fluorescent in situ hybridization (FISH). These foci, known as dysfunctional telomere induced DNA damage foci (TIFs), mark dysfunctional telomeres. They provide an opportunity to quantify the extent of telomere dysfunction in all cell types and to monitor the DDR pathways activated by dysfunctional telomeres [6, 7].

---

2   Materials

2.1   Cell Culture

1. Dulbecco's Modified Eagle's Medium (DMEM) supplemented with 10 % fetal bovine serum (FBS, Sigma), OPTI-MEM (Gibco).

2. 293T (ATCC) and Mouse Embryonic Fibroblast (MEFs) Cells.

3. 0.25 % Trypsin.

4. Phosphate-buffered saline (PBS).

2.2   Retroviral Production and Infection

1. pCL Eco, Empty pBabe, p-Babe shTRF2, Empty pQCXIP, pQCXIP TPP1$^{\Delta RD}$ [8].

2. Polybrene Stock 6 mg/ml. Filter through a 0.2 μm filter, aliquot, and store at −20 °C.

3. Lipofectamine Plus Reagent (Invitrogen), Fugene 6 (Roche).

4. 0.45 μm syringe filters (Millipore).

2.3   Immunofluo-rescence-Telomere FISH

1. Nunc Lab-Tek 8 well slide chambers (Nalgene Nunc, 12-565-1), Microscope coverslips 18×18-1 (Fisher-12-548-A), Microscope Slides (Fisher 12-544-3).

2. Phosphate-buffered saline (PBS): Prepare 10× stock with 1.37 M NaCl, 27 mM KCl, 100 mM Na2HPO4, 18 mM KH_2PO_4 (adjust to pH 7.4 with HCl if necessary) and autoclave before storage at room temperature. Prepare working solution by dilution of one part with nine parts water.

3. Fix Solution: 2 % paraformaldehyde/2 % sucrose.

4. Blocking Solution PBG: 0.2 % fish gelatin (Sigma), 0.5 % BSA (Sigma). Aliquot PBG and store at –20 °C.

5. Permeabilization Buffer: 0.5 % (v/v) Nonidet-P40 in PBS.

6. TBST: 1× PBS with 0.1 % Triton.

7. Primary antibodies: 53BP1 and γ-H2AX antibodies (Upstate).

8. Secondary antibodies: Alexa Fluor 568 goat anti-mouse IgG {H + L} (Molecular Probes A-11004).

9. 20× SSC (3.0 M NaCl and 0.3 M sodium citrate, pH 7.0).

10. Formamide (Fisher).

11. TelC-TAMRA, TAMRA-OO-(CCCTAA)3 Peptide Nucleic Acid (PNA) Probe (Pan agene-F2002). Stock solution 1 µg/µl in H_2O.

12. Yeast tRNA (Invitrogen). Stock solution 1 mg/ml in H_2O.

13. Wash Solution I: (70 % formamide, 0.1 % Tween-20, 0.1 % BSA, 10 mM Tris–HCl, pH 7.5).

14. Wash Solution II: (50 mM Tris–HCl, pH 7.5, 150 mM NaCl, 0.1 % BSA, 0.1 % Tween-20).

15. Mounting Medium with Antifate: DAPI (Vectashield H-1200).

---

3 Methods

TIFs can sometimes be detected in human or mouse cells which have experienced natural telomere attrition. However, robust TIF formation is accompanied by the disruption of normal telomere structure through depletion of TRF2, or removal of the TPP1-POT1a/b complex from telomeres [4–9]. To accomplish efficient induction of TIFs in Mouse Embryonic Fibroblasts (MEFs), depletion of TRF2 using shRNA against TRF2 [4] or overexpression of TPP1$^{\Delta RD}$ (a TPP1 mutant lacking the POT1 interaction domain) to disrupt endogenous TPP1-POT1a/b interactions [9] is performed. Induction of TIFs in human cells can be achieved similarly [8]. For infecting MEFs, use the pCL-ECO packaging plasmid, and for infecting human cells, use VSV-G/Gag-Pol packaging constructs for generating high titer shTRF2 or TPP1$^{\Delta RD}$ retroviral particles [8]. To achieve high titer retroviral particles, use early passage 293T cells and high quality DNA preparations. Cells with ≥5 53BP1 or γ-H2AX signals co-localized with telomere signals are considered TIF-positive. Score at least 100–200 TIFs positive cells to reach statistical significance.

3.1 Retrovirus Production in 293T Cells

1. *Day 0*: On the day before transfection, plate 0.5–1×10⁶ 293T cells into a 6 cm tissue culture dish in 4.0 ml DMEM supplemented with 10 % FBS (*see* **Note 1**). The cells are ready for transfection after 18–20 h, or when they are about 60–70 % confluent. Plate slightly more cells when making VSV-G pseudotyped viruses.

2. *Day 1*: Aspirate the medium and replace the cells with 2.0 ml DMEM without FBS or any antibiotic. Transfect 293T cells with 2.0 µg pCL-ECO and 4.0 µg of transfer vectors (p-Babe shTRF2, pQXCIP TPP1ᐃᴿᴰ) using Lipofectamine Plus Reagent following the manufacturer's protocol. For making VSV-G retroviruses by triple transfection, use 0.9 µg Gag/Pol expression vector, 0.1 µg VSV-G expression vector, and 1.0 µg transfer vector. For making VSV-G pseudotype viruses, use Fugene 6 following the manufacturer's protocol.

3. Change the medium 5–7 h after transfection with 4.0 ml of fresh medium (*see* **Note 2**).

4. *Day 3*: Harvest the viral supernatants at 48 h post-transfection. Filter the viral supernatant with a 0.45 µm syringe filter. Add 10 ml of fresh DMEM medium supplemented with 10 % FBS to the cells.

5. *Day 4*: Harvest the viral supernatant at 72 h of post-infection as above.

3.2 Retroviral Infection

1. *Day 2*: Grow 20 % confluent target cells either on coverslips in 6-well plates or in 8-well slide chambers (*see* **Note 3**).

2. *Day 3*: Infect the cells with retroviral particles harvested at 48 h. Add 2.0 ml viral particles (1:1 diluted in DMEM/10%FBS) in a 6-well plate and 500 µl in 8-well chambers to infect MEFs/Human cells. Add 6 µg/ml polybrene for infecting MEFs and 4 µg/ml polybrene for infecting Hela or U2OS cells (*see* **Note 4**).

3. *Day 4*: After 24 h, reinfect the cells with the 72 h harvest of retroviral particles.

4. *Day 5*: Replace the cells with fresh medium (*see* **Note 5**).

3.3 Immunofluorescence-Telomere FISH

1. *Day 6*: Aspirate the medium and wash the cells twice for 5 min each with 1× PBS at room temperature (RT).

2. Fix the cells with 2 % paraformaldehyde/2 % sucrose for 10 min at RT.

3. Wash the fixed cells twice for 5 min each with 1× PBS.

4. Permeabilize the cells with 0.5 % Nonidet-P40 for 10 min at RT.

5. Wash the cells thrice for 5 min with 1× PBS.

6. Incubate the cells with PBG for 1 h to block nonspecific binding.

7. Incubate the cells with the primary antibody diluted in PBG (1:2000 53BP1 or γ-H2AX) overnight at 4 °C in a humidified chamber (*see* **Note 6**). Add 60 µl antibody for 8-well chambers, and 30–50 µl for cells on coverslips. For cells on coverslips, drop antibodies on paraffin film and gently place coverslips with cells facing down on top of antibody drop.

8. *Day 7*: Wash the cells thrice for 5 min each with PBST followed by 5 min blocking with PBG.

9. Incubate the cells with appropriate secondary antibody diluted in PBG (1:2000) for 1 h at RT. Incubation should be performed in the dark.

10. Wash the cells thrice for 5 min each with 1× PBST.

11. Post-fix the secondary antibody to primary antibody by incubating the cells in 4 % paraformaldehyde for 10 min at room temperature (*see* **Note 7**).

12. Wash the cells twice for 5 min each with PBS, RT.

13. Add freshly prepared PNA-FISH hybridization mix: (30 µl/coverslip, face down on paraffinized slides; 60 µl per eight chamber slide). PNA-hybridization mix recipe:

H_2O	2.85 µl
2 % BSA	1.5 µl
100 µg/ml tRNA	0.15 µl
0.6× SSC	3.0 µl
100 % Formamide	21.0 µl
10 ng/µl PNA Probe	1.5 µl
Total	30.0 µl

14. Denature the slide at 85 °C on a hot plate for 3 min; place the slide in the dark overnight in a humidified chamber (*see* **Note 8**).

15. *Day 8*: Wash twice for 15 min each in Wash Solution I. For slides use a Coplin jar, for coverslips use a 6-well plate.

16. Wash thrice for 5 min each in Wash Solution II.

17. Ethanol dehydrate the slides for 2 min each with 70, 85, and 95 % Ethanol.

18. Counterstain with DAPI and seal with nail vanish. The coverslip should be carefully inverted to a drop of mounting medium on a microscope slide. For 8-well chambers, carefully remove the gasket and place a few drops of mounting medium and cover with coverslips (*see* **Note 9**). The slides can be viewed immediately when the varnish is dried or can be stored in the dark at 4 °C for up to a month.

19. Visualize and image under a fluorescent microscope.

4 Notes

1. It is very important to have single cell suspensions (trypsinize well) and evenly distributed cells.

2. 293T cells detach easily, be careful with all media changes.

3. Coverslips must be autoclaved or sterilized by flaming with 95 % alcohol. Place the coverslips in 6-well plates to cool down.

4. Polybrene enhances the rate of infection.

5. Visualize any GFP control plates under the fluorescent microscope to be sure the cells are expressing GFP. If they are, you can assume the cells have taken in the DNA and are producing virus.

6. Make sure cells are covered and will not dry out.

7. It is critical to post-fix the secondary antibody to primary antibody using paraformaldehyde in order to retain the primary antibody signals.

8. Make absolutely sure that the temperature is exactly 85 °C using a thermometer.

9. Air bubbles are undesirable in the mounting medium.

References

1. Cosme-Blanco W, Shen MF, Lazar A et al (2007) Telomere dysfunction suppresses spontaneous tumorigenesis *in vivo* by activating p53-mediated cellular senescence. EMBO Rep 8:497–503

2. de Lange T (2005) Shelterin: the protein complex that shapes and safeguards human telomeres. Genes Dev 19:2100–2110

3. Deng Y, Chan SS, Chang S (2008) Telomere dysfunction and tumour suppression: the senescence connection. Nat Rev Cancer 8:450–458

4. Deng Y, Guo X, Ferguson DO et al (2009) Multiple roles for MRE11 at uncapped telomeres. Nature 460:914–918

5. Rai R, Zheng H, He H et al (2010) The function of classical and alternative non-homologous end-joining pathways in the fusion of dysfunctional telomeres. EMBO J 29:2598–2610

6. d'Adda di Fagagna F, Reaper PM, Clay-Farrace L et al (2003) A DNA damage checkpoint response in telomere initiated senescence. Nature 426:194–198

7. Takai H, Smogorzewska A, de Lange T (2003) DNA damage foci at dysfunctional telomeres. Curr Biol 13:1549–1556

8. Liu D, Safari A, O'Connor MS et al (2004) PTOP interacts with POT1 and regulates its localization to telomeres. Nat Cell Biol 6:673–680

9. Guo X, Deng Y, Lin Y et al (2007) Dysfunctional telomeres activate an ATM-ATR-dependent DNA damage response to suppress tumorigenesis. EMBO J 26:4709–4719

Chapter 15

Single-Cell Analysis of T-Cell Receptor αβ Repertoire

Pradyot Dash*, George C. Wang*, and Paul G. Thomas

Abstract

The unbiased, paired analysis of T-cell receptor (TCR) α- and β-chain usage at the single-cell level provides a valuable window of understanding into the TCR repertoire and the nature of the immune response. Earlier technologies for TCR repertoire analysis were often limited to examining TCR complementarity-determining region 3 (CDR3) β expression or required in vitro cloning procedures that can artificially skew the TCR repertoire from its in vivo state. We describe here a direct ex vivo, single-cell-based strategy for the clonotypic analysis of TCRαβ repertoires that utilizes multiplexed panels of TCRα and TCRβ-specific primers in a nested PCR to amplify expressed transcripts from individual, epitope-specific T cells. This strategy yields the paired TCRαβ sequences of any given population of αβ T cells of interest.

Key words T-cell receptor repertoire, Complementarity-determining region 3, TCR alpha, TCR beta, TCR diversity, Single-cell analysis, Unbiased repertoire, Paired analysis, Clonotype, Epitope

1 Introduction

The ability to characterize the repertoire of a population of T cells responding to an epitope, whether pathogen- or host-derived, offers unique insights into the immune response. The T-cell receptor (TCR) αβ heterodimer binds to peptides presented in the context of self major histocompatibility complex (MHC) glycoproteins on cell membranes. The third complementarity-determining region (CDR3) of the TCR, which interacts specifically with the MHC-bound peptide [1], is primarily responsible for the variations in TCR structure that enable T cells to bind to unique peptide-MHC (pMHC) complexes. The uniqueness of each CDR3 derives from somatic rearrangements within the variable (V) and joining (J) gene segments of the TCRα chain and the V, D (diversity), and J gene segments of the TCRβ chain [1–3].

Historically, the tools for studying epitope-specific TCR repertoires can be categorized by their level of resolution. Flow cytometry-based TCR Vβ frequency analysis [4] and spectratyping

---

*These authors made equal contributions to this work.

Albert C. Shaw (ed.), *Immunosenescence: Methods and Protocols*, Methods in Molecular Biology, vol. 1343,
DOI 10.1007/978-1-4939-2963-4_15, © Springer Science+Business Media New York 2015

181

[5] offer limited-resolution snapshots of the TCR repertoire by examining percentages of T cells expressing particular Vβ chains and distributions in CDR3 size, respectively. Various molecular cloning and sequencing methods provide clonotype-level resolution of the TCR repertoire, ranging from establishment of cell lines [6, 7] to direct sequencing by anchored polymerase chain reaction (PCR) of cells ex vivo [8]. Any procedure that involves in vitro cloning of T cells can potentially artificially skew the TCR repertoire from its in vivo state. Additionally, any bulk amplification of RNA may be biased by variation between cells in RNA levels. Thus, recent advances in high-throughput sequencing of TCR clonotypes primarily focus on genomic DNA in order to maintain relative quantification [9, 10]. This bulk-sequencing approach does not currently allow the concurrent characterization of CDR3α and CDR3β sequences or knowledge of allelic expression, a component required for an assessment of the true repertoire structure and diversity that only a single-cell, RNA-based approach can provide.

Therefore, we developed a method for the unbiased, paired analysis of epitope-specific TCRαβ repertoire at the single-cell level, using multiplexed panels of CDR3α- and CDR3β-specific primers in a nested PCR to amplify the expressed CDR3α and CDR3β segments from individual T cells [11, 12]. The co-expression data of CDR3α and CDR3β sequences are then obtained by nucleotide sequencing of the single-cell-derived, amplified CDR3 products. This strategy can be used on any given population of αβ T cells of interest (e.g., epitope-specific CD4+ or CD8+ T cells), from mice [11] or humans [12], thus allowing cloning and expression of paired TCR for further characterization. Subsequently, other investigators have used a different single-cell approach to study TCRαβ chains in human CD8+ T cells [13]. This chapter focuses on the analysis of human T cells. An example is given in Subheadings 2 and 3 whereby cytomegalovirus (CMV) epitope-specific human T cells are the cells of interest and are isolated via tetramer staining and flow cytometry-based single-cell sorting. This method can be applied to other cell populations single-cell sorted via other strategies.

2 Materials

2.1 Cell Sorting Reagents and Instrument

1. Human peripheral blood mononuclear cells (PBMC): Fresh or frozen PBMC isolated by density gradient (e.g., GE Healthcare Ficoll-Paque PLUS) centrifugation from peripherally withdrawn venous whole blood collected into sodium heparin-coated collection tubes. Frozen PBMC should be cryopreserved in liquid nitrogen.

2. Fluorochrome-conjugated monoclonal antibodies and tetramer: The following list of reagents is used for the isolation

of human leukocyte antigen (HLA) A*0201-restricted CMV pp65$_{495-503}$ NLVPMVATV (CMV-NLV) CD8+ T cells. (Use other reagents and/or cell-identification strategies as appropriate for the isolation of other cell populations). Live dead discrimination dye (LIVE/DEAD Fixable Aqua Dead Cell Stain Kit, for 405 nm excitation), FITC-conjugated anti-human CD3 (e.g., BD 349201), PE-Cy7-conjugated anti-human CD8 (e.g., BD 557746), PE-conjugated anti-human CD14 (e.g., BD 340683), and APC-conjugated, peptide-loaded pMHCI tetramer (e.g., HLA-A*0201-CMV pp65 (NLVPMVATV), Beckman Coulter, T01023). The antibodies and tetramer should be titrated to determine the optimal dilution required for staining with minimal background. Store the antibodies and tetramer at +4 °C in the dark.

3. Sort buffer: PBS containing 0.1 % BSA, fraction V (Life Technologies). Make a fresh batch and filter sterilize before each sorting experiment.

4. RNase inhibitor: Add 200 U/ml RNAsin (Promega) to sort buffer to be used for final resuspension of cells prior to sorting.

5. Polypropylene DNase- and RNase-free 96-well PCR plates (Eppendorf) and adhesive sealing films (MicroAmp, Applied Biosystems).

6. Centrifuge with a plate carrier.

7. MoFlo, iCyt, or equivalent flow cytometric cell sorter with a single-cell sorting module.

2.2 RT-PCR and Gel Electrophoresis

1. Multichannel pipette and tips: 12-channel (5–50 μl) and 8-channel (0.5–10 μl) pipettes, 10, 20, and 200 μl DNase- and RNase-free barrier tips.

2. Individually wrapped sterile reservoir boats.

3. Reverse transcription kit: iScript cDNA Synthesis Kit (Bio-Rad) containing 5× iScript reaction mix and iScript reverse transcriptase.

4. Triton X-100, molecular biology grade (Sigma).

5. PCR kit: Taq polymerase-based PCR kit (Qiagen) with 10× PCR buffer containing 15 mM $MgCl_2$, CoralLoad buffer (10×) containing 15 mM $MgCl_2$, 10 mM dNTP and Taq DNA polymerase (5 U/μl).

6. Oligonucleotide primers (Table 1) (*see* **Note 1**):

   Stock dilution: Resuspend primers to 200 μM using 1× TE buffer (low EDTA; 10 mM Tris–HCl, 0.1 mM EDTA, pH 8.0; USB). Store the stock dilutions in –20 °C.

Table 1
Primers targeting T-cell receptor alpha (TRA) and beta (TRB) genes

TRA gene(s) targeted by primer	External primer sequence (EXT)	Internal primer sequence (INT)
TRAV1	5′ AACTGCACGTACCAGACATC 3′	5′ GCACCCACATTTCTKTCTTAC 3′
TRAV2	5′ GATGTGCACCAAGACTCC 3′	5′ CACTCTGTGTCCAATGCTTAC 3′
TRAV3	5′ AAGATCAGGTCAACGTTGC 3′	5′ ATGCACCTATTCAGTCTCTGG 3′
TRAV4	5′ CTCCATGGACTCATATGAAGG 3′	5′ ATTATATCACGTGGTACCAACAG 3′
TRAV5	5′ CTTTTCCTGAGTGTCCGAG 3′	5′ TACACAGACAGCTCCTCCAC 3′
TRAV6	5′ CACCCTGACCTGCAACTATAC 3′	5′ TGGTACCGACAAGATCCAG 3′
TRAV7	5′ AGCTGCACGTACTCTGTCAG 3′	5′ ACAATTTGCAGTGGTACAGG 3′
TRAV8-1	5′ CTCACTGGAGTTGGGATG 3′	5′ GTCAACACCTTCAGCTTCTC 3′
TRAV8-2, 8-4	5′ GCCACCCTGGTTAAAGG 3′	5′ AGAGTGAAACCTCCTTCCAC 3′
TRAV8-3	5′ CACTGTCTCTGAAGGAGCC 3′	5′ TTTGAGGCTGAATTTAAGAGG 3′
TRAV8-6	5′ GAGCTGAGGTGCAACTACTC 3′	5′ AACCAAGGACTCCAGCTTC 3′
TRAV8-7	5′ CTAACAGAGGCCACCCAG 3′	5′ ATCAGAGGTTTTGAGGCTG 3′
TRAV9-1, 9-2	5′ TGGTATGTCCAATATCCTGG 3′	5′ GAAACCACTTCTTTCCACTTG 3′
TRAV10	5′ CAAGTGGAGCAGAGTCCTC 3′	5′ GAAAGAACTGCACTCTTCAATG 3′
TRAV12-1, 12-2, 12-3	5′ CARTGTTCCAGAGGGAGC 3′	5′ AAGATGGAAGGTTTACAGCAC 3′
TRAV13-1	5′ CATCCTTCAACCCTGAGTG 3′	5′ TCAGACAGTGCCTCAAACTAC 3′
TRAV13-2	5′ CAGCGCCTCAGACTACTTC 3′	5′ CAGTGAAACATCTCTCTCTGC 3′
TRAV14	5′ AAGATAACTCAAACCCAACCAG 3′	5′ AGGCTGTGACTCTGGACTG 3′
TRAV16	5′ AGTGGAGCTGAAGTGCAAC 3′	5′ GTCCAGTACTCCAGACAACG 3′
TRAV17	5′ GGAGAAGAGGATCCTCAGG 3′	5′ CCACCATGAACTGCAGTTAC 3′
TRAV18	5′ TCCAGTATCTAAACAAAGAGCC 3′	5′ TGACAGTTCCTTCCACCTG 3′
TRAV19	5′ AGGTAACTCAAGCGCAGAC 3′	5′ TGTGACCTTGGACTGTGTG 3′
TRAV20	5′ CACAGTCAGCGGTTTAAGAG 3′	5′ TCTGGTATAGGCAAGATCCTG 3′
TRAV21	5′ TTCCTGCAGCTCTGAGTG 3′	5′ AACTTGGTTCTCAACTGCAG 3′
TRAV22	5′ GTCCTCCAGACCTGATTCTC 3′	5′ CTGACTCTGTGAACAATTTGC 3′
TRAV23	5′ TGCTTATGAGAACACTGCG 3′	5′ TGCATTATTGATAGCCATACG 3′
TRAV24	5′ CTCAGTCACTGCATGTTCAG 3′	5′ TGCCTTACACTGGTACAGATG 3′
TRAV25	5′ GGACTTCACCACGTACTGC 3′	5′ TATAAGCAAAGGCCTGGTG 3′

(continued)

Table 1
(continued)

TRA gene(s) targeted by primer	External primer sequence (EXT)	Internal primer sequence (INT)
TRAV26-1	5′ GCAAACCTGCCTTGTAATC 3′	5′ CGACAGATTCACTCCCAG 3′
TRAV26-2	5′ AGCCAAATTCAATGGAGAG 3′	5′ TTCACTTGCCTTGTAACCAC 3′
TRAV27	5′ TCAGTTTCTAAGCATCCAAGAG 3′	5′ CTCACTGTGTACTGCAACTCC 3′
TRAV29	5′ GCAAGTTAAGCAAAATTCACC 3′	5′ CTGCTGAAGGTCCTACATTC 3′
TRAV30	5′ CAACAACCAGTGCAGAGTC 3′	5′ AGAAGCATGGTGAAGCAC 3′
TRAV34	5′ AGAACTGGAGCAGAGTCCTC 3′	5′ ATCTCACCATAAACTGCACG 3′
TRAV35	5′ GGTCAACAGCTGAATCAGAG 3′	5′ ACCTGGCTATGGTACAAGC 3′
TRAV36	5′ GAAGACAAGGTGGTACAAAGC 3′	5′ ATCTCTGGTTGTCCACGAG 3′
TRAV38-1, 38-2	5′ GCACATATGACACCAGTGAG 3′	5′ CAGCAGGCAGATGATTCTC 3′
TRAV39	5′ CTGTTCCTGAGCATGCAG 3′	5′ TCAACCACTTCAGACAGACTG 3′
TRAV40	5′ GCATCTGTGACTATGAACTGC 3′	5′ GGAGGCGGAAATATTAAAGAC 3′
TRAV41	5′ AATGAAGTGGAGCAGAGTCC 3′	5′ TTGTTTATGCTGAGCTCAGG 3′
TRAC	5′ GACCAGCTTGACATCACAG 3′	5′ TGTTGCTCTTGAAGTCCATAG 3′

TRB gene(s) targeted by primer	External primer sequence (EXT)	Internal primer sequence (INT)
TRBV2	5′ TCGATGATCAATTCTCAGTTG 3′	5′ TTCACTCTGAAGATCCGGTC 3′
TRBV3-1	5′ CAAAATACCTGGTCACACAG 3′	5′ AATCTTCACATCAATTCCCTG 3′
TRBV4-1, 4-2, 4-3	5′ TCGCTTCTCACCTGAATG 3′	5′ CCTGCAGCCAGAAGACTC 3′
TRBV5-1, 5-3, 5-4	5′ GATTCTCAGGKCKCCAGTTC 3′	5′ CTTGGAGCTGGRSGACTC 3′
TRBV5 5, 5-6, 5-7, 5-8	5′ GTACCAACAGGYCCTGGGT 3′	5′ TCTGAGCTGAATGTGAACG 3′
TRBV6-1, 6-2, 6-3, 6-5, 6-6, 6-7, 6-8, 6-9	5′ ACTCAGACCCCAAAATTCC 3′	5′ GTGTRCCCAGGATATGAACC 3′

(continued)

Table 1
(continued)

TRB gene(s) targeted by primer	External primer sequence (EXT)	Internal primer sequence (INT)
TRBV6-4	5′ ACTGGCAAAGGAGAAGTCC 3′	5′ TGGTTATAGTGTCTCCAGAGC 3′
TRBV7-1, 7-2, 7-3	5′ TRTGATCCAATTTCAGGTCA 3′	5′ TCYACTCTGAMGWTCCAGCG 3′
TRBV7-4, 7-6, 7-7, 7-8, 7-9	5′ GSWTCTYTGCAGARAGGCC 3′	5′ TGRMGATYCAGCGCACA 3′
TRBV9	5′ GATCACAGCAACTGGACAG 3′	5′ GTACCAACAGAGCCTGGAC 3′
TRBV10-1, 10-2, 10-3	5′ TGTWCTGGTATCGACAAGACC 3′	5′ TCCYCCTCACTCTGGAGTC 3′
TRBV11-1, 11-2, 11-3	5′ CGATTTTCTGCAGAGACGC 3′	5′ GACTCCACTCTCAAGATCCA 3′
TRBV12-3, 12-4, 12-5	5′ ARGTGACAGARATGGGACAA 3′	5′ CYACTCTGARGATCCAGCC 3′
TRBV13	5′ AGCGATAAAGGAAGCATCC 3′	5′ CATTCTGAACTGAACATGAGC 3′
TRBV14	5′ CCAACAATCGATTCTTAGCTG 3′	5′ ATTCTACTCTGAAGGTGCAGC 3′
TRBV15	5′ AGTGACCCTGAGTTGTTCTC 3′	5′ ATAACTTCCAATCCAGGAGG 3′
TRBV16	5′ GTCTTTGATGAAACAGGTATGC 3′	5′ GAAAGATTTTCAGCTAAGTGCC 3′
TRBV17	5′ CAGACCCCCAGACACAAG 3′	5′ TGTTCACTGGTACCGACAG 3′
TRBV18	5′ CATAGATGAGTCAGGAATGCC 3′	5′ CGATTTTCTGCTGAATTTCC 3′
TRBV19	5′ AGTTGTGAACAGAATTTGAACC 3′	5′ TTCCTCTCACTGTGACATCG 3′
TRBV20-1	5′ AAGTTTCTCATCAACCATGC 3′	5′ACTCTGACAGTGACCAGTGC 3′
TRBV23-1	5′ GCGATTCTCATCTCAATGC 3′	5′ GCAATCCTGTCCTCAGAAC 3′
TRBV24-1	5′ CCTACGGTTGATCTATTACTCC 3′	5′ GATGGATACAGTGTCTCTCGA 3′
TRBV25-1	5′ ACTACACCTCATCCACTATTCC 3′	5′ CAGAGAAGGGAGATCTTTCC 3′
TRBV27, 28	5′ TGGTATCGACAAGACCCAG 3′	5′ TTCYCCCTGATYCTGGAGTC 3′
TRBV29-1	5′ TTCTGGTACCGTCAGCAAC 3′	5′ TCTGACTGTGAGCAACATGAG 3′
TRBV30	5′ TCCAGCTGCTCTTCTACTCC 3′	5′ AGAATCTCTCAGCCTCCAGAC 3′
TRBC	5′ TAGAACTGGACTTGACAGCG 3′	5′ TTCTGATGGCTCAAACACAG 3′

Primers targeting TRAV and TRBV genes are sense. Primers targeting TRAC and TRBC genes are antisense. *TRAV* T-cell receptor Vα, *TRAC* T-cell receptor Cα, *TRBV* T-cell receptor Vβ, *TRBC* T-cell receptor Cβ

Working dilution: TRAV-EXT (cocktail of external TCRα primers): Mix 25 μl of each TRAV-EXT forward primers (40 of them, 200 μM stock) and make up the volume to 1000 μl with 1× TE buffer (low EDTA; 10 mM Tris–HCl, 0.1 mM EDTA, pH 8.0) to achieve a working stock of 5 pmol/μl for each primer in the cocktail.

TRBV-EXT (cocktail of external TCRβ primers): Mix 25 μl of each TRBV-EXT forward primers (27 of them, 200 μM stock) and make up the volume as above to 1000 μl of diluted primer cocktail with each primer at 5 pmol/μl working concentration.

TRAV-INT (cocktail of internal TCRα primers): Mix 25 μl of each TRAV-INT forward primer (40 of them, 200 μM stock) and make up the volume as above to 1000 μl of diluted primer cocktail with each primer at 5 pmol/μl working concentration.

TRBV-INT (cocktail of internal TCRβ primers): Mix 25 μl of each TRBV-INT forward primers (27 of them, 200 μM stock) and make up the volume as above to 1000 μl of diluted primer cocktail with each primer at 5 pmol/μl working concentration.

Resuspend all four reverse primers (TRAC-EXT, TRAC-INT, TRBC-EXT, TRBC-INT) to 20 μM working stocks (*see* **Note 2**).

7. Thermocyclers with heated lid.

8. Agarose gel electrophoresis instrument: e.g., Owl™ A3-1 Large-Gel Electrophoresis System with 50-well microwell combs. The microwell-format combs provide rapid sample loading with a multichannel pipette. Up to six 96-well plates worth of samples can be analyzed at the same time.

9. 1× TAE buffer: 0.04 M Tris-acetate with 0.001 M EDTA.

10. GelRed nucleic acid stain, 10,000× (Biotium).

11. Imager: e.g., Bio-Rad Geldoc system.

2.3 Sequencing and Analysis

1. PCR product purification: Exonuclease I (USB), Shrimp Alkaline Phosphatase (SAP, 7 USB), Tris–Cl, 50 mM, pH 8.0.

2. Big Dye® Terminator (v3.1) kit (Life technologies) and 3730XL DNA Analyzers (Applied Biosystems).

3. Software: Chromas chromatogram viewer (Technelysium) and MegAlign DNA sequence alignment and analysis program (DNASTAR Laser gene).

4. Macro-enabled, customized Microsoft Excel analysis sheet.

5. St. Jude TCR web application: https://tcr.stjude.org/tcr/. Access to the application can be acquired through correspondence with the authors.

3 Methods

***3.1 Immunofluo-
rescence Staining***

The following subsection provides an example of immunofluorescence staining for the identification and sorting of HLA A*0201-restricted CMV-NLV CD8+ T cells. For the identification of other cell populations, use other established procedures accordingly.

1. After isolating fresh PBMC or after thawing and washing cryopreserved PBMC according to established procedures, resuspend the isolated PBMC in 1 ml of D-PBS-Ca++Mg++ with no extraneous proteins.

2. Stain cells with LIVE/DEAD Fixable Aqua Dead Cell Stain for 30 min at room temperature in the dark.

3. At the end of the incubation, wash two times with sort buffer by centrifuging at $350 \times g$ and +4 °C for 5 min.

4. Resuspend the cells in 200 μl sort buffer containing APC-conjugated, peptide-loaded pMHCI tetramer, FITC-conjugated anti-human CD3, PE-Cy7-conjugated anti-human CD8, and PE-conjugated anti-human CD14 in appropriate dilutions. Incubate the cells at room temperature in the dark for 30 min.

5. Wash the cells twice in sort buffer.

***3.2 Single-Cell
Sorting***

1. Resuspend the cells in 0.5 ml of sort buffer containing RNase inhibitor at a concentration of 200 U/ml (*see* **Note 3**).

2. Filter the cell suspension through a 40 μm cell strainer.

3. (This step describes the gating strategy for the sorting of tetramer + CD8+ cells. Substitute appropriate gating strategies for other cell populations accordingly.) Gate the lymphocytes first on their scatter properties based on an FSC-A/SSC-A plot. From the probable lymphocyte population, select the live cells based on Live/Dead staining and CD14 negativity. Then gate on CD3⁺CD8⁺ cells to enrich the tetramer⁺ cells for sorting.

4. Set the parameter on MoFlo to "single cell 1" with a drop envelope of 1 (or corresponding parameter on other cell sorters) to ensure stringency for single-cell only sorting. Additional crosschecks for single-cell deposition accuracy should be carried out by the users by visualization under light microscopy of single cells in 96-well culture plates and by confirmation of clonality in single-cell sorted hybridomas from mixed cultures.

5. Sort the cells of interest into each well in Columns 1–10 of a 96-well polypropylene PCR plate (Eppendorf). Leave Columns 11 and 12 empty. Column 12 will be the negative (no template) control. Following the sort, seal the plate with adhesive plate seal. Make sure that the edges of the adhesive

seal are pressed thoroughly using an applicator or similar blunt end object (e.g., round edge of a marker pen) to ensure a proper seal. Place the plate on ice. After the sort is completed, spin the plates briefly to settle the contents to the bottom of the wells and store at –80 °C until ready to perform reverse transcription and PCR.

3.3 Reverse Transcription (RT)

The reverse transcription of the TCRα and β mRNA is carried out directly on the lysed cells in the 96-well plate without any RNA extraction step. Lysis is achieved by the combination of freeze-thaw cycle and inclusion of a detergent, Triton X-100, in the RT mixture.

1. Remove the plate from –80 °C and thaw on ice.

2. Centrifuge the plate at $500 \times g$ for 2 min and keep on ice.

3. Prepare master mix for RT. We have reduced the final volume of RT mix to one-eighth of the manufacturer's recommendation (from 20 to 2.5 µl) for single-cell reactions with a modification where we add Triton-X 100 to a final concentration of 0.1 % (*see* **Note 4**).

	Per well (µl)	1 plate (88 ± 22 = 110 reactions) (µl)
5× RT Buffer	0.5	55
iScript RT enzyme	0.125	13.25
Water, Nuclease free	1.6	178.75
Triton-X100 (1 %)	0.25	27.5

4. Keep 8-channel (0.5–10 µl) pipette, barrier tips (10 µl), reagent reservoir, adhesive plate seal, and its applicator ready. Take the plate containing single cells from ice, hold down firmly, and remove the adhesive seal carefully. Add 2.5 µl of RT master mix to each well using a multichannel pipette, changing tips for each column. Work quickly to avoid evaporation. Add to Columns 1–10 (samples) and 12 (negative control).

5. Seal the plate with a new adhesive plate film thoroughly and centrifuge at $500 \times g$ for 2 min.

6. Run cDNA synthesis program on a thermocycler as follows: 5 min at 25 °C; 45 min at 42 °C; 5 min at 85 °C; hold at 4 °C.

7. Store the plate at –20 °C if you would like to proceed to the next step later.

3.4 Nested PCR

Carry out a nested PCR protocol as described below for amplifying the TCRα and β chain from single cells. A schematic for the PCR is shown in Fig. 1.

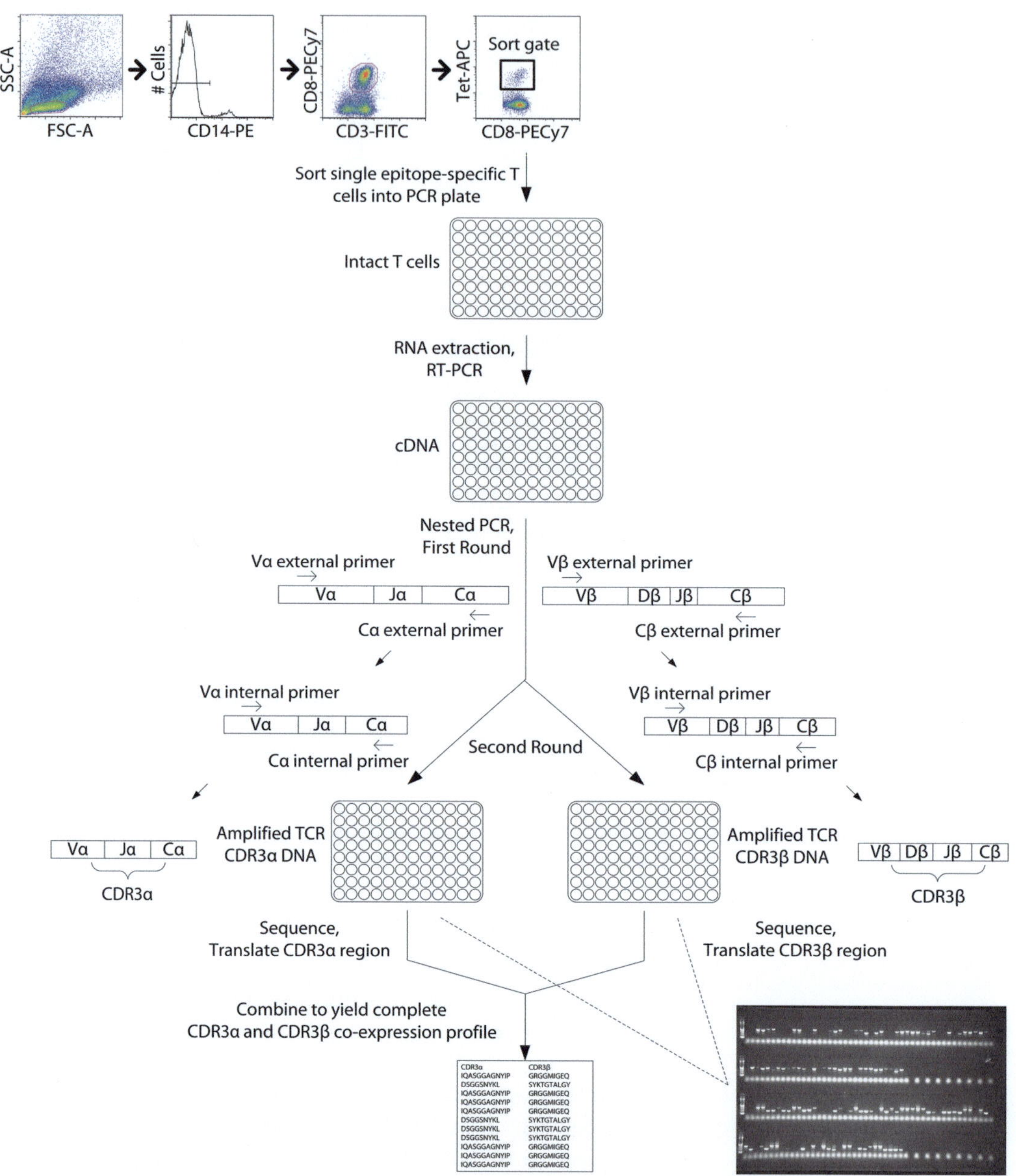

Fig. 1 Overview of single-cell multiplex clonotypic analysis of epitope-specific T cells. Single epitope-specific CD8+ T cells are sorted on a flow cytometric cell sorter into 96-well PCR plates. RT-PCR is performed on the individual cells. The resultant cDNA is subjected to two rounds of nested PCR. In the first round, CDR3α and CDR3β transcript amplification is achieved with the use of a multiplexed, comprehensive panel of external sense Vα and Vβ and antisense Cα and Cβ segment-specific primers. First-round PCR products are subjected to two separate second-round PCRs, incorporating, respectively, a multiplexed panel of external sense Vα and antisense Cα or external sense Vβ and antisense Cβ segment-specific primers. PCR products thus derived are sequenced and translated to yield paired CDR3αβ repertoire data. Inset: Nucleotide products from nested PCR performed on cDNA derived from single CMV-NLV-specific CD8+ T cells from a young adult donor, incorporating TCRα- (*top two rows*) and TCRβ-specific primers (*bottom two rows*). Reproduced with permission from Wang et al., 2012 [12]

1. *First-round PCR*: Prepare a reaction master fix as follows (*see* **Note 4**):

	Per well (µl)	1 plate (88 ± 12 = 100 reactions) (µl)
Nuclease-free water	17.35	1735
PCR buffer, 10×	2.5	250
(Containing 15 mM MgCl₂)		
dNTP, 10 mM	0.5	50
TRAC-EXT (20 µM)	0.5	50
TRAV-EXT	0.5	50
(Cocktail of α primers)		
TRBC-EXT (20 µM)	0.5	50
TRBV-EXT	0.5	50
(Cocktail of β primers)		
Taq DNA Polymerase	0.15	15
Total	22.5	2250

2. Remove the plate seal carefully and add 22.5 µl of master mix to all samples and control wells using a 12-channel pipette (5–50 µl) (*see* **Note 5**).

3. Reseal the plate thoroughly with a new adhesive plate seal, ensuring the edges are sealed tightly, and centrifuge the plate to settle the contents to the bottom of wells.

4. Perform PCR in a thermocycler as follows:

    Initial denaturation, 5 min at 95 °C; denaturation, 20 s at 95 °C; primer annealing, 2 0 s at 52 °C; polymerase extension, 45 s at 72 °C; repeat denaturation to extension step 34 times; final extension, 7 min at 72 °C; and hold at +4 °C. The plates can be stored at −20 °C until the next step.

5. *Second-round PCR*: At this point, you will set up TCRα and TCRβ PCRs separately. Thus, identical wells of α and β plates will be derived from single cells. For example, well position A1 of the α plate will pair with A1 of the β plate. Prepare two reaction master mixes (α and β) as follows (*see* **Note 4**):

	Per well (µl)	1 plate (88 ± 12 = 100 reactions) (µl)
Nuclease-free water	18.35	1835
CoralLoad PCR buffer, 10X	2.5	250

(continued)

	Per well (µl)	1 plate (88 ± 12 = 100 reactions) (µl)
(Containing 15 mM MgCl$_2$)		
dNTP, 10 mM	0 .5	50
TRAC-INT (20 µM) *OR* TRBC-INT (20 µM)	0.5	50
TRAV-INT *OR* TRBV-INT	0.5	50
(Cocktail of TCRα or β primers)		
Taq DNA Polymerase	0.15	15
Total	22.5	2250

6. Add 22.5 µl of the respective master mix to each well of new plates labeled α and β in the hood or similar dedicated space for PCR work.

7. Add 2.5 µl of the product from the first-round PCR plate to each well of both α and β plates containing their respective master mix (*see* **Note 5**).

8. Seal the plates thoroughly with adhesive plate seals, ensuring the edges are sealed tightly, and centrifuge the plates briefly to settle the contents to the bottom of wells.

9. Perform PCR in a thermocycler as described above (**step 4**). The plates can be stored at 4 °C (short term) or –20 °C (long term) until analysis of the samples by agarose gel electrophoresis.

3.5 Agarose Gel Electrophoresis

1. Cast a 2 % agarose gel in 1× TAE buffer using the tray and combs described in Subheading 2.2.

2. Using an 8-channel micropipette (0.5–10 µl), load the gel wells with 5 µl of PCR products. The CoralLoad buffer contains gel-loading dye, thus allowing direct loading of the PCR reactions into the wells of the agarose gel.

3. Perform electrophoresis at 175 V for 40 min to separate the PCR products.

4. At the end of the electrophoresis, visualize and record the image of the agarose gel using a Bio-Rad or similar gel documentation system.

5. Count the number of bands and verify the negative controls (*see* **Note 6**).

3.6 Sequencing

Following a successful PCR reaction, the PCR products can be purified and sequenced by standard procedures. For example, the PCR products can be purified using a silica-based column purification system (Wizard SV96 PCR purification kit, Promega) as described [11, 12]. Recently, we have adopted an Exonuclease I and Shrimp

Alkaline Phosphatase (SAP) based enzymatic purification method as a low cost option, which is described below.

1. Prepare a master mix for the purification of the PCR products as follows.

	Per reaction (µl)	1 plate (100 reactions) (µl)
Shrimp alkaline phosphatase (SAP, USB)	0.2	20
Exonuclease I (ExoI) (USB)	0.2	20
Tris–HCl, 50 mM, pH 8	4.6	460
Total	5	500

2. Distribute 5 µl of the Exo/SAP master mix to a 96-well PCR plate.

3. Using a multichannel pipette (0.5–10 µl), add 1 µl of the PCR product from the second-round PCR plate.

4. Seal the plate with adhesive plate seal, centrifuge, and incubate at 37 °C for 15 min followed by 80 °C for 15 min.

5. Chill the plate on ice. Prepare the primer master mix for the sequencing reaction as described in the following table.

Primer mix	Per reaction (µl)	Per plate (100 reactions) (µl)
TRAC INT REV (20 µM) OR TRBC INT REV (20 µM)	0.25	25
Water, Nuclease free	5.75	575
Total	6	600

6. Remove the plate seal carefully and add 6 µl of appropriate primer mix to the α and β plates (*see* **Note** 7).

7. The purified PCR product and primer mix is then sequenced using Big Dye® Terminator (v3.1) Chemistry on a 3730XL DNA Analyzers (Applied Biosystems). Sequence data are confirmed by inspection of chromatograms using a trace viewer such as Chromas (Technelysium).

3.7 Sequence Data Analysis

We analyze the sequence data using a custom-made Microsoft Excel analysis spreadsheet that utilizes macros obtained from http://www.bioc.uzh.ch/antibody and ref. 14 and a TCR web application https://tcr.stjude.org/tcr/ [11] that queries the international ImMunoGeneTics information system (IMGT) database [15].

The output returns the CDR3α and CDR3β nucleotide and amino acid sequence information and their frequencies, paired expression profile, TRAV, TRAJ, TRBV, TRBJ, and TRBD usage data in the same Excel spreadsheet, thus allowing further downstream calculations and statistics. The Excel spreadsheet consists of three worksheets for CDR3α and three worksheets for CDR3β analysis. The data are summarized in the data summary worksheet. The next two worksheets integrate the TRAV, TRAJ, TRBV, TRBJ, and TRBD assignments derived from the TCR web application, https://tcr.stjude.org/tcr/. The next two worksheets consist of pivot tables that summarize the pairing data for CDR3, TRAV-TRAJ and TRBV-TRBJ. A template for the customized, macro-enabled Excel analysis spreadsheet is available from the authors upon request.

1. Download the sequence data in .ab1 and .seq format.

2. Using MegAlign software (DNASTAR Lasergene), import the .ab1 files.

3. Copy the alignment report and paste into Cell A1 of the "DNA seqs-Valpha" worksheet of the Excel spreadsheet.

4. Select Cells B5–B85 and run the reverse complement macro ("revcomp.revcomp"). Over the next seven columns (C–H), the nucleotide sequences (64 nt) are then pruned to extract the CDR3 region (V end-CDR3-J-C beginning) and summarized in Columns K, L, and M of the worksheet.

5. In the "Parsed-Valpha" worksheet, the extracted nucleotide sequences are converted into amino acid sequences. Select Cells A4–A83 and run the "AA_Parse_3Letter" macro. The 64 nucleotides of the CDR3 region are then parsed into three letter blocks in Columns B4–V4.

6. Select Cells B4–V83 and run the "AA_Convert_NtoAA" macro to derive the amino acid sequences.

7. In the "AA seqs-Valpha" worksheet, the amino acid sequence data of the CDR3 region are further processed to extract the exact CDR3 sequences, and their frequencies are calculated.

8. The exact same steps are followed for the analysis of the TCRβ sequences to extract CDR3β data in the next three worksheets.

9. The data are then summarized to derive paired CDR3αβ expression in the "Data Summary" worksheet.

10. To assign the TRAV-TRAJ and TRBV-TRBD-TRBJ nomenclature, a compressed file of the .seq files is uploaded to the https://tcr.stjude.org/tcr/ web application written in PHP 5 and MySQL 5 [11]. This interface allows users to upload individual FASTA files or zipped archives of multiple FASTA files and queries them against the IMGT online database using PHP cUrl. The resulting output containing receptor family names,

an amino acid translation of the receptor, and nucleotide sequence of the translation can be downloaded in .csv format.

11. The TRAV-TRAJ and TRBV-TRBD-TRBJ data can then be copied into the analyzed Excel spreadsheet (in the "Data Summary" worksheet) and are then summarized in subsequent worksheets.

4   Notes

1. IMGT nomenclature of TCRα and β variable, junctional, and diversity family notation is used throughout the text.

2. Recently, we preferred diluting primers in TE buffer instead of water to increase the stability of the primers in storage. The final concentration of EDTA in the diluted primer cocktail in the PCR mix is well below the inhibitory level.

3. Single-cell sorting can be done by two methods: (a) by directly sorting into empty PCR plate so each well contains cell with approximately 1/1000th of a μl of sort buffer. (b) The PCR plates can be preloaded with 2.5 μl of reverse transcription mix before sorting single cells into each well. The former method is cost effective in comparison to the preloading method as multiple plates can be sorted and stored as backup from same sample without the need to use expensive reverse transcription reagents. However, the latter method of preloading the PCR plate with reverse transcription mix gives approximately 5 % more bands in single-cell PCR. If the preloading method is used, there is no need of using RNAsin in sort buffer prior to sorting as the Reverse transcription kit usually contains RNAse inhibitor as a component.

4. Because of the small volume used per well for RT and PCR, an additional 22 or 12 reactions, respectively, are taken to account for pipetting error and evaporation.

5. To avoid contamination, the master mix should be prepared in a dedicated space with dedicated pipettes for PCR. Barrier tips should be used for all pipetting. The master mix should be added to the cDNA plate away from the PCR station on a bench.

6. In a multiplex PCR, it is critical to prevent aerosol contamination. In our protocol, we have eight negative control wells (Column 12) separated by an empty column (Column 11) from the samples (Column 1–10). In the event that a band (even a weak 1) appears in the gel products from the control wells, we remake the primer stock, replace the working PCR reagents, and decontaminate the PCR workstation and pipettes with DNA Zap (Life Technologies). It also helps to prevent

contamination by separating the PCR setup area (RT and PCR) from the post-PCR processing (gel electrophoresis and sequencing reactions) and routinely cleaning all work and storage areas with DNA Zap.

7. The sequencing reaction will have a red tinge from the CoralLoad PCR buffer of the nested PCR reaction. This should not be a problem for sequencing, as the dye will be removed following post-sequencing reaction cleanup.

Acknowledgments

This work was supported by NIH—National Institute of Allergy and Infectious Diseases grants AI077714 and AI107625, the American Syrian Lebanese Associated Charities, NIH—National Institute on Aging grant AG033113, Atlantic Philanthropies, American Geriatrics Society, the John A. Hartford Foundation, and the Association of Subspecialty Professors.

References

1. Jorgensen JL, Esser U, de St F, Groth B, Reay PA, Davis MM (1992) Mapping T-cell receptor-peptide contacts by variant peptide immunization of single-chain transgenics. Nature 355:224–230

2. Davis MM, Bjorkman PJ (1988) T-cell antigen receptor genes and T-cell recognition. Nature 334:395–402

3. Blackwell TK, Alt FW (1989) Molecular characterization of the lymphoid V(D)J recombination activity. J Biol Chem 264:10327–10330

4. Valmori D, Dutoit V, Lienard D, Lejeune F, Speiser D, Rimoldi D, Cerundolo V, Dietrich PY, Cerottini JC, Romero P (2000) Tetramer-guided analysis of TCR beta-chain usage reveals a large repertoire of melan-A-specific CD8+ T cells in melanoma patients. J Immunol 165:533–538

5. Pannetier C, Even J, Kourilsky P (1995) T-cell repertoire diversity and clonal expansions in normal and clinical samples. Immunol Today 16:176–181

6. Trautmann L, Rimbert M, Echasserieau K, Saulquin X, Neveu B, Dechanet J, Cerundolo V, Bonneville M (2005) Selection of T cell clones expressing high-affinity public TCRs within Human cytomegalovirus-specific CD8 T cell responses. J Immunol 175:6123–6132

7. Argaet VP, Schmidt CW, Burrows SR, Silins SL, Kurilla MG, Doolan DL, Suhrbier A, Moss DJ, Kieff E, Sculley TB, Misko IS (1994) Dominant selection of an invariant T cell antigen receptor in response to persistent infection by Epstein-Barr virus. J Exp Med 180:2335–2340

8. Price DA, Brenchley JM, Ruff LE, Betts MR, Hill BJ, Roederer M, Koup RA, Migueles SA, Gostick E, Wooldridge L, Sewell AK, Connors M, Douek DC (2005) Avidity for antigen shapes clonal dominance in CD8+ T cell populations specific for persistent DNA viruses. J Exp Med 202:1349–1361

9. Wang C, Sanders CM, Yang Q, Schroeder HW Jr, Wang E, Babrzadeh F, Gharizadeh B, Myers RM, Hudson JR Jr, Davis RW, Han J (2010) High throughput sequencing reveals a complex pattern of dynamic interrelationships among human T cell subsets. Proc Natl Acad Sci U S A 107:1518–1523

10. Sherwood AM, Desmarais C, Livingston RJ, Andriesen J, Haussler M, Carlson CS, Robins H (2011) Deep sequencing of the human TCRγ and TCRβ repertoires suggests that TCRβ rearranges after αβ and γδ T Cell commitment. Sci Transl Med 3:90ra61

11. Dash P, McClaren JL, Oguin TH III, Rothwell W, Todd B, Morris MY, Becksfort J, Reynolds C, Brown SA, Doherty PC, Thomas PG (2011) Paired analysis of TCRα and TCRβ chains at the single-cell level in mice. J Clin Invest 121:288–295

12. Wang GC, Dash P, McCullers JA, Doherty PC, Thomas PG (2012) T cell receptor αβ diversity inversely correlates with pathogen-specific antibody levels in human cytomegalovirus infection. Sci Transl Med 4:128ra42

13. Sun X, Saito M, Sato Y, Chikata T, Naruto T, Ozawa T, Kobayashi E, Kishi H, Muraguchi A, Takiguchi M (2012) Unbiased analysis of TCRα/β chains at the single-cell level in human CD8+ T-cell subsets. PLoS One 7:e40386

14. Ewert S, Huber T, Honegger A, Pluckthun A (2003) Biophysical properties of human antibody variable domains. J Mol Biol 325: 531–553

15. Lefranc MP, Giudicelli V, Ginestoux C, Jabado-Michaloud J, Folch G, Bellahcene F, Wu Y, Gemrot E, Brochet X, Lane J, Regnier L, Ehrenmann F, Lefranc G, Duroux P (2009) IMGT, the international ImMunoGeneTics information system. Nucleic Acids Res 37:D1006–D1012

Chapter 16

Assessment of B Cell Repertoire in Humans

Yu-Chang Wu, David Kipling, and Deborah Dunn-Walters

Abstract

The B cell receptor (BCR) repertoire is highly diverse. Repertoire diversity is achieved centrally by somatic recombination of immunoglobulin (Ig) genes and peripherally by somatic hypermutation and Ig heavy chain class-switching. Throughout these processes, there is selection for functional gene rearrangements, selection against gene combinations resulting in self-reactive BCRs, and selection for BCRs with high affinity for exogenous antigens after challenge. Hence, investigation of BCR repertoires from different groups of B cells can provide information on stages of B cell development and shed light on the etiology of B cell pathologies. In most instances, the third complementarity determining region of the Ig heavy chain (CDR-H3) contributes the majority of amino acids to the antibody/antigen binding interface. Although CDR-H3 spectratype analysis provides information on the overall diversity of BCR repertoires, this fairly simple technique analyzes the relative quantities of CDR-H3 regions of each size, within a range of approximately 10–80 bp, without sequence detail and thus is limited in scope. High-throughput sequencing (HTS) techniques on the Roche 454 GS FLX Titanium system, however, can generate a wide coverage of Ig sequences to provide more qualitative data such as V, D, and J usage as well as detailed CDR3 sequence information. Here we present protocols in detail for CDR-H3 spectratype analysis and HTS of human BCR repertoires.

Key words B cell, B cell receptor, Immunoglobulin, Antibody, Repertoire, High-throughput sequencing, Next generation sequencing, Spectratyping

1 Introduction

There are a number of processes that contribute to B cell diversity. B cell receptors (BCR), or immunoglobulins (Ig), are comprised of heavy and light chain proteins encoded by genes that undergo rearrangement during B cell development in the bone marrow. Rearrangement of Ig heavy chain genes (*IGH*), in which *variable* (*IGHV*), *diversity* (*IGHD*), and *joining* (*IGHJ*) genes are randomly selected and joined together occurs first [1]. During the process of somatic recombination in the *IGH*, further BCR diversity is introduced by imprecise insertion and deletion of nucleotides at the junctions of the rearranged genes, resulting in

Albert C. Shaw (ed.), *Immunosenescence: Methods and Protocols*, Methods in Molecular Biology, vol. 1343, DOI 10.1007/978-1-4939-2963-4_16, © Springer Science+Business Media New York 2015

the third complementarity determining (CDR-H3) region. The CDR-H3 serves as a genetic fingerprint for an individual B cell clone throughout its development. There is further random assortment of pairing between the *IGH* and the light chain genes. Light chain proteins consist of either kappa or lambda isotypes; kappa (*IGK*) or lambda (*IGL*) genes are formed as a result of rearrangement of variable and joining region genes (either *IGKV* to *IGKJ* or *IGLV* to *IGLJ*).

The diverse repertoire created by these mechanisms can then be shaped by events external to the cell. Negative selection to remove cells with self-reactive BCRs occurs, and positive selection to expand cells reactive to exogenous pathogen challenge also occurs. Upon activation by exogenous antigens in the periphery, the B cell repertoire is further diversified by processes of somatic hypermutation (SHM), heavy chain class switch recombination (CSR), and affinity maturation of the rearranged Ig genes. Due to the constant selection pressures on the B cell repertoire, the quality and diversity of *IGH*, *IGK*, and *IGL* repertoires may reflect B cell development [2–4], the history of antigen challenge [5, 6], the ageing process [7, 8], and many pathological conditions [9, 10].

The complexity and diversity of the BCR repertoire has previously made it difficult to analyze in great detail. Initially, a polymerase chain reaction (PCR)-based method that amplifies the Ig gene fragment across the CDR-H3 region, termed CDR-H3 spectratype analysis, made it possible to examine global changes of BCR repertoires with ageing [9] and in response to vaccination [6]. CDR-H3 spectratyping has also been a useful tool to detect expansion of a particular clone such as might be seen in lymphomas. However, spectratyping is limited to the measurement of CDR-H3 size and cannot provide additional information on BCR repertoires, e.g., the usage of different Ig genes, the extent of hypermutation, and the exact sequence of CDR-H3. Although the traditional Sanger sequencing technique can overcome the limitations of CDR-H3 spectratyping with respect to providing detailed sequence information, it does not have the advantage that spectratyping has, of being able to easily evaluate sufficient numbers of Ig sequences with coverage that could reflect the diversity of the BCR repertoire in humans. With advances in next generation sequencing (NGS) technologies, several platforms have been developed that yield large numbers of reads that Sanger sequencing techniques cannot deliver [11]. Currently, there are two main competitors in NGS technologies: Illumina and Roche 454 platforms. As compared with the Illumina MiSeq platform with a capacity of 15×10^6 reads per run and a maximum read length of 250 bp, the upgraded Roche 454 GS FLX+ system is able to produce long-read sequences up to 1000 bp—albeit with a smaller coverage of 1×10^6 reads per run. Since the length of an Ig gene from the beginning of the Ig gene, through the CDR-H3 region, to the constant region is 400–500 bp, this longer read length makes the 454 GS FLX+ system ideal for high-throughput sequencing (HTS) of human Ig genes. By incorporating Multiplex Identifier (MID)-containing adaptors into 454 NGS technology, several BCR repertoire libraries can be multiplexed in order to reduce cost [12].

We have previously used CDR-H3 spectratype analysis in conjunction with HTS techniques on the 454 GS FLX Titanium system to demonstrate temporal and age-related changes in human peripheral blood *IGH* repertoires in response to vaccination [6, 7]. We have also shown that *IGH* repertoires in different B cell subsets can be distinguished from one another by HTS techniques [13, 14]. Here we describe detailed protocols for CDR-H3 spectratyping on the ABI 3730*xl* DNA Analyzer system and HTS from *IGH* and *IGK* or *IGL* repertoires on the 454 GS FLX Titanium system using human cDNA.

2   Materials

Analyses of gene families by methods that use PCR are particularly at risk for cross contamination, especially for low abundance targets such as in single cell analyses. UV isolation cabinets should be used and different steps in the protocol should be carried out in different areas of the lab, or in different rooms, wherever possible. A DNA/RNA-free UV isolation hood with dedicated pipettes should be reserved for preparation of Sort-Lysis Reverse Transcription (SLyRT) buffers and PCR mixes. Areas where PCR products are analyzed by electrophoresis should be as far away from sample preparation areas as possible. PCR-grade water should be used throughout for all sample preparation.

2.1 Components for Direct cDNA Synthesis from Cells

Sort-Lysis Reverse Transcription (SLyRT) buffer and SuperScript III Reverse Transcription (RT) enzyme allow direct cDNA synthesis from cells. The buffer lyses the cells, stabilizes the mRNA, and bypasses mRNA purification steps, allowing synthesis of cDNA from low cell numbers or single cells. This does, however, mean that contaminants such as protein and genomic DNA are present along with cDNA (*see* **Note 1**).

1. Polymerase chain reaction (PCR)-grade H_2O.

2. Detergents Triton X-100: 5 % in PCR-grade H_2O (*see* **Note 2**).

3. dNTP mix: 20 mM each of dATP, dTTP, dCTP, dGTP in PCR-grade H_2O (*see* **Note 3**).

4. Random hexamers pd(N)$_6$: diluted to 50 ng/μl in PCR-grade H_2O (Qiagen, UK).

5. RiboSafe RNase inhibitor: 40 U/μl (Bioline, UK).

6. 0.1 M dithiothreitol (DTT).

7. 5× First-Strand RT buffer: 250 mM Tris–HCl (pH 8.3 at RT), 375 mM KCl, 15 mM MgCl₂ (supplied with SuperScript III RT enzyme; Invitrogen, UK).

8. 25 U/μl SuperScript III RT enzyme (Invitrogen, UK): diluted from 200 U/μl with PCR-grade H₂O.

9. 200 μl PCR tubes.

10. PCR thermal cycler.

2.2 Components for Polymerase Chain Reaction

PCR components listed below are used to generate products for CDR-H3 spectratyping and HTS, using appropriate primers as indicated in different sections.

1. PCR-grade H₂O.

2. dNTP mix: 20 mM each of dATP, dTTP, dCTP, dGTP in PCR-grade H₂O.

3. Phusion High-Fidelity polymerase (NEB, UK) diluted in PCR-grade water.

4. 5× GC buffer (supplied with Phusion High-Fidelity polymerase; NEB, UK).

5. Complete primer mix: choose accordingly as indicated [6, 15].

6. cDNA (*see* Subheading 3.1).

7. 96-well PCR plates.

8. PCR thermal cyclers.

9. Thermal seals.

2.3 Components for HTS of Human Immuno globulin Genes

1. Multiplex Identifier (MID)-tagged amplicons of human immunoglobulin genes (*see* Subheading 3.3).

2. Agarose gels: Dissolve 1.5 g of agarose powder in 100 ml of 1× TAE buffer in a microwave. Once the agarose solution is cooled to 55 °C, add 10 μl of 10,000× GelStar Nucleic Acid Gel Stain (final concentration = 1×; Lonza, UK) or 1 μl of 10 mg/ml ethidium bromide (EtBr; final concentration = 0.1 μg/ml), as indicated.

3. 1X Tris-Acetate-EDTA (TAE) running buffer: 40 mM Tris-acetate and 1 mM EDTA at pH 8.3 in distilled water (*see* **Note 4**).

4. Hyper Ladder IV Ladder (Bioline, UK).

5. Horizontal electrophoresis system (e.g., multiSUB-4 (Wolflabs, UK)).

6. 6× Orange G loading dye: 10 mM Tris–HCl (pH 7.6), 0.15 % orange G, 60 % glycerol, 60 mM EDTA in distilled water (*see* **Note 5**).

7. 15 ml Falcon tubes.

8. Disposable scalpels.

9. DarkReader 46B Transilluminator instrument (LabTech, UK).

10. QIAquick gel purification kit (Qiagen, UK).

11. Qubit 2.0 Fluorometer and Qubit dsDNA HS Assay Kits (Invitrogen, UK).

12. QIAquick PCR purification kit (Qiagen, UK).

2.4 Components for Spectratype Analysis of Human Immunoglobulin CDR-H3

1. PCR products of human immunoglobulin genes (*see* Subheading 3.2).

2. Highly deionized (Hi-Di) formamide (AppliedBiosystems, UK).

3. GeneScan 350 TAMRA Size Standard (AppliedBiosystems, UK).

4. Non-skirted, 96-well PCR plate.

5. Applied Biosystems 3730*xl* DNA Analyzer system (AppliedBiosystems, UK).

6. GeneMapper software (AppliedBiosystems, UK).

3 Methods

3.1 Direct cDNA Synthesis from Cells

1. Assemble the components of SLyRT buffer as listed in Table 1. Keep SLyRT buffer on ice for immediate use or store at −20 °C.

2. Aliquot 36 μl of the SLyRT buffer into PCR tubes.

3. Deposit 1000–10,000 B cells from the flow cytometry sorter directly into PCR tubes containing 36 μl of SLyRT buffer.

Table 1
SLyRT buffer

Reagents	Initial concentration	1 reaction volumes (μl)	50 reaction volumes (μl)	Final reaction concentration[a]
First-Strand RT buffer	5×	8	400	1×
pd(N)$_6$	50 ng/μl	12	600	15 ng/μl
Triton X	5 %	1	50	0.13 % (v/v)
RiboSafe RNase inhibitor	40 U/μl	2.5	125	2.5 U/μl
DTT	0.1 M	4.5	225	11.25 mM
dNTP mix	10 mM each	2	100	500 μM
PCR-graded H$_2$O	NA	6	300	NA

[a]The final reaction concentration indicates the concentration in a total reaction volume of 40 μl after cDNA, Superscript III RT enzyme, and primers are added

Table 2
Reverse transcriptase reaction conditions

Steps	Temperatures (°C)	Time (min)
Denaturation	42	10
Annealing	25	10
RT (extension)	55	60
RT termination	72	15

4. Invert PCR tubes several times to ensure all cells are immersed in SLyRT buffer. Briefly centrifuge the PCR tubes at 3000 rpm in a microfuge for 2 min.

5. Add 4 μl of SuperScript III RT enzyme at 25 U/μl, final reaction concentration 2.5 U/μl.

6. Carry out the RT reaction on the thermal cycler, programmed as in Table 2.

7. Once the RT reaction is complete, centrifuge the PCR tubes at 13,000 rpm in a microfuge for 5 min. Immediately transfer 35 μl of the reaction mix to a clean PCR tube without disturbing any cell debris at the bottom of the tube. This step reduces cellular contaminants from being carried forward to downstream applications.

8. Add 70 μl of PCR-grade H_2O to 35 μl of the reaction mix and pipette several times to mix (*see* **Note 1**).

9. Store samples at –20 °C.

3.2 Spectratype Analysis of Human Immunoglobulin CDR-H3 Regions

Spectratype analysis allows investigation of BCR repertoires by measuring relative quantities of different sizes of CDR-H3 regions. It is relatively cheap and quick compared to HTS techniques. If HTS is employed the information will be in the sequencing data and spectratyping will not be necessary. This section includes generation of PCR products, which span across human immunoglobulin CDR-H3 regions and into the 5′-end of the constant region (Fig. 1), and preparation of samples prior to fragment size analysis on the Applied Biosystems 3730*xl* DNA Analyzer system.

1. Assemble reagents for PCR master mix and vortex to mix thoroughly. Change the 3′-end primer for different isotypes of the heavy chains. The concentration for each reagent is shown in Table 3.

2. Aliquot the PCR master mix to a 96-well plate, 23 μl per well.

3. Add cDNA to the 96-well PCR1 plate, 2 μl per well (*see* **Note 7**; *see* Subheading 3.1).

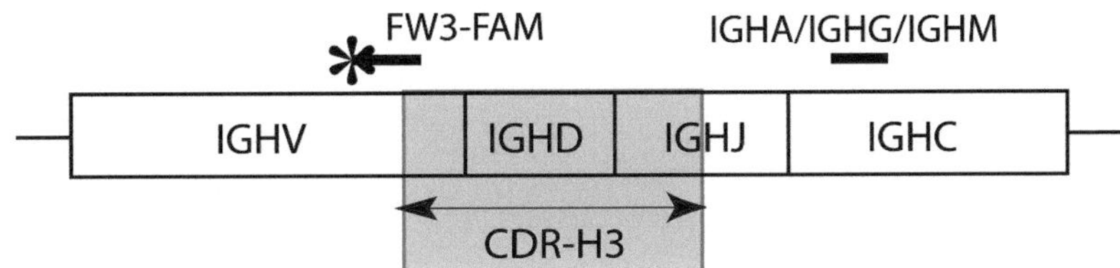

Fig. 1 Schematic presentation of immunoglobulin gene cDNA showing the primer binding sites for CDR-H3 spectratyping

Table 3
Spectratype PCR reaction mix (25 μl per reaction)

Reagents	Initial concentration	1 reaction volumes (μl)	110 reaction volumes (μl)	Final reaction concentration[a]
GC buffer	5×	5	550	1×
1:20 Phusion polymerase	0.25 U/μl	2	220	0.02 U/μl
dNTP mix	20 mM each	0.5	55	400 μM each
5′-end FW3-FAM primer[b]	10 μM	1	110	400 nM
3′-end constant primer[b]	10 μM	1	110	400 nM
PCR-grade H$_2$O	NA	13.5	1485	NA

[a]The final reaction concentration indicates the concentration after cDNA is added
[b]*See* **Note 6**

Table 4
PCR thermal cycling conditions

Steps		Temperature (°C)	Time (s)
Initial denaturation		95	60
15 cycles	Denaturation	95	45
	Annealing	61 (IgA); 55 (IgG and IgM)	45
	Extension	72	45
Final extension		72	600

4. Seal PCR plates with thermal seals and carry out PCR reaction on the thermal cycler programmed as Table 4.

5. Briefly centrifuge the PCR plate to collect the content.

6. In a non-skirted PCR plate, add 3 μl of the PCR products to 1.5 μl GeneScan 350 TAMRA Size Standard and 13.5 μl Hi-Di formamide per well. Pipette up and down a couple of times to mix thoroughly (*see* **Note 8**).

7. Centrifuge the PCR plate to collect the content and ensure no air bubbles are present.

8. Place the plate on the *3730xl* DNA Analyzer system for spectratyping (*see* **Note 9**).

9. Collect and analyze the data on the GeneMapper software according to the manufacturer's instructions (*see* **Note 10**).

3.3 HTS of Human Immuno globulin Genes

HTS allows analysis of BCR repertoires in detail, including the distribution of CDR-H3 sizes. This section includes production of immunoglobulin gene amplicons, gel purification of amplicons, assembly of multiple amplicons (up to 12 MID barcodes per sequencing sample), and enrichment of pooled amplicons. Sequencing on the 454 GS FLX Titanium instrument is performed by LGC Genomics, where each sequencing sample (containing 12 MIDS) is run on 1/16th of a chip. Take care to avoid cross contamination between samples. Each research (cDNA) sample that is required to be distinguishable from other research samples needs to be amplified with its own MID tag. Within that MID tag it is possible to combine three different isotypes of heavy chains, and kappa and lambda light chains for that particular research sample, since these can be distinguished later by their sequence (*see* **Note 11**).

1. To generate MID-tagged amplicons, perform semi-nested PCR reactions (Fig. 2).

2. Assemble reagents for PCR1 master mix (Table 5), and vortex to mix thoroughly. Change primer mix accordingly to produce different types of amplicons (different heavy chain classes or kappa light chain or lambda light chains).

3. Aliquot the PCR1 master mix into a 96-well PCR1 plate, 22 µl per well.

4. Add 1:3 diluted cDNA (*see* Subheading 3.1) to the 96-well PCR1 plate, 3 µl per well. Use one PCR plate for each type of amplicon (i.e., either IgA, IgG, IgM, IgK, or IgL) and perform eight PCR1 reactions for each sample.

5. Seal PCR plates with thermal seals and carry out PCR1 reaction on the thermal cycler programmed as in Table 6.

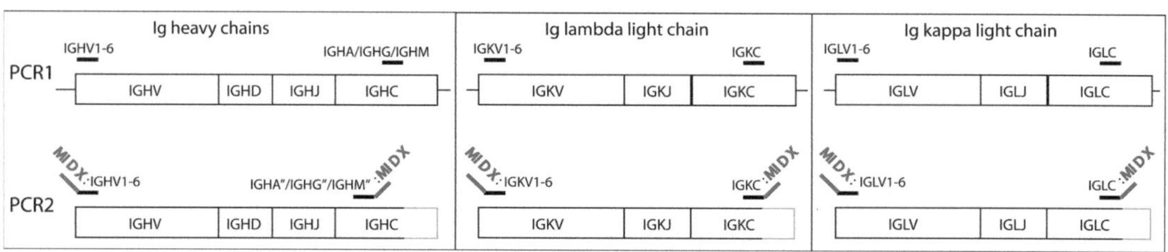

Fig. 2 Schematic representation of immunoglobulin gene cDNA and primer binding sites for HTS, semi-nested PCR

Table 5
HTS PCR1 reaction mix (25 μl per reaction)

Reagents	Initial concentration	1 reaction volume (μl)	110 reaction volumes (μl)	Final reaction concentration[a]
GC buffer	5×	5	550	1×
1:40 Phusion polymerase	0.125 U/μl	5	550	0.025 U/μl
dNTP mix	20 mM each	0.25	27.5	200 μM each
Primer mix[b]		1.25	125	
5′-end variable primers	835 nM each			41.75 nM each
3′-end constant primer	5 μM			250 nM
PCR-grade H$_2$O	NA	10.5	1155	NA

[a]The final reaction concentration indicates the concentration after cDNA and primers are added
[b]*See* **Note 12**

Table 6
PCR1 thermal cycling conditions

Steps		Temperature (°C)	Time (s)
Initial denaturation		98	30
15 cycles	Denaturation	98	10
	Annealing	58	15
	Extension	72	30
Final extension		72	600

6. Briefly centrifuge plates to collect the contents and store the plate at –20 °C.

7. Assemble reagents for PCR2 master mix (110 reactions), and vortex to mix thoroughly. Concentrations for each reagent are shown in Table 7.

    (a) Aliquot the PCR2 master mix to 96-well PCR plates, 17 μl per well.

    (b) Add MID-containing primer mix (*see* **Note 13**) to the 96-well PCR2 plate, 1 μl per well.

    (c) Add 2 μl per well of PCR1 products accordingly to the 96-well PCR plate. For each PCR1 product, perform duplicate of PCR2 reactions. This results in 16 wells of final PCR product per amplicon type and research sample to be purified for sequencing. This, together with the short PCR amplification reactions, is designed such that larger

Table 7
HTS PCR2 reaction mix (20 µl per reaction)

Reagents	Initial concentration	1 reaction volume (µl)	110 reaction volumes (µl)	Final reaction concentration[a]
GC buffer	5×	4	440	1×
1:20 Phusion polymerase	0.25 U/µl	2	220	0.025 U/µl
dNTP mix	20 mM each	0.2	22	200 µM each
PCR-grade H₂O	NA	10.8	1188	NA

[a]The final reaction concentration indicates the concentration after sample and primers are added

Table 8
PCR2 thermal cycling conditions

Steps		Temperature (°C)	Time (s)
Initial denaturation		98	30
20 cycles	Denaturation	98	10
	Annealing	58	15
	Extension	72	30
Final extension		72	600

amounts of product for sequencing can be obtained while at the same time maximizing the representation of in vivo diversity over in vitro PCR amplification processes.

(d) Seal PCR plates with thermal seals and carry out the PCR2 reaction on the thermal cycler programmed as in Table 8.

(e) Briefly centrifuge plates to collect the contents and store the plate until required at –20 °C.

8. Combine all 16 wells of PCR2 products (20 µl per well; 320 µl in total) into one 15 ml Falcon tube. Each 15 ml Falcon tube therefore contains 320 µl of PCR2 products in total per amplicon type (having the same MID and type of Ig gene amplified from the same research sample).

9. Add 64 µl of 6× orange G loading dye per tube to the combined PCR2 products.

10. Preheat samples at 98 °C on a heat block for 5–10 min.

11. Place 1.5 % agarose/TAE gels containing 1× GelStar Nucleic Acid Gel Stain in the horizontal electrophoresis apparatus filled with 1× TAE buffer.

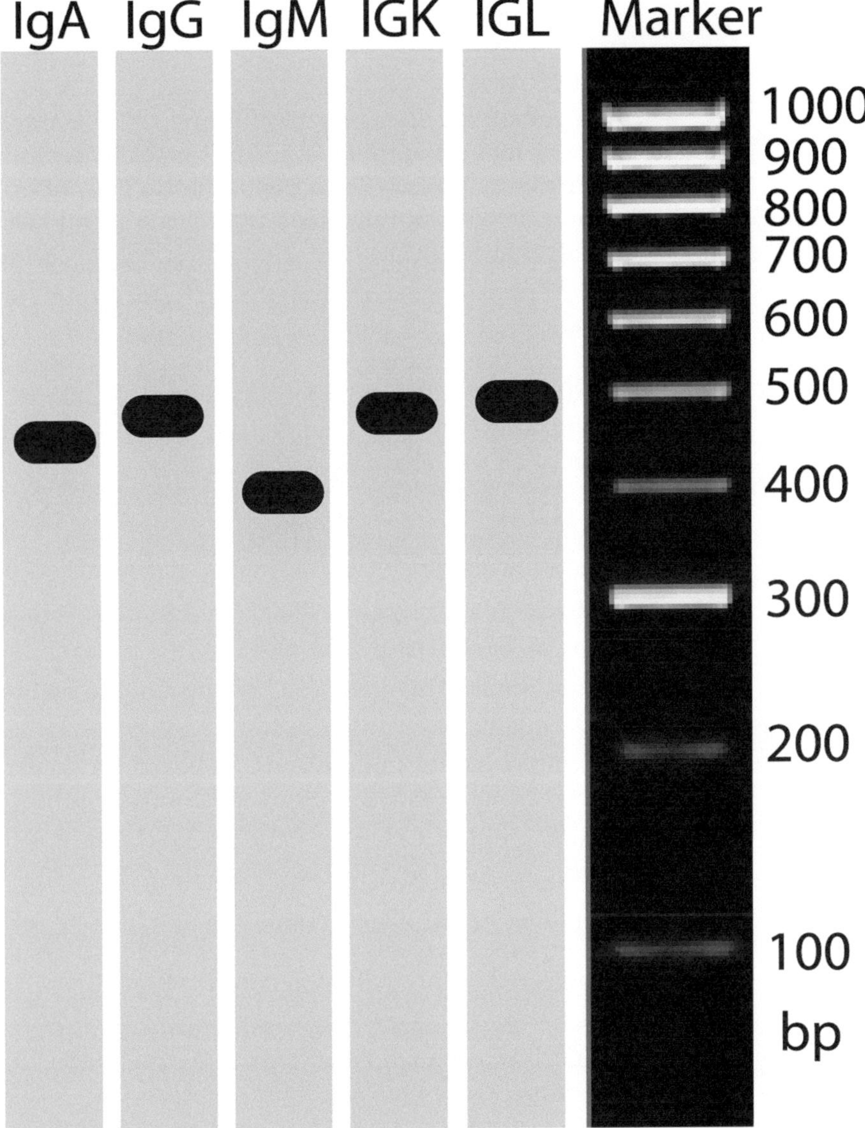

Fig. 3 Diagram to illustrate the PCR amplicon sizes of different *IGH* isotypes, *IGL* and *IGK,* in relation to the Hyperladder IV DNA size marker, on a 1.5 % TAE agarose gel

12. Load the preheated samples on the gel and use 5 μl of Hyper Ladder IV Ladder. Separate DNA fragments by electrophoresis at 100 V for 60 min.

13. Visualize DNA fragments using the DarkReader 46B Transilluminator instrument.

14. Excise fragments of the right size (Fig. 3), using sterile scalpels and transfer gel slices into 15 ml Falcon tubes.

15. Extract DNA using the QIAquick gel purification kit, according to the manufacturer's instructions, except for the following changes:

    (a) Incubate gel slices in 5 ml of Buffer QG per amplicon type in 15 ml Falcon tubes at 55 °C. Vortex frequently until gel slices are melted. Expect approximately 6 ml of the solutions in total per amplicon type in the 15 ml Falcon tube.

    (b) Use one QIAquick spin column per amplicon type: apply 750 μl of the solution to the QIAquick spin column and centrifuge at 13,000 rpm in a microfuge for 30 s. Collect, rather than discard, the flow-through in a separate 15 ml Falcon tube. Repeat this process until all mixture has been applied to the same column, spun and recollected in a separate 15 ml Falcon tube.

    (c) Apply the flow-through (750 μl at a time) back to the same spin column, spin at 13,000 rpm, and discard the second flow-through.

    (d) Wash the spin column with 750 μl Buffer PE by centrifuging at 13,000 rpm for 1 min.

    (e) Add 55 μl PCR-grade H_2O to the column membrane and leave at RT for 3 min.

    (f) Centrifuge the column at 13,000 rpm for 1 min and collect the elution in 1.5 ml microcentrifuge tube.

    (g) Add additional 55 μl of PCR-grade water to the same column membrane and leave at RT for 3 min.

    (h) Spin to collect the elution in the same 1.5 ml microcentrifuge tube. In total, approximately 100 μl of elution will be collected in one 1.5 ml microcentrifuge tube.

16. Measure the concentration and quality of the gel-purified products for each amplicon type using the Qubit dsDNA HS Assay Kits on the Qubit 2.0 Fluorometer.

17. Assemble the multiple amplicons into one sequencing sample.

    When 12 MID barcodes are used, transfer 900 ng of products per MID to a clean 1.5 ml microcentrifuge tube, i.e., a total of 10,800 ng are pooled from 12 MID types (*see* **Note 14**). If amplicons of multiple isotypes of heavy chain and light chains are allocated to the same MID barcode, divide 900 ng equally. Examples for the amount (in ng) of gel-purified products for pooling multiple amplicon types are listed in Table 9.

18. Enrich pooled products using the QIAquick PCR purification kit, according to the manufacturer's instructions. This step is carried out in a similar way as **step 9**, except Buffer PBI is used to mix with the pooled gel-purified solutions. Elute products in two lots of 55 μl PCR-grade water as **step 9**.

Table 9
Assembly of sequencing samples

	IgA	IgG	IgM	IgK	IgL	Total (ng/MID)
MID 1	900	NA	NA	NA	NA	900
MID 2	300	300	300	NA	NA	900
MID 3	NA	NA	NA	450	450	900
MID 4	180	180	180	180	180	900
MID 5	NA	450	NA	NA	450	900
MID 6	225	225	225	NA	225	900
MID 7	180	180	180	180	180	900
MID 8	180	180	180	180	180	900
MID 9	180	180	180	180	180	900
MID 10	180	180	180	180	180	900
MID 11	180	180	180	180	180	900
MID 12	180	180	180	180	180	900
Total = 10,800 ng per 1/16th microtitre chip						

19. Measure the concentration and quantity of the pooled mixture as **step 10**. The pooled mixture for the final sequencing sample needs to be a total of at least 5 μg at a concentration of 100 ng/μl.

20. Analyze 100 ng of the final sequencing sample on 1.5 % agarose/TAE/EtBr gel to check that all primers have been removed before HTS is carried out. Samples are sent for sequencing according to the instructions from the contractor (LGC Genomics).

21. Sequence data are output as the .FASTA format and the raw FASTA files are analyzed in a three-stage approach [6, 15].

    (a) First, individual potential IGH sequences are subjected to a series of quality control (QC) assessments with the aim of identifying sequences that are implausible from a biological perspective (e.g., an interval between the two Ig primers that is too short based on known Ig gene sequences, or an arrangement or spacing of internal Ig motifs that is incompatible with known Ig gene sequences), contain evidence of PCR or library construction artifacts (such as internal MID sequences, or mis-matches between the start and finish MID motifs), or are too short to provide data on isotype or CDR-H3 region. Sequences that fail this initial QC step are excluded from further analysis.

(b) Sequences that pass this quality control are then edited to remove any terminal adapter and MID sequences added as part of the sequencing protocol, and each sequence is renamed so as to capture and embed sample information based on the MID tag. Sequences are then passed in bulk to HighV-QUEST [16, 17]. This is a freely available online resource (http://www.imgt.org/HighV-QUEST/index.action) that analyzes each sequence with reference to a database of human Ig sequences and returns a summary file cataloguing a range of outputs for each sequence including V, D, and J gene usage and CDR-H3 sequence and length.

(c) The V-QUEST output file is then parsed locally to further summarize the data for each sequence regarding gene usage. The amino acid sequence of the CDR-H3 junction peptide is extracted and analyzed for a range of physico-chemical properties (hydrophobicity, charge, amino acid use, and so forth) using a locally scripted version of the ProtParam tool that is available on the ExPASy server [18]. In addition, the DNA sequence of the CDR3 region is used, in combination with hierarchical clustering and tree cutting, to identify clusters ("clones") of sequences that share related CDR-H3 sequences. Further analysis highlights clones that span multiple isotypes (indicative of class switching). Finally, a single sequence from each clone is identified that represents the most common pattern of gene usage as a reference sequence for further analysis, such as regarding overall repertoire (*see* **Note 15**).

4   Notes

1. At low cell numbers this is not an issue but if high cell numbers (over 6000 cells) are used, the subsequent PCR steps may be more efficient if the cDNA sample synthesized using SLyRT buffer is diluted 1 in 3 (35+70 μl) with PCR-grade water.

2. 100 % Triton is difficult to pipette due to high viscosity so it may be helpful to cut the end of the pipette tip with a scalpel to make it wider, and pipette slowly.

3. Add 200 μl each of dATP, dTTP, dCTP, dGTP (20 mM each; Promega, UK) to 200 μl DNase/RNase-free H_2O and vortex to mix.

4. 1× TAE running buffer contained 40 mM Tris-borate and 1 mM EDTA. To make 50× TAE, 242 g Tris base, 57.1 ml glacial acetic acid (Merck, UK), and 100 ml EDTA (pH 8.0)

Table 10
Spectratyping primers

	Sequence (5′–3′)
5′-end primer	
FW3-FAM	ACACGGCTGTGTATTACTGT
In combination with	
3′-end primer	
IGHA or	GGAAGAAGCCCTGGACCAGGC
IGHG or	CACCGTCACCGGTTCGG
IGHM	CAGGAGACGAGGGGGAA

were dissolved in 1 l distilled water, and then filtered to steril-ize. 1 volume of 50× TAE was then diluted with 49 volumes of distilled water to make 1× TAE.

5. To make 6× Orange loading dye, add 0.25 g Orange G (Sigma Aldrich, UK) to 30 ml glycerol and 70 ml distilled water in a 50 ml Falcon tube and vortex to mix thoroughly.

6. Primers for spectratyping are listed in Table 10 below.

7. cDNA can be either obtained using SLyRT buffer or commercially available kits, e.g., RNeasy Mini kit (Qiagen, UK) in conjunction with First-Strand cDNA synthesis kit (Invitrogen, UK). The amount of cDNA used for PCR should be optimized.

8. If necessary, PCR products for spectratype analysis can be analyzed on 10 % polyacrylamide gels to check before running on the analyser.

9. FW3-FAM primers are light sensitive and should avoid exposure to the light. PCR products for spectratyping should not be kept in the fridge longer than 3 days before analysis, as the signals from the 3730*xl* DNA Analyzer system could be reduced.

10. The primers for the C regions in the different isotypes do not all bind at the same distance away from the joining region. Therefore a correction will need to be applied to normalize the data. To get the actual CDR-H3 size without primer sequences, subtract 70 bp (IGHM primers) or 146 bp (IGHG primers) or 126 bp (IGHA primers).

11. An example of experimental organization for HTS samples is shown in Table 11, where 12 research samples are multiplexed as one sequencing sample.

Table 11
Example of multiplex sequencing sample assembly

Patient	Tissue	Cell type	IgM	IgG	IgA	kappa	lambda	Multiplex ID
A	Blood	Transitional B cell	×	NA	NA	×	×	MID1
	Blood	Naive B cell	×	NA	NA	×	×	MID2
	Blood	Memory B cell	×	×	×	×	×	MID3
	Blood	Plasma cell	×	×	×	×	×	MID4
B	Blood	Transitional B cell	×	NA	NA	×	×	MID5
	Blood	Naive B cell	×	NA	NA	×	×	MID6
	Blood	Memory B cell	×	×	×	×	×	MID7
	Blood	Plasma cell	×	×	×	×	×	MID8
C	Blood	Transitional B cell	×	NA	NA	×	×	MID9
	Blood	Naive B cell	×	NA	NA	×	×	MID10
	Blood	Memory B cell	×	×	×	×	×	MID11
	Blood	Plasma cell	×	×	×	×	×	MID12

12. PCR1 primer mix (Table 12) contains 5′-end multiplex primers that anneal to all families of the variable regions and 3′-end primers that anneal to the constant region. 1.25 μl of the primer mix, containing 835 nM each of 5′-end primers and 5 μM 3′-end primer, is used in a final reaction volume of 25 μl, to give the final concentrations at 41.75 nM each and 250 nM, respectively.

13. PCR2 primers are comprised of gene-specific sequences and non-gene-specific, 10-base MID sequence motifs. PCR2 primer mix contains 5′-end multiplex MID-containing primers that anneal to all families of the variable regions and 3′-end MID-containing primers that anneal to the constant region. 1 μl of the MID-containing primer mix, containing 835 nM each of 5′-end primers and 5 μM 3′-end primer, is used in a final reaction volume of 20 μl, to give the final concentrations at 41.75 nM each and 250 nM, respectively. Each primer mix contains only one MID barcode for amplification from one research sample and a total of 12 different MID barcodes can be used for 12 different research samples (Table 13).

The gene-specific sequences of 5′-end primers for the heavy and light chains and 3′-end primers for the light chains are same as PCR1. The gene-specific sequences in the 3′-end primers of the heavy chains anneal for PCR2 reactions (Table 14) to the template more upstream to those used in PCR1.

For space consideration, MID1-containing primers for IgA are shown as an example (Table 15).

14. Although it only requires 5 ng (50 ng/μl) in total of the purified pooled mixture to be sequenced as one sequencing sample using a 1/16th microchip on the 454 GS FLX Titanium

Table 12
PCR1 primer mix

5′-end primer	Sequence (5′–3′)	3′-end primers	Sequence (5′–3′)	Amplicon type
IGHV1	CCTCAGTGAAGGTCTCCTGCAAGG	combined with IGHA	GGCTCCTGGGGGAAGAAGCC	IgA
IGHV2	TCCTGCGCTGGTGAAACCCACACA		or	
IGHV3	GGTCCCTGAGACTCTCCTGTGCA	IGHG	GCGCCTGAGTTCCACGACAC	IgG
IGHV4	TCGGAGACCCTGTCCCTCACCTGC		or	
IGHV5	CAGTCTGGAGCAGAGGTGAAA	IGHM	GGGGAATTCTCACAGGAGAC	IgM
IGHV6	CCTGTGCCATCTCCGGGGACAGTG			
IGKV1	CATCCAGWTGACCCAGTCTCC	combined with		
IGKV2	GATATTGTGATGACCCAGWCT			
IGKV3	GACRCAGTCTCCAGCCACCCTG	IGKC	CCTTCCACTGTACTTTGGCCTC	Kappa heavy chain
IGKV4	GACATCGTGATGACCCAGTCT			
IGKV5	GAAACGACACTCACGCAGTCT			
IGKV6	GAAATTGTGCTGACTCAGTCT			
IGLV1	CAGTCTGTGCTGACKCAGCC	combined with		
IGLV2	CAGTCTGCCCTGACTCAGCC			
IGLV3	CCTATGAGCTGACWCAGCCAC	IGLC	GCCACTGTCACRGCTCCCGGG	Lambda light chain
IGLV4/5	CAGCCTGTGCTGACTCARYC			
IGLV6	CCAGNCTGTGSTGACTCAG			

Table 13
PCR2 primer mix

	Sequence (5′–3′)
MID 1	acgagtgcgt
MID 2	acgctcgaca
MID 3	agacgcactc
MID 4	agcactgtag
MID 5	atcagacacg
MID 6	atatcgcgag
MID 7	cgtgtctcta
MID 8	ctcgcgtgtc
MID 9	tagtatcagc
MID 10	tctctatgcg
MID 11	tgatacgtct
MID 12	tactgagcta

Table 14
3′ Heavy chain primers

	Sequence (5′–3′)
IGHA″	GGAAGAAGCCCTGGACCAGGC
IGHG″	CACCGTCACCGGTTCGGGG
IGHM″	CAGGAGACGAGGGGGAAAAGG

Table 15
MID1-containing IgA primers

5′-end primer	Sequence (5′–3′)		3′-end primer Sequence (5′–3′)
MID1:IGHV1	acgagtgcgtCCTCAGTGAA GGTCTCCTGCAAGG	combined with	MID1:IGHA″ acgagtgcgtGGCTCCTGG GGGAAGAAGCC
MID1:IGHV2	acgagtgcgtTCCTGCGCTG GTGAAACCCACACA		
MID1:IGHV3	acgagtgcgtGGTCCCTG AGACTCTCCTGTGCA		
MID1:IGHV4	acgagtgcgtTCGGAGAC CCTGTCCCTCACCTGC		
MID1:IGHV5	acgagtgcgtCAGTCTG GAGCAGAGGTGAAA		
MID1:IGHV6	acgagtgcgtCCTGTGCCA TCTCCGGGGACAGTG		

platform, a significant amount of products can be lost during the gel purification and enrichment steps. It is therefore ideal to prepare more products than 5 ng in total before gel purification and enrichment steps and then dilute final sequencing sample to the concentration of 50 ng/µl.

15. All the analyses (other than online submission to HighV-Quest) are performed using custom scripts written in the open-source R language [19] using additional packages, notable Biostrings, from the Bioconductor project [20]. All the R/Bioconductor packages are open source and freely available. A full work flow, including custom R scripts to perform the pre-V-QUEST quality control filtering and editing, the parsing of the V-QUEST output files and ProtParam analysis, and the clustering-based clone identification, is available from the authors (KiplingD@cardiff.ac.uk) upon request.

References

1. Sanz I (1991) Multiple mechanisms participate in the generation of diversity of human H chain CDR3 regions. J Immunol 147:1720–1729

2. Tonegawa S (1983) Somatic generation of antibody diversity. Nature 302:575–581

3. Raaphorst FM, Raman CS, Tami J, Fischbach M, Sanz I (1997) Human Ig heavy chain CDR3 regions in adult bone marrow pre-B cells display an adult phenotype of diversity: evidence for structural selection of DH amino acid sequences. Int Immunol 9:1503–1515

4. Volpe JM, Kepler TB (2008) Large-scale analysis of human heavy chain V(D)J recombination patterns. Immunome Res 4:3

5. Larimore K, McCormick MW, Robins HS, Greenberg PD (2012) Shaping of human germline IgH repertoires revealed by deep sequencing. J Immunol 189:3221–3230

6. Ademokun A, Wu YC, Martin V, Mitra R, Sack U, Baxendale H, Kipling D, Dunn-Walters DK (2011) Vaccination-induced changes in human B-cell repertoire and pneumococcal IgM and IgA antibody at different ages. Aging Cell 10:922–930

7. Wu YC, Kipling D, Dunn-Walters DK (2012) Age-related changes in human peripheral blood IGH repertoire following vaccination. Front Immunol 3:193

8. Cuisinier AM, Guigou V, Boubli L, Fougereau M, Tonnelle C (1989) Preferential expression of VH5 and VH6 immunoglobulin genes in early human B-cell ontogeny. Scand J Immunol 30:493–497

9. Gibson KL, Wu YC, Barnett Y, Duggan O, Vaughan R, Kondeatis E, Nilsson BO, Wikby A, Kipling D, Dunn-Walters DK (2009) B-cell diversity decreases in old age and is correlated with poor health status. Aging Cell 8:18–25

10. Tschumper RC, Asmann YW, Hossain A, Huddleston PM, Wu X, Dispenzieri A, Eckloff BW, Jelinek DF (2012) Comprehensive assessment of potential multiple myeloma immunoglobulin heavy chain V-D-J intraclonal variation using massively parallel pyrosequencing. Oncotarget 3:502–513

11. Warsame AA, Aasheim HC, Nustad K, Troen G, Tierens A, Wang V, Randen U, Dong HP, Heim S, Brech A, Delabie J (2011) Splenic marginal zone lymphoma with VH1-02 gene rearrangement expresses poly- and self-reactive antibodies with similar reactivity. Blood 118:3331–3339

12. Luo C, Tsementzi D, Kyrpides N, Read T, Konstantinidis KT (2012) Direct comparisons of Illumina vs. Roche 454 sequencing technologies on the same microbial community DNA sample. PLoS One 7:e30087

13. Meyer M, Stenzel U, Myles S, Prufer K, Hofreiter M (2007) Targeted high-throughput sequencing of tagged nucleic acid samples. Nucleic Acids Res 35, e97

14. Wu YC, Kipling D, Dunn-Walters DK (2011) The relationship between CD27 negative and positive B cell populations in human peripheral blood. Front Immunol 2:81

15. Wu YC, Kipling D, Leong HS, Martin V, Ademokun AA, Dunn-Walters DK (2010)

High-throughput immunoglobulin repertoire analysis distinguishes between human IgM memory and switched memory B-cell populations. Blood 116:1070–1078

16. Alamyar E, Duroux P, Lefranc MP, Giudicelli V (2012) IMGT® tools for the nucleotide analysis of immunoglobulin (IG) and T cell receptor (TR) V-(D)-J repertoires, polymorphisms, and IG mutations: IMGT/V-QUEST and IMGT/HighV-QUEST for NGS. Methods Mol Biol 882:569–604

17. Alamyar E, Giudicelli V, Li S, Duroux P, Lefranc MP (2012) IMGT/HIGHV-QUEST: the IMGT® web portal for immunoglobulin (Ig) or antibody and T cell receptor (TR) analysis from NGS high throughput and deep sequencing. Immunome Res 8:26

18. Gasteiger E, Hoogland C, Gattiker A, Duvaud S, Wilkins MR, Appel RD, Bairoch A (2005) Protein Identification and Analysis Tools on the ExPASy Server. In: Walker JM (ed) The proteomics protocols handbook. Humana Press, Clifton, UK, pp 571–607

19. R Development Core Team, R Foundation for Statistical Computing, Vienna, Austria (2010) ISBN 3-900051-07-0

20. Gentleman RC, Carey VJ, Bates DM, Bolstad B, Dettling M, Dudoit S, Ellis B, Gautier L, Ge Y, Gentry J, Hornik K, Hothorn T, Huber W, Iacus S, Irizarry R, Leisch F, Li C, Maechler M, Rossini AJ, Sawitzki G, Smith C, Smyth G, Tierney L, Yang JY, Zhang J (2004) Bioconductor: open software development for computational biology and bioinformatics. Genome Biol 5:R80

Laboratory and Data Analysis Methods for Characterization of Human B Cell Repertoires by High-Throughput DNA Sequencing

Chen Wang, Yi Liu, Krishna M. Roskin, Katherine J.L. Jackson, and Scott D. Boyd

Abstract

High-throughput DNA sequencing techniques have greatly accelerated the pace of research into the repertoires of antibody and T cell receptor gene rearrangements that confer antigen specificity to adaptive immune responses. Studies of aging-related changes in human B cell repertoires have benefited from the ability to detect and quantify thousands to millions of B cell clones in human samples, and study the mutational lineages and isotype switching relationships within each clonal lineage. Correlation of repertoire analysis with antibody gene data from antigen-specific B cells is poised to give much greater insight into clinically relevant B cell responses and memory storage. Here, we describe strategies for preparing and analyzing human antibody gene libraries for studying B cell repertoires.

Key words Antibody, Immunoglobulin, High-throughput DNA sequencing, Deep sequencing, Repertoire, Immunome, Aging

1 Introduction

The antigen receptors expressed by human B cells and T cells provide the basis for recognition of diverse antigens by the adaptive immune system, and are the molecular basis for antigen-specific immune system memory. The immunoglobulins (Ig) expressed by B cells, and T cell receptors (TCR) expressed by T cells, are encoded by some of the more complicated regions of the human genome, in which an array of potential variable (V), diversity (D), and joining (J) gene segments are arranged in series. During the formation of new B cells, the genomic DNA at the immunoglobulin heavy chain (IGH), and the kappa or lambda light chain (IGK, IGL) loci, is physically rearranged by the RAG protein complex to bring together single V, D, and J gene segments (for IGH) or V and J segments (for IGK and IGL), with additional diversification of the

Albert C. Shaw (ed.), *Immunosenescence: Methods and Protocols*, Methods in Molecular Biology, vol. 1343, DOI 10.1007/978-1-4939-2963-4_17, © Springer Science+Business Media New York 2015

junctions between gene segments mediated by variable degrees of exonuclease digestion of segment ends, and addition of non-templated nearly random junctional nucleotides (N nucleotides) [1]. The combinatorial diversity resulting from V, D, and J segment choice, and the additional diversity due to exonuclease digestion of segment ends and addition of randomized nucleotides, results in a vast potential repertoire of expressed Ig receptors, each containing two molecules of the B cell's IGH product paired with the IGK or IGL product.

Although the genetic mechanisms responsible for generating Ig receptors have been studied for more than three decades, the advent of "next-generation" DNA sequencing has enabled rapid progress in the comprehensive study of immunoglobulin gene rearrangements [2, 3]. This methodology permits tracking of B cell populations involved in normal physiological responses to pathogens and vaccinations, and study of the alterations seen in immune-mediated diseases and immune deficiencies, including the immune system impairments that accompany human aging. Current high-throughput DNA sequencing (HTS) technologies enable measurement of thousands to millions of Ig or TCR sequences at costs that are orders of magnitude lower than Sanger sequencing [3–12]. The power of these new sequencing methods is enhanced if experimental design and sequencing library preparation are guided by the data analysis plans for the questions that are of greatest interest in the experiment.

HTS of Ig gene rearrangements generates rich and complex data sets, with data analysis typically including one or more of the following approaches: analysis of overall repertoire features or repertoire features associated with particular antibody isotypes; detection and analysis of Ig expressed by clonally expanded B cell populations; and detection of Ig sequences known to be of biological interest, identified by selection of B cells that specifically bind a particular antigen, or B cells from a particular functional subset defined by cell surface markers or other phenotypic features. Overall repertoire features include the frequency of usage of particular V, D, and J segments; numbers of bases removed from segment ends by exonuclease digestion, and the number of non-templated bases added; length and amino acid usage of the complementarity-determining region 3 (CDR3); frequency and distribution of somatic hypermutation; isotype usage for particular VDJ rearrangements, and measurement of the number of distinct sequences obtained from a sample of known B cell number; and evidence of unusual sequence features such as receptor editing or rare large-scale mutations such as insertions or deletions within gene segments [3, 13, 14]. It can be very informative to analyze the Ig sequences expressed by B cells that have undergone clonal expansion to the extent that more than one member of the clone is captured in the sample studied, particularly in cases where there is an acute stimulation such as vaccination. Finally, detection of members of clonal populations for which functional data are available (such as antigen-specific B cells isolated by flow cytometric sorting, or B cells cultured at limiting dilution under conditions where the binding activity of their secreted antibodies can be measured), followed by IGH and IGK/L determination by single-cell PCR and sequencing, has proved to be a powerful method for studying the evolution of HIV-specific or other pathogen-specific B cell responses in humans [14, 15].

The major decision points in preparing HTS libraries for Ig sequencing are (1) choice of template (genomic DNA or cDNA), (2) choice of gene-specific primers in amplifying V(D)J rearrangements, versus a method such as 5′ rapid amplification of cDNA ends (5′RACE), and (3) choice of sequencing platform.

The advantage of genomic DNA (gDNA) as template for PCR amplification is that each B cell only contributes a single-template molecule to its productive IGH and IGK/L rearrangements; thus, separately amplified library pools made from different aliquots of gDNA can be considered as samplings of separate cell populations, if the productive gene rearrangements are analyzed. cDNA templates, in contrast, provide numerous and generally unknown numbers of template molecules from each B cell, such that generation of replicate sequence libraries from a sample must begin with separation of different cell aliquots and isolation of RNA from each separately prior to cDNA synthesis. Despite this disadvantage, constant (C) gene-specific primers can be used to amplify cDNA templates to identify IGH from each antibody isotype, providing valuable functional information about the B cell from which a given transcript was isolated. In addition, cDNA templates facilitate the use of 5′ primers complementary to the leader exon sequences that lie upstream of a short intron preceding each V gene; such leader sequences are less affected by somatic hypermutation than the V gene, and primers targeting the leader sequence may permit amplification of heavily mutated IGH which would fail to amplify with V segment-specific primers [16].

A number of primer sets have been designed to amplify human IGH and IGK/L gene rearrangements. Our group has typically used IGHV gene framework 1 (FR1) and framework 2 (FR2) primers, paired with a single IGHJ primer, based on the BIOMED-2 set that was devised for clinical lab diagnostic use, as well as primers targeting the V gene leader sequences, paired with primers specific for antibody isotype sequences in the first exon of the constant chain [3, 14, 16, 17]. We usually generate several libraries using each primer set from each sample, to avoid missing sequences that amplify poorly with any one primer set. An alternate approach is to use a 5′RACE protocol with the initial reverse transcription step of the protocol primed with constant chain primers for each isotype. The 5′RACE method does not rely on 5′-end gene-specific primers, so it is likely to be an effective way of detecting heavily mutated antibody gene sequences, although it has so far not been widely applied to HTS library generation [18].

The following protocols focus on preparation of libraries for sequencing with the 454 platform (Roche, Basel, Switzerland), but similar methods can be used for Illumina MiSeq or HiSeq library preparation (Illumina, San Diego, CA). These instruments have been the most popular choices of investigators working in this area. The 454 platform provides long single-read lengths (~500 bases) and moderate throughput (one million reads per run), but is more expensive than the Illumina platform which gives higher through-put (tens to hundreds of millions of reads per run) for comparable cost, but shorter single-read lengths (currently up to 250 base reads from each end of a DNA molecule). The ability of the 454 instrument to sequence nearly the full length of an IGH VDJ sequence in a single read facilitates analysis of hypermutation patterns, but as the read lengths of Illumina sequencing have increased to their current levels, the relative advantage of 454 in these analyses has been decreasing [3, 5, 7, 9, 15, 19, 20]. The Illumina platform is well suited to TCR sequencing, where somatic hypermutation is not present [4, 8, 21].

2 Materials

1. RNA and DNA template isolation: All-prep DNA/RNA mini kit, or separate DNA/RNA prep kits (Qiagen).

2. Reverse transcription: SuperScript III Reverse Transcriptase kit (Invitrogen); Random hexamer primers (Promega).

3. PCR Primers: Primers are ordered as standard quality synthesis, or as "ultramer" higher quality synthesis (Integrated DNA Technologies), without additional purification.

4. PCR amplification: AmpliTaq Gold polymerase (Applied Biosystems) with "buffer II" that comes with that polymerase (adding Mg^{2+} to give a final concentration of 1.5 mM in each reaction); dNTP (Roche).

5. Agarose gel electrophoresis: Agarose (Invitrogen).

6. Tris-acetate-EDTA buffer: Tris 40 mM, acetic acid 20 mM, EDTA 1 mM, pH 8.0.

7. DNA ladder for product size determination: Quick-load 100 bp ladder (New England Biolabs).

8. Gel extraction: gel extraction kit (Qiagen).

9. Qubit DNA quantitation: Qubit DNA kit (Invitrogen).

3 Methods

3.1 Primer Design and Barcoding

1. For 454 library preparation, forward and reverse PCR primers are designed with the following elements in 5′–3′ order: 454 instrument-specific primer regions (required for emulsion PCR and initiation of sequencing in the instrument protocols), followed by a 10-base "barcode" sequence that encodes the sample identity and PCR replicate library identity, followed by the IGHV or IGHJ gene-specific primer sequence. Primer sequences and barcodes are indicated in Tables 1 and 2.

3.2 Template Preparation

1. Genomic DNA and RNA are isolated from peripheral blood mononuclear cell samples, or purified B cell samples using the standard protocols in the Qiagen All-Prep kit.

2. cDNA synthesis is carried out with priming by random hexamer primers at 20 ng/µl final concentration, following the manufacturer's protocol for reverse transcription (Invitrogen). The RNase H RNA hydrolysis step following cDNA synthesis does not appear to be necessary for subsequent Ig PCR amplifications.

3.3 PCR Amplification of Ig Gene Rearrangements, and Analysis by Gel Electrophoresis

1. We typically amplify up to 250 ng of genomic DNA template in a 30 µl reaction. Depending on the amount of template available from a sample, we will set up 6 replicate PCR per sample, with 100 ng or 200 ng of PBMC-derived genomic DNA template per replicate.

2. The IGHV primers for each barcoded reaction should be combined to make the FR1 mix (containing 6 primers), the FR2 mix (containing 7 primers), or the leader primer set. The concentrations listed below (3.3 µM) are for the sum of all the primers in the V primer mixes.

3. PCR is set up in 96-well plates on ice, with primers being added to each well first, followed by template, followed by the master mix containing all the remaining components of the PCR reaction (*see* **Note 1**). Mix by pipetting up and down several times gently (*see* **Note 2**).

4. PCR mixture components are:

   Template: 100–200 ng genomic DNA, or cDNA from 100 to 200 ng total RNA

   3.3 µM V Primer mix (FR1, FR2, or leader primers): 3 µl

   3.3 µM J Primer or Constant region primer: 3 µl

   10× PCR buffer: 3 µl

   $MgCl_2$: 1.8 µl

Table 1
Primer sequences for PCR amplification of gDNA library 1st reaction. The 5′-end primers consist of adapter sequences for 454 platform (454-A), barcodes encoding sample identity, and sequences complementary to the FR1 or FR2 regions of different V-gene families [3, 7, 17]. The 3′-end primers consist of adapter 454-B, barcodes encoding replicate identity, and sequence complementary to the J region

Primer name	454 adapter_[barcode]_gene-specific sequence
V-FR1-primer	
454A_VH1-FR1	cgtatcgcctccctcgcgccatcag_[barcode]_GGCCTCAGTGAAGGTCTCCTGCAAG
454A_VH2-FR1	cgtatcgcctccctcgcgccatcag_[barcode]_GTCTGGTCCTACGCTGGTGAAACCC
454A_VH3-FR1	cgtatcgcctccctcgcgccatcag_[barcode]_CTGGGGGGTCCCTGAGACTCTCCTG
454A_VH4-FR1	cgtatcgcctccctcgcgccatcag_[barcode]_CTTCGGAGACCCTGTCCCTCACCTG
454A_VH5-FR1	cgtatcgcctccctcgcgccatcag_[barcode]_CGGGGAGTCTCTGAAGATCTCCTGT
454A_VH6-FR1	cgtatcgcctccctcgcgccatcag_[barcode]_TCGCAGACCCTCTCACTCACCTGTG
V-FR2-primer	
454A_VH1-FR2	cgtatcgcctccctcgcgccatcag_[barcode]_CTGGGTGCGACAGGCCCCTGGACAA
454A_VH2-FR2	cgtatcgcctccctcgcgccatcag_[barcode]_TGGATCCGTCAGCCCCCAGGGAAGG
454A_VH3-FR2	cgtatcgcctccctcgcgccatcag_[barcode]_GGTCCGCCAGGCTCCAGGGAA
454A_VH4-FR2	cgtatcgcctccctcgcgccatcag_[barcode]_TGGATCCGCCAGCCCCCAGGGAAGG
454A_VH5-FR2	cgtatcgcctccctcgcgccatcag_[barcode]_GGGTGCGCCAGATGCCCGGGAAAGG
454A_VH6-FR2	cgtatcgcctccctcgcgccatcag_[barcode]_TGGATCAGGCAGTCCCCATCGAGAG
454A_VH7-FR2	cgtatcgcctccctcgcgccatcag_[barcode]_TTGGGTGCGACAGGCCCCTGGACAA
J-primer	
454B_J	ctatgcgccttgccagcccgctcag_[barcode]_CTTACCTGAGGAGACGGTGACC

2 mM dNTP: 3 µl

AmpliTaq Gold (5 U/µl): 0.3 µl

Water to 30 µl

5. Although the AmpliTaq Gold is a hot-start polymerase, we keep the PCR plate on ice until the thermocycler block has reached 95 °C, and then add the plate to the thermocycler.

6. The PCR program is as follows: Denaturation 95 °C for 7 min; 35 cycles of 95 °C for 30 s, 60 °C for 45 s, and 72 °C for 90 s; and final extension: 72 °C for 10 min. If the PCR will run overnight, we set the thermocycler to keep the plate at 10 °C indefinitely after the run is complete.

7. Products of PCR are analyzed by 1.5 % agarose gels with 1×TAE running buffer, using ethidium bromide for DNA visualization under ultraviolet light (ethidium bromide is added to running buffer as well as the TAE used to make the gel). We usually use the NEB Quick-load 100 bp ladder for size comparison.

Table 2
**Examples of sequence barcodes in the IGHJ primer being used to indicate the sample (Sample 1–
Sample 4) from which a library was generated, while barcodes in the IGHV FR1 and FR2 primer sets
are used to label the different replicate libraries generated by PCR of distinct aliquots of genomic
DNA template from the sample (replicate libraries R1–R6 for each sample). Different replicate
libraries from the same sample share the J-barcode and are distinguished by V-barcodes**

	V-barcode	J-barcode		V-barcode	J-barcode
Sample 1			*Sample 3*		
R1	TTATGCCAGG		R1	TTATGCCAGG	
R2	TCCTGCCAGG		R2	TCCTGCCAGG	
R3	CCTTCCTAAG	TAGAAGCAAG	R3	CCTTCCTAAG	CGGAAGCAAG
R4	AGCTCCTAAG		R4	AGCTCCTAAG	
R5	ACGTCCTAAG		R5	ACGTCCTAAG	
R6	TAGTGCCAGG		R6	TAGTGCCAGG	
Sample 2			*Sample 4*		
R1	TTATGCCAGG		R1	TTATGCCAGG	
R2	TCCTGCCAGG		R2	TCCTGCCAGG	
R3	CCTTCCTAAG	TGTAAGCAAG	R3	CCTTCCTAAG	CCTAAGCAAG
R4	AGCTCCTAAG		R4	AGCTCCTAAG	
R5	ACGTCCTAAG		R5	ACGTCCTAAG	
R6	TAGTGCCAGG		R6	TAGTGCCAGG	

3.4 Library Pooling and Gel Purification

1. Based on the intensities of amplified bands from each PCR reaction, we pool the barcoded products in approximately equimolar amounts (or with greater representation of particular samples, if more reads are wanted from them).

2. Run the pooled library on a new 1.5 % agarose gel in 1×TAE buffer (using a comb with several teeth taped together to give a broad single well), and cut out the gel slice containing the desired PCR bands, being generous in the cutting to include some gel above the highest band and below the lowest band. We exclude the tips of the band from the excised slice, as "smiling" of the band can cause the separation to be poorer at the ends.

3. DNA is isolated from the gel slice using a Qiagen gel purification kit, and eluted in TE buffer. The final gel-purified library band is run on a final analytical 1.5 % agarose 1×TAE gel (*see* **Note 3**).

4. Quantitation of the pooled gel-extracted library is conducted with Nanodrop spectrometry or Qubit fluorimetry.

3.5 High-Throughput DNA Sequencing

1. The 454 libraries are sequenced using 454 Titanium chemistry, with amplicon sequencing reagents, and only from the "B" side. Using the primer design presented here, the sequencing reads start from the J segment end of the amplicon, and the Ig gene rearrangement is sequenced as the reverse complement of the mRNA sequence. The advantage of sequencing starting from the J segment is that the VDJ junctional region is measured early in the sequencing run when the read quality is highest.

2. Illumina libraries are sequenced with the MiSeq instrument, using paired 250 bp read reagent kits. Using the primer design presented here, the J segment end of the amplicon is sequenced in the first read, while the second read begins from the V segment.

3.6 DNA Sequence Data Analysis

1. There are a large number of options for processing and filtering DNA sequence data. Our data analysis pipeline is integrated with a PostgreSQL database for maintaining analysis results in a consistent and orderly format, and to facilitate comparison between sequences obtained from different experiments and different sequencing runs. The components of the data analysis pipeline are carried out sequentially as indicated below.

2. Identifying which sequences in the 454 instrument output files came from each sample and each replicate sequence library from that sample is carried out by searching for exact matches to the "barcode" sequences encoded in the forward and reverse PCR primers for each sample and replicate library. In addition to matching the barcode sequence perfectly, the 7 bases of gene-specific primer that follow the barcode sequence are required to match exactly. This criterion enables the use of pooled libraries in which the same barcode sequence can be used with different primer sets, such as IGH primers and T cell receptor primers, in the same sequencing run.

3. Gene-specific primer sequences are trimmed from the sequence reads, to avoid incorporating primer-encoded sequence into the later steps in the data analysis. For IGH amplicons that are to be further analyzed with the iHMMune-align algorithm, we do not trim the IGHJ primer, as the program requires the additional length of IGHJ sequence to function. In this particular case, downstream data analysis does not make use of apparent hypermutation positions that occur in the IGHJ primer-encoded parts of the sequence.

4. Alignment of Ig gene products to germline V, D, and J gene segments can be carried out with a variety of different programs. We have used iHMMune-align (www.ihmmune. unsw.edu.au), IgBLAST (www.ncbi.nlm.nih.gov/igblast/), and IMGT/V-QUEST (www.imgt.org) in the past [22–24].

We currently use iHMMune-align as the main sequence alignment program in the analysis pipeline as the program builds a probabilistic model of VDJ rearrangement with alignments performed against the model rather than as independent local sequence alignments for each gene segment set, as is the case for IgBLAST and IMGT/V-QUEST. The probabilistic model accounts for the mutation state of V gene segment in determining the most likely D gene segment, and considers the interplay between nucleotide addition, removal, and mutation in determining the processing of the gene segment ends and the extent of non-template-encoded bases at the V-D and D-J junctions. The output of each of these alignment programs provides the predicted germline V, D, and J gene segments used in each Ig rearrangement, non-templated junctional nucleotides, positions of mutations compared to the predicted germline gene segments, predicted amino acid sequences of the encoded protein, including the CDR3 region, and a number of other metrics.

5. Summary measures of the sequences obtained from a sample, such as the frequency of rearrangements using each V, D, and J segment, extent of exonuclease digestion and non-templated base addition, length and amino acid usage of the CDR3, and frequency and distribution of somatic hypermutation changes, can be readily calculated from the sequence parsing output from iHMMune-align or other alignment programs. Our laboratory uses a variety of scripts in the Python scripting language (www.python.org) or the R statistical language (http://www.r-project.org/) to aggregate these data, perform statistical tests, and generate plots for data visualization. In experiments where multiple replicate libraries have been generated from either gDNA template or cDNA from distinct cell aliquots, it is often advisable to "collapse" sequences within each replicate library if they share identical V(D)J segment usage and non-templated bases, as variations in sequence count for different species within a replicate library are usually the result of differences in PCR amplification efficiency for templates which were each derived from one cell (*see* **Note 4**). Analysis of B cell repertoire features in a sample can be affected by many variables, such as the proportion of naïve vs. memory B cells or the proportion of B cells expressing various switched antibody isotypes. It is advisable to compare similar kinds of sequence data sets between healthy controls and experimental subjects, where the data have been generated using the same library generation approach, and sequenced with the same sequencing platform, preferably within the same instrument run (*see* **Note 5**).

6. Identification of clonally related sequences within a data set can be carried out with various degrees of strictness, and is impacted by the extent of somatic hypermutation within the clone of B cells, and the differences in mutation levels between clone members. To avoid being overly sensitive to the effects of hypermutation on allele calling for V or J segments, and to permit some hypermutation changes in the VDJ junctional regions, we usually search for sequences that share the same V and J segment calls (omitting the allele call) and have CDR3 regions of the same length that are 80 % identical at the amino acid level. The threshold for CDR3 similarity is a parameter that can be adjusted according to the experimental question being asked. For example, if the goal is to detect all potentially related members of a clone that contains highly hypermutated members as well as near-germline members, then a more permissive threshold for CDR3 similarity would help to prevent false-negative results.

7. Quantitation of the degree of B cell clonality observed in a sample has not been standardized within the HTS literature, but is an important measure. Simple approaches such as counting the number of unique sequences detected within a given number of total sequences can be strongly affected by both biological and experimental parameters, such as the expression level of an Ig transcript in experiments where HTS libraries are generated from cDNA template, or differences in PCR amplification efficiency. A primary benefit of preparing independent replicate sequencing libraries from each sample is that it enables a more accurate identification of sequences that are derived from clonally expanded B cells. In such experimental designs, an IGH sequence is designated as evidence of a clonally expanded B cell population only if it is observed in more than a single replicate library from the sample. With this approach, a "clonality score" normalized for the depth of sequencing performed on each library can be calculated.

   We represent the clonality score as a ratio of a numerator against a normalizing denominator. The numerator counts the total number of unordered pairings of reads, in which the two reads arise from different replicate libraries, but belong to the same clone. The denominator normalizes the numerator against the sequencing depth in each replicate library by counting the number of such pairwise comparisons made. For each pair of distinct replicate libraries, the number of comparisons made is the number of reads in one replicate library multiplied by the number of reads in the other replicate library. The denominator counts the total number of comparisons made, across all unordered pairings of replicate libraries. When the clonality score is viewed as a fraction, it can be interpreted as the probability that two random and independently drawn reads from a given sample would belong to the same clone.

Therefore, the clonality score is calculated as follows: sum of $N_{ij} \times N_{ik}$ ($j \neq k$) over i, j, k divided by the sum of $T_j \times T_k$ ($j \neq k$) over j, k, where N_{ij} and N_{ik} are the copy numbers of clone i observed in independent replicate PCR libraries j and k generated from independent aliquots of template DNA, or from RNA isolated from separate cell aliquots from the sample. T_j and T_k are total read numbers in the corresponding replicate libraries.

Empirically, the clonality scores across different samples tend to follow a lognormal distribution. Thus, it is often sensible to apply t-tests to the logarithms of the clonality scores during data analysis. Taking logarithms requires us to systematically address the occasions where no pair of replicate libraries shares any reads. This issue is frequently encountered and well discussed in various branches of the machine learning literature. We apply Laplace smoothing, which involves adding 1 to the numerator and 2 to the denominator, to avoid this problem [25].

The clonality score is simple to interpret, and the specific procedure provided above is unbiased. In part due to this estimator's simplicity, not all the known subtleties of the experimental reality are directly addressed; for example, some replicate libraries may contain fewer B cells, or experience more variation during PCR or sequencing. In addition, the presence of a single large clonal population, or many smaller clones, can give rise to equivalent clonality scores, so graphical visualization of the number and size of expanded clones detected in a sample is helpful for further exploration of the data.

8. Estimation of the diversity of a B cell population based on HTS Ig repertoire data is more challenging than the estimation of clonality. If "diversity" is taken to mean the true number of distinct species within a population, then current experimental methods are still somewhat underpowered to obtain the correct answer, and ethical limits on human subjects research present a more significant barrier to collecting samples containing enough cells to permit accurate determination of the answer. Most estimates of "diversity" in the published literature on lymphocyte populations are in fact estimates of the lower limit of diversity, not the upper limit or the most likely value [3, 4, 26]. There are approximately one to two billion circulating B cells in healthy individuals' blood, and probably tens to hundreds of billions of B cells in the entire human body [27–29]. Experiments sampling thousands or millions of cells from these much larger pools have limited ability to assess the number and size of rare clonal populations, which may make up most of the actual diversity of a sample. In contrast, a metric such as the clonality score that emphasizes the quantification of large clonal populations is more easily reproducible because it relies little on contributions from the rare members of the population.

4 Notes

1. It is convenient to create stock primer plates containing pre-aliquoted barcoded IGHV and IGHJ or Ig constant region primer combinations, and then to use a multichannel micropipettor to create a number of replica plates from the stock plate, so that primers do not have to be separately aliquoted for each experiment. Such primer plates can be stored for several months at –80 °C.

2. PCR contamination is a danger in any experiment using common PCR primers to amplify similar kinds of amplicons in successive experiments, and HTS is an excellent way to be able to detect such contaminants. Maintaining strict separation of separate laboratory rooms for pre-PCR experimental work, and post-PCR analysis of products, pooling of libraries, and other manipulations is essential.

3. In this analytical gel of the pooled library, we usually also run a titration of the 100 bp ladder (four different concentrations of the ladder) to confirm the proportions of the library components, and for comparison with the concentration values given by spectrophotometric or fluorimetric measurement methods.

4. Exceptions to this rule would include samples in which there are large clonal B cell populations, such that many or most replicate libraries generated from the sample contain instances of the IGH expressed by the clone, in which case the proportion of that IGH sequence in each replicate library is likely to be more meaningful.

5. As one example of potentially confounding variables that can affect B cell repertoire analysis, IGH rearrangements using some V segments tend to be under- or overrepresented in the memory B cell pool (such as the lower frequency of IGHV1-69 in memory B cells) [13]. Therefore, if two samples differ in the proportion of memory B cells that are present, it would be expected that V1-69 usage would appear to differ between the samples as well. Comparing only sequences that are hypermutated, or are not hypermutated, between different samples would help to correct for this source of error.

References

1. Jung D, Alt FW (2004) Unraveling V(D)J recombination; insights into gene regulation. Cell 116(2):299–311

2. Hozumi N, Tonegawa S (1976) Evidence for somatic rearrangement of immunoglobulin genes coding for variable and constant regions. Proc Natl Acad Sci U S A 73(10):3628–3632

3. Boyd SD, Marshall EL, Merker JD, Maniar JM, Zhang LN, Sahaf B, Jones CD, Simen BB, Hanczaruk B, Nguyen KD, Nadeau KC, Egholm M, Miklos DB, Zehnder JL, Fire AZ (2009) Measurement and clinical monitoring of human lymphocyte clonality by massively parallel VDJ pyrosequencing. Sci Transl Med 1(12):12–23

4. Robins HS, Campregher PV, Srivastava SK, Wacher A, Turtle CJ, Kahsai O, Riddell SR, Warren EH, Carlson CS (2009) Comprehensive assessment of T-cell receptor beta-chain diversity in alphabeta T cells. Blood 114(19):4099–4107, doi: blood-2009-04-217604 [pii]10.1182/blood-2009-04-217604

5. Campbell PJ, Pleasance ED, Stephens PJ, Dicks E, Rance R, Goodhead I, Follows GA, Green AR, Futreal PA, Stratton MR (2008) Subclonal phylogenetic structures in cancer revealed by ultra-deep sequencing. Proc Natl Acad Sci U S A 105(35):13081–13086, doi: 0801523105 [pii]10.1073/pnas.0801523105

6. Wang C, Sanders CM, Yang Q, Schroeder HW Jr, Wang E, Babrzadeh F, Gharizadeh B, Myers RM, Hudson JR Jr, Davis RW, Han J (2010) High throughput sequencing reveals a complex pattern of dynamic interrelationships among human T cell subsets. Proc Natl Acad Sci U S A 107(4):1518–1523, doi: 0913939107 [pii]10.1073/pnas.0913939107

7. Margulies M, Egholm M, Altman WE, Attiya S, Bader JS, Bemben LA, Berka J, Braverman MS, Chen YJ, Chen Z, Dewell SB, Du L, Fierro JM, Gomes XV, Godwin BC, He W, Helgesen S, Ho CH, Irzyk GP, Jando SC, Alenquer ML, Jarvie TP, Jirage KB, Kim JB, Knight JR, Lanza JR, Leamon JH, Lefkowitz SM, Lei M, Li J, Lohman KL, Lu H, Makhijani VB, McDade KE, McKenna MP, Myers EW, Nickerson E, Nobile JR, Plant R, Puc BP, Ronan MT, Roth GT, Sarkis GJ, Simons JF, Simpson JW, Srinivasan M, Tartaro KR, Tomasz A, Vogt KA, Volkmer GA, Wang SH, Wang Y, Weiner MP, Yu P, Begley RF, Rothberg JM (2005) Genome sequencing in microfabricated high-density picolitre reactors. Nature 437(7057):376–380, doi: nature03959 [pii]10.1038/nature03959

8. Freeman JD, Warren RL, Webb JR, Nelson BH, Holt RA (2009) Profiling the T-cell receptor beta-chain repertoire by massively parallel sequencing. Genome Res 19(10):1817–1824, doi: gr.092924.109 [pii]10.1101/gr.092924.109

9. Wu YC, Kipling D, Leong HS, Martin V, Ademokun AA, Dunn-Walters DK (2010) High-throughput immunoglobulin repertoire analysis distinguishes between human IgM memory and switched memory B-cell populations. Blood 116(7):1070–1078, doi: blood-2010-03-275859 [pii]10.1182/blood-2010-03-275859

10. Venturi V, Quigley MF, Greenaway HY, Ng PC, Ende ZS, McIntosh T, Asher TE, Almeida JR, Levy S, Price DA, Davenport MP, Douek DC (2011) A mechanism for TCR sharing

between T cell subsets and individuals revealed by pyrosequencing. J Immunol 186(7):4285–4294, doi: jimmunol.1003898 [pii]10.4049/jimmunol.1003898

11. Glanville J, Zhai W, Berka J, Telman D, Huerta G, Mehta GR, Ni I, Mei L, Sundar PD, Day GM, Cox D, Rajpal A, Pons J (2009) Precise determination of the diversity of a combinatorial antibody library gives insight into the human immunoglobulin repertoire. Proc Natl Acad Sci U S A 106(48):20216–20221, doi: 0909775106 [pii]10.1073/pnas.0909775106

12. Bentley DR, Balasubramanian S, Swerdlow HP, Smith GP, Milton J, Brown CG, Hall KP, Evers DJ, Barnes CL, Bignell HR, Boutell JM, Bryant J, Carter RJ, Keira Cheetham R, Cox AJ, Ellis DJ, Flatbush MR, Gormley NA, Humphray SJ, Irving LJ, Karbelashvili MS, Kirk SM, Li H, Liu X, Maisinger KS, Murray LJ, Obradovic B, Ost T, Parkinson ML, Pratt MR, Rasolonjatovo IM, Reed MT, Rigatti R, Rodighiero C, Ross MT, Sabot A, Sankar SV, Scally A, Schroth GP, Smith ME, Smith VP, Spiridou A, Torrance PE, Tzonev SS, Vermaas EH, Walter K, Wu X, Zhang L, Alam MD, Anastasi C, Aniebo IC, Bailey DM, Bancarz IR, Banerjee S, Barbour SG, Baybayan PA, Benoit VA, Benson KF, Bevis C, Black PJ, Boodhun A, Brennan JS, Bridgham JA, Brown RC, Brown AA, Buermann DH, Bundu AA, Burrows JC, Carter NP, Castillo N, Chiara ECM, Chang S, Neil Cooley R, Crake NR, Dada OO, Diakoumakos KD, Dominguez-Fernandez B, Earnshaw DJ, Egbujor UC, Elmore DW, Etchin SS, Ewan MR, Fedurco M, Fraser LJ, Fuentes Fajardo KV, Scott Furey W, George D, Gietzen KJ, Goddard CP, Golda GS, Granieri PA, Green DE, Gustafson DL, Hansen NF, Harnish K, Haudenschild CD, Heyer NI, Hims MM, Ho JT, Horgan AM, Hoschler K, Hurwitz S, Ivanov DV, Johnson MQ, James T, Huw Jones TA, Kang GD, Kerelska TH, Kersey AD, Khrebtukova I, Kindwall AP, Kingsbury Z, Kokko-Gonzales PI, Kumar A, Laurent MA, Lawley CT, Lee SE, Lee X, Liao AK, Loch JA, Lok M, Luo S, Mammen RM, Martin JW, McCauley PG, McNitt P, Mehta P, Moon KW, Mullens JW, Newington T, Ning Z, Ling Ng B, Novo SM, O'Neill MJ, Osborne MA, Osnowski A, Ostadan O, Paraschos LL, Pickering L, Pike AC, Chris Pinkard D, Pliskin DP, Podhasky J, Quijano VJ, Raczy C, Rae VH, Rawlings SR, Chiva Rodriguez A, Roe PM, Rogers J, Rogert Bacigalupo MC, Romanov N, Romieu A, Roth RK, Rourke NJ, Ruediger ST, Rusman E, Sanches-Kuiper RM, Schenker MR, Seoane JM, Shaw RJ, Shiver MK, Short SW, Sizto NL, Sluis JP, Smith MA, Ernest Sohna Sohna J,

Spence EJ, Stevens K, Sutton N, Szajkowski L, Tregidgo CL, Turcatti G, Vandevondele S, Verhovsky Y, Virk SM, Wakelin S, Walcott GC, Wang J, Worsley GJ, Yan J, Yau L, Zuerlein M, Mullikin JC, Hurles ME, McCooke NJ, West JS, Oaks FL, Lundberg PL, Klenerman D, Durbin R, Smith AJ (2008) Accurate whole human genome sequencing using reversible terminator chemistry. Nature 456(7218):53–59, doi: nature07517 [pii]10.1038/nature07517

13. Glanville J, Kuo TC, von Budingen HC, Guey L, Berka J, Sundar PD, Huerta G, Mehta GR, Oksenberg JR, Hauser SL, Cox DR, Rajpal A, Pons J (2011) Naive antibody gene-segment frequencies are heritable and unaltered by chronic lymphocyte ablation. Proc Natl Acad Sci U S A 108(50):20066–20071, doi: 1107498108 [pii]10.1073/pnas.1107498108

14. Liao HX, Lynch R, Zhou T, Gao F, Alam SM, Boyd SD, Fire AZ, Roskin KM, Schramm CA, Zhang Z, Zhu J, Shapiro L, Becker J, Benjamin B, Blakesley R, Bouffard G, Brooks S, Coleman H, Dekhtyar M, Gregory M, Guan X, Gupta J, Han J, Hargrove A, Ho SL, Johnson T, Legaspi R, Lovett S, Maduro Q, Masiello C, Maskeri B, McDowell J, Montemayor C, Mullikin J, Park M, Riebow N, Schandler K, Schmidt B, Sison C, Stantripop M, Thomas J, Thomas P, Vemulapalli M, Young A, Mullikin JC, Gnanakaran S, Hraber P, Wiehe K, Kelsoe G, Yang G, Xia SM, Montefiori DC, Parks R, Lloyd KE, Scearce RM, Soderberg KA, Cohen M, Kamanga G, Louder MK, Tran LM, Chen Y, Cai F, Chen S, Moquin S, Du X, Joyce MG, Srivatsan S, Zhang B, Zheng A, Shaw GM, Hahn BH, Kepler TB, Korber BT, Kwong PD, Mascola JR, Haynes BF (2013) Co-evolution of a broadly neutralizing HIV-1 antibody and founder virus. Nature 496(7446):469–476. doi:10.1038/nature12053

15. Liao HX, Chen X, Munshaw S, Zhang R, Marshall DJ, Vandergrift N, Whitesides JF, Lu X, Yu JS, Hwang KK, Gao F, Markowitz M, Heath SL, Bar KJ, Goepfert PA, Montefiori DC, Shaw GC, Alam SM, Margolis DM, Denny TN, Boyd SD, Marshal E, Egholm M, Simen BB, Hanczaruk B, Fire AZ, Voss G, Kelsoe G, Tomaras GD, Moody MA, Kepler TB, Haynes BF (2011) Initial antibodies binding to HIV-1 gp41 in acutely infected subjects are polyreactive and highly mutated. J Exp Med 208(11):2237–2249. doi:10.1084/jem.20110363

16. Scheid JF, Mouquet H, Feldhahn N, Seaman MS, Velinzon K, Pietzsch J, Ott RG, Anthony RM, Zebroski H, Hurley A, Phogat A, Chakrabarti B, Li Y, Connors M, Pereyra F, Walker BD, Wardemann H, Ho D, Wyatt RT, Mascola JR, Ravetch JV, Nussenzweig MC (2009) Broad diversity of neutralizing antibodies isolated from memory B cells in HIV-infected individuals. Nature 458(7238):636–640. doi:10.1038/nature07930

17. van Dongen JJ, Langerak AW, Bruggemann M, Evans PA, Hummel M, Lavender FL, Delabesse E, Davi F, Schuuring E, Garcia-Sanz R, van Krieken JH, Droese J, Gonzalez D, Bastard C, White HE, Spaargaren M, Gonzalez M, Parreira A, Smith JL, Morgan GJ, Kneba M, Macintyre EA (2003) Design and standardization of PCR primers and protocols for detection of clonal immunoglobulin and T-cell receptor gene recombinations in suspect lymphoproliferations: report of the BIOMED-2 Concerted Action BMH4-CT98-3936. Leukemia 17(12):2257–2317. doi:10.1038/sj.leu.2403202

18. Tobisawa Y, Maruyama T, Tanikawa T, Nakanishi K, Kurohane K, Imai Y (2011) Establishment of recombinant hybrid-IgG/IgA immunoglobulin specific for Shiga toxin. Scand J Immunol 74(6):574–584. doi:10.1111/j.1365-3083.2011.02617.x

19. Weinstein JA, Jiang N, White RA 3rd, Fisher DS, Quake SR (2009) High-throughput sequencing of the zebrafish antibody repertoire. Science 324(5928):807–810, doi: 324/5928/807 [pii]10.1126/science.11700

20. Wu X, Zhou T, Zhu J, Zhang B, Georgiev I, Wang C, Chen X, Longo NS, Louder M, McKee K, O'Dell S, Perfetto S, Schmidt SD, Shi W, Wu L, Yang Y, Yang ZY, Yang Z, Zhang Z, Bonsignori M, Crump JA, Kapiga SH, Sam NE, Haynes BF, Simek M, Burton DR, Koff WC, Doria-Rose NA, Connors M, Mullikin JC, Nabel GJ, Roederer M, Shapiro L, Kwong PD, Mascola JR (2011) Focused evolution of HIV-1 neutralizing antibodies revealed by structures and deep sequencing. Science 333(6049):1593–1602, doi: science.1207532 [pii]10.1126/science.1207532

21. Robins H, Desmarais C, Matthis J, Livingston R, Andriesen J, Reijonen H, Carlson C, Nepom G, Yee C, Cerosaletti K (2011) Ultrasensitive detection of rare T cell clones. J Immunol Methods 375(1-2):14–19, doi: S0022-1759(11)00246-8 [pii]10.1016/j.jim.2011.09.001

22. Brochet X, Lefranc MP, Giudicelli V (2008) IMGT/V-QUEST: the highly customized and integrated system for IG and TR standardized V-J and V-D-J sequence analysis. Nucleic Acids Res 36(Web Server issue):503–508. doi:10.1093/nar/gkn316

23. Giudicelli V, Brochet X, Lefranc MP (2011) IMGT/V-QUEST: IMGT standardized analysis of the immunoglobulin (IG) and T cell

receptor (TR) nucleotide sequences. Cold Spring Harb Protoc 2011(6):695–715. doi:10.1101/pdb.prot5633

24. Gaeta BA, Malming HR, Jackson KJ, Bain ME, Wilson P, Collins AM (2007) iHMMune-align: hidden Markov model-based alignment and identification of germline genes in rearranged immunoglobulin gene sequences. Bioinformatics 23(13):1580–1587, doi: btm147 [pii]10.1093/bioinformatics/btm147

25. Russell SJ, Norvig P (2003) Artificial intelligence: a modern approach. Pearson Education, Upper Saddle River, NJ

26. Arstila TP, Casrouge A, Baron V, Even J, Kanellopoulos J, Kourilsky P (1999) A direct estimate of the human alphabeta T cell receptor diversity. Science 286(5441):958–961, doi: 7939 [pii]

27. Ganusov VV, De Boer RJ (2007) Do most lymphocytes in humans really reside in the gut? Trends Immunol 28(12):514–518, doi: S1471-4906(07)00231-1 [pii]10.1016/j.it.2007.08.009

28. Greer JP, Foerster J, Rodgers GM, Paraskevas F, Glader B, Arber DA, Means RT (2008) Wintrobe's clinical hematology, vol 1. Lippincott Williams & Wilkins, Philadelphia, PA

29. Morbach H, Eichhorn EM, Liese JG, Girschick HJ (2010) Reference values for B cell subpopulations from infancy to adulthood. Clin Exp Immunol 162(2):271–279. doi:10.1111/j.1365-2249.2010.04206.x

Chapter 18

Discovery of Novel microRNAs in Aging *Caenorhabditis elegans*

Alexandre de Lencastre and Frank Slack

Abstract

The rapid development of deep sequencing technologies over the last few years and concomitant increases in sequencing depth and cost efficiencies have opened the door to a ever-widening range of applications in biology—from whole-genome sequencing, to ChIP-seq analysis, epigenomic and RNA transcriptome surveys. Here we describe the application of deep sequencing to the discovery of novel microRNAs and characterization of their differential expression during adulthood in *Caenorhabditis elegans*.

Key words *Caenorhabditis elegans*, microRNA, Differential gene expression, Deep sequencing

1   Introduction

microRNAs (miRNAs) are short, endogenous RNAs with functions in post-transcriptional regulation in a wide variety of eukaryotes [1]. As a novel class of gene regulatory elements, miRNAs have been implicated in a wide variety of functions during development in plants and animals and accumulating evidence points to functions of certain miRNAs as oncogenes and tumor suppressors [2]. Recent breakthroughs expand the repertoire of post-developmental functions for miRNAs and suggest that alteration of miRNA levels can directly affect the health span and longevity of organisms. In work pioneered in *C. elegans* we have shown that mutations to certain miRNAs can significantly lengthen or shorten nematode life-span [3, 4]. At least four of these miRNAs were first identified as miRNAs that are up-regulated during adulthood in *C. elegans* [4]. Importantly, these miRNAs function in longevity at least partially through conserved pathways such as the insulin-like and DNA damage response pathways. We have shown that these functions are at least partially mediated by miRNA repression of genes in these pathways, consistent with stereotypical miRNA-mediated regulation. These results expand the universe of known

Albert C. Shaw (ed.), *Immunosenescence: Methods and Protocols*, Methods in Molecular Biology, vol. 1343,
DOI 10.1007/978-1-4939-2963-4_18, © Springer Science+Business Media New York 2015

functions for miRNAs but it is clear that much remains to be discovered. Surveys of miRNA mutations in *C. elegans* have so far identified only a handful of miRNAs with obvious phenotypes, and the vast majority of miRNAs have unknown functions [5–7]. Furthermore, many other miRNAs remain undiscovered. In our deep sequencing surveys of aged nematodes, we identified and validated the expression of 17 novel miRNAs [4, 8]. Finally, miR-NAs have the potential to target a vast number of genes. Together, these results suggest possible functional roles of many new miR-NAs during adulthood and emphasize the power of deep sequencing technologies in uncovering these new regulatory factors or their targets. Here we discuss methods for discovery and differential expression analysis of miRNAs during adulthood in *C. elegans*.

2   Materials

2.1   *C. elegans* Maintenance and Growth

1. Strains: Obtain *C. elegans* strains from the *Caenorhabditis Genetics Center (CGC)*. Some useful strains for the discovery of novel miRNAs during aging: wild-type N2 (Bristol), *daf-2(e1370)* and *alg-1(gk214)*. All mutant strains are backcrossed against the reference N2 strain at least three times before further characterization.

2. Nematode growth medium (NGM): Mix 6 g NaCl, 34 g agar and 5 g BACTO peptone in 2 L of water. After autoclaving, let cool to 55 °C in a water bath for 15 min and then mix the following, in order, allowing each to mix completely: 50 ml 1 M potassium phosphate pH 6.0 (108.3 g KH_2PO_4, 35.6 g K_2HPO_4, in 1 L of water); 2 ml 5 mg/ml cholesterol, 2 ml 1 M $MgSO_4$ and 2 ml 1 M $CaCl_2$. Finally, dispense the NGM solution into petri dishes. Fill plates 2/3 full of agar (for small 6 cm plates, that would be about 10 ml of NGM).

3. M9 buffer: Mix 3 g of KH_2PO_4, 5 g NaCl, and 6 g Na_2HPO_4 in 1 L water. After autoclaving, add 1 ml 1 M $MgSO_4$.

4. FUDR: Prepare 40× stock solution of 5′-fluoro-2′deoxyuridine (Roche) in water (4 mg/ml) and filter-sterilize through 0.2 μm filter discs. Store individual aliquots at 20 °C. Once thawed, discard unused FUDR solution.

2.2   RNA Isolation, Cloning, Deep Sequencing, and qRT-PCR

1. Siliconized, RNase/DNase-free microcentrifuge tubes.
2. TRIzol reagent (Roche).
3. miRVana miRNA isolation kit (Ambion).
4. Superscript III Reverse Transcriptase (Invitrogen).
5. Turbo DNAfree kit (Ambion).
6. DGE-Small RNA Sample Prep Kit ver. 1.0 (Illumina).

7. Taqman miRNA Assays (Applied Biosystems).

8. Custom Taqman miRNA Assays (Applied Biosystems).

9. Taqman miRNA Reverse Transcription Kit (Applied Biosystems), containing Multi-scribe RT (50 U/μl), RNase Inhibitor (20 U/μl), 10 mM dNTP mix.

10. TaqMan® Universal PCR Master Mix, No AmpErase® UNG (Applied Biosystems).

11. miScript II RT Kit (Qiagen), containing 5× miScript HiFlex Buffer.

12. miScript Primer Assays (Qiagen), including RNA6B control.

13. miScript SYBR Green PCR Kit (Qiagen).

2.3 Bioinformatic Analysis

1. Required input files:

   C. elegans genome: cel_ws201.fa from wormbase: ftp://ftp.wormbase.org/pub/wormbase/genomes/c_elegans/sequences/dna/

   C. elegans mature miRNA sequences, mature_cel.fa in fasta format obtained from miRBase (mirbase.org):

   C. elegans precursor miRNA sequences, mature_other.fa, obtained from miRBase.

   mature miRNA sequences of other species, precursor_cel.fa, obtained from miRBase.

   Deep sequencing reads, in fastq or fasta format.

2. Software packages:

   Differential expression of miRNAs and novel miRNA discovery: miRDeep2 [9]. Other prerequisite software can be installed automatically or manually (*see* miRDeep2 documentation and tutorial).

   Statistical analysis of differential expression: Any of a number of software packages: DESeq, DEGseq, edgeR, baySeq, mirZ, or SAMseq [10–15].

3 Methods

3.1 RNA Isolation from Synchronized Populations of Adult C. elegans

Routine *C. elegans* culture procedures are carried using standard, published protocols [16].

1. Allow animals to grow for at least three generations on *E. coli* strain OP50 without starvation. In order to obtain 15–20 μg of RNA, a mixed population of animals (medium density population, unstarved, on a NGM plate) are harvested from 10 to 20 small (6 cm) NGM plates or 1–2 large (15 cm) NGM plates using 10–15 ml of M9 buffer (*see* **Note 1**). The worm pellets

are washed 3–4 times with M9 to remove OP50. These animals are then bleach-treated in 0.1 % (vol/vol) sodium hypochlorite and 0.5 M NaOH in total volume of 5 ml in a 15 ml falcon tube for a maximum of 5 min and washed with M9 buffer 5–6 times (*see* **Note 2**). The remaining eggs are then resuspended in 20–50 ml of M9 buffer and incubated overnight at 20 °C (or appropriate temperature for temperature sensitive mutants) with gentle shaking/nutation in a 200 ml Erlenmeyer flask covered loosely with aluminum foil (to prevent hypoxia).

2. Synchronized, starved L1-stage larvae are plated on large NGM plates containing OP50 and grown at 20 °C (or appropriate temperature) until late L4-early adulthood stage. At this point, animals are transferred using M9 to plates containing 5′-fluoro-2′-deoxyuridine (FUDR) (0.1 mg/ml) (to prevent progeny production) and maintained at 20 °C (or appropriate temperature). At selected time points of adulthood, animals are harvested using M9, washed 6 times with M9 buffer, flash frozen in liquid N2, and stored at –80 °C for later analysis.

3. Worm lysis for RNA extraction: Worms can be lysed by traditional mortar and pestle grinding of frozen worm pellets or by alternative methods. Currently, we lyse worm preps using Zirconia beads (1 mm, Biospec) in a Fastprep24 homogenizer (MP Biomedicals), which permits rapid and uniform lysis of multiple *C. elegans* samples at one time.

4. Small RNA extraction: Isolate total RNA by guanidine thiocyanate hydrochloride/phenol method or using the commercial TRIzol reagent (Roche) (*see* **Note 3**). Small RNAs can be harvested from total RNA by size selection in the presence of ^{32}P-labeled RNA oligonucleotide size markers using polyacrylamide gel electrophoresis (PAGE) [4, 17]. Alternatively, isolate small RNAs using specialized commercial kits, such as the miRVana miRNA isolation kit (Ambion) following the manufacturer's protocols. We have had good success extracting RNA enriched for small RNAs by either method [4, 8].

5. Small RNA cloning: cDNA libraries of small RNAs are prepared using the DGE-Small RNA Sample Prep Kit ver. 1.0 (Illumina) following the manufacturer's recommended protocols. Small RNAs corresponding to sizes of 10–30 nucleotides are selectively purified and ligated to adapters and amplified by RT-PCR (*see* **Notes 4** and **5**). Consider the use of multiplexing in order to substantially decrease the cost of sequencing and increase the number of samples to be sequenced [18]. Purified DNA is then loaded on an Illumina Flow Cell for cluster generation and sequenced according to the manufacturer's instructions. For miRNA sequencing, 36-cycle, single-end read sequencing is appropriate—following the manufacturer's protocols for the DGE-Small RNA Cluster Generation Kit and 36 Cycle Solexa (Illumina) Sequencing Kit.

3.2 Analysis Using miRDeep2

1. Collect sequencing data and ensure that it is in a format that is compatible with miRDeep2 [9]. Typically, sequencing data from Illumina will be in fastq format, which is compatible with miRDeep2. However, if necessary (*see* miRDeep2 documentation for information on compatible input formats), convert the sequencing file into an acceptable input format using any number of appropriate tools—one option is the online web server, Galaxy [19].

2. To facilitate sequence alignment, obtain the *C. elegans* genome from Wormbase and build an index of it using Bowtie and the Bowtie-build command included in miRDeep2: bowtie-build cel_genome.fa cel_genome

   This will generate several .ebwt files which miRDeep2 will use.

3. Create a text file, config.txt, containing the filenames of your samples, and a chosen sample ID (three-letter format), with one sample per line, in the general format:

Filename	SamplenameID (3 letter format)
N2_young.fa	N2y
N2_old.fa	N2o
daf2_young.fa	d2y
daf2_old.fa	d2o

4. Collapse deep sequencing reads and map against reference genome by running script "mapper.pl" (part of miRDeep2 package) from command line:

   mapper.pl config.txt -d -k AGCAGTGACGTGTGTGTGT -c -m -i -j -l 17/-p genome_cel -s reads.fa -t reads_vs_genome.arf

   Explanation of parameters:

   config.txt contains list of samples (*see* Subheading 3.3, **step 3**).

   -d tells mapper to use config file for names of input files to process.

   -c specifies that read samples are in fasta format.

   -m collapses the reads.

   -k trims the 3′ adapter sequence.

   -i converts rna to dna.

   -j removes any sequence other than ATGC.

   - l 17 removes any sequences shorter than 17 bases.

-p genome_cel specifies the reference genome.

-s reads.fa specifies the filename of the output.

-t prints read mappings to this file (which is used in subsequent steps).

The output of this mapping procedure will be a "reads.fa" file (or whatever was chosen as the output filename) containing all the reads that match the reference genome in collapsed format. The name of each read will contain the samplenameID and a_x index, where x represents the number of identical, collapsed reads found in the sequencing data.

5. To determine differential expression, run the miRDeep2 script "quantifier.pl":

quantifier.pl -p precursor-cel.fa -m mature12-cel.fa -r reads.fa -c config.txt -g 1 -t cel

where -p precusor-cel.fa specifies the file containing known miRNA precursors from mirbase.

-m mature-cel.fa specifies the file containing mature miRNA sequences.

-r reads.fa specifies the input file of deep sequencing reads (generated by mapper.pl).

-c config.txt contains list of samples and sample code (3-letter).

-g 1 allows one mismatch.

-t cel specifies the reference genome (3-letter species code).

As output, the quantifier.pl script will generate a file named expression.html which is viewable in a browser and contains a summary of the data and links to pdfs that show the miRNA mappings, with pileup of reads, read counts, frequency diagrams, and signature and secondary structure of the precursor hairpins (Fig. 1). Optional parameters can be used in quantifier.pl to report mismatches, take star sequences into consideration, or alter the mapping parameters to the precursors sequences (*see* **Note 6**). The expression tables generated by quantifier.pl script will include both raw number of reads as well as normalized reads. It is important to consider which normalization method is appropriate to the biological question being studied (*see* **Note 7**) and to ensure that proper biological controls and replicates are integrated into the study design (*see* **Note 8**). The quantifier.pl program will also generate a .csv file with full read counts for all known miRNAs which can be exported to spreadsheet programs and/or to various packages for further statistical analysis (*see* **Note 9**).

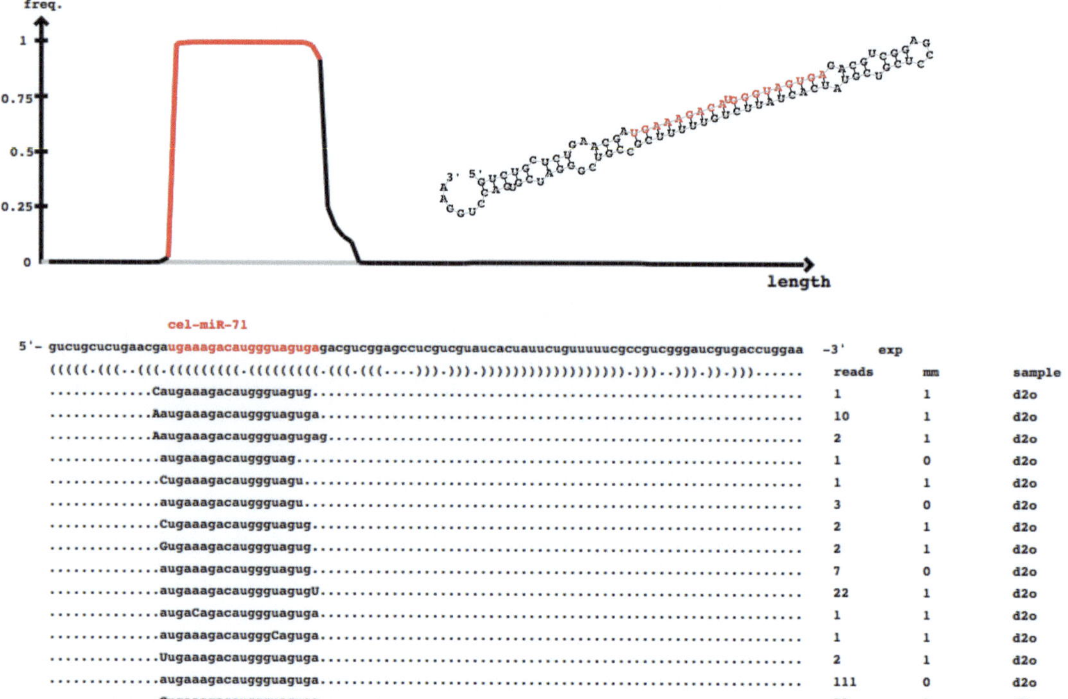


```
5'- gucugcucugaacgaugaaagacauggguagugagacgucggagccucgucguaucacuauucuguuuuucgccgucgggaucgugaccuggaa  -3'    exp
    (((((.(((..(((.((((((((((.((((((((((.(((.(((....))).))).)))))))))))))))))))).))).)))).)).))).......   reads    mm        sample
.............Caugaaagacauggguagug...........................................................................    1        1         d2o
............Aaugaaagacauggguaguga...........................................................................   10        1         d2o
............Aaugaaagacauggguagugag..........................................................................    2        1         d2o
.............augaaagacauggguag..............................................................................    1        0         d2o
............Cugaaagacauggguagu..............................................................................    1        1         d2o
.............augaaagacauggguagu.............................................................................    3        0         d2o
............Cugaaagacauggguagug.............................................................................    2        1         d2o
............Gugaaagacauggguagug.............................................................................    2        1         d2o
.............augaaagacauggguagug............................................................................    7        0         d2o
.............augaaagacauggguagugU...........................................................................   22        1         d2o
............augaCagacauggguaguga............................................................................    1        1         d2o
............augaaagacaugggCaguga............................................................................    1        1         d2o
...........Uugaaagacauggguaguga.............................................................................    2        1         d2o
.............augaaagacauggguaguga...........................................................................  111        0         d2o
............Cugaaagacauggguaguga............................................................................   53        1         d2o
```

Fig. 1 Analysis of deep sequencing reads of known miRNAs using miRDeep2. Frequency diagram, pileup of reads, identification of mismatches (mm), 2° structure of precursor, and mature sequence highlighted in *red*

6. To identify novel miRNAs, use the "miRDeep2.pl" script:

   miRDeep2.pl reads.fa genome_cel.fa reads_vs_genome.arf mature-cel.fa \

   mature-other.fa precursors-cel.fa -t cel -b -2 2>report.log

   where reads.fa and reads_vs_genome.arf represent the files generated by mapper.pl; genome_cel.fa is the reference genome; and mature-cel.fa and precursors-cel.fa are the *C. elegans* mature miRNAs and precursors from miRBase. The file mature-other.fa contains miRNA sequences for other species, with potential overlap or homology with new candidate miRNAs.

   -b minimum cutoff score for predicted novel miRNAs to be displayed in table. Default is 0. Adjust or -1 or -2 to identify more candidates (including more false positives).

   The miRDeep2.pl script will generate various output files, including a table in html format that summarizes the information for the top candidate novel miRNAs identified by the program, including miRDeep score, *p*-values, read counts

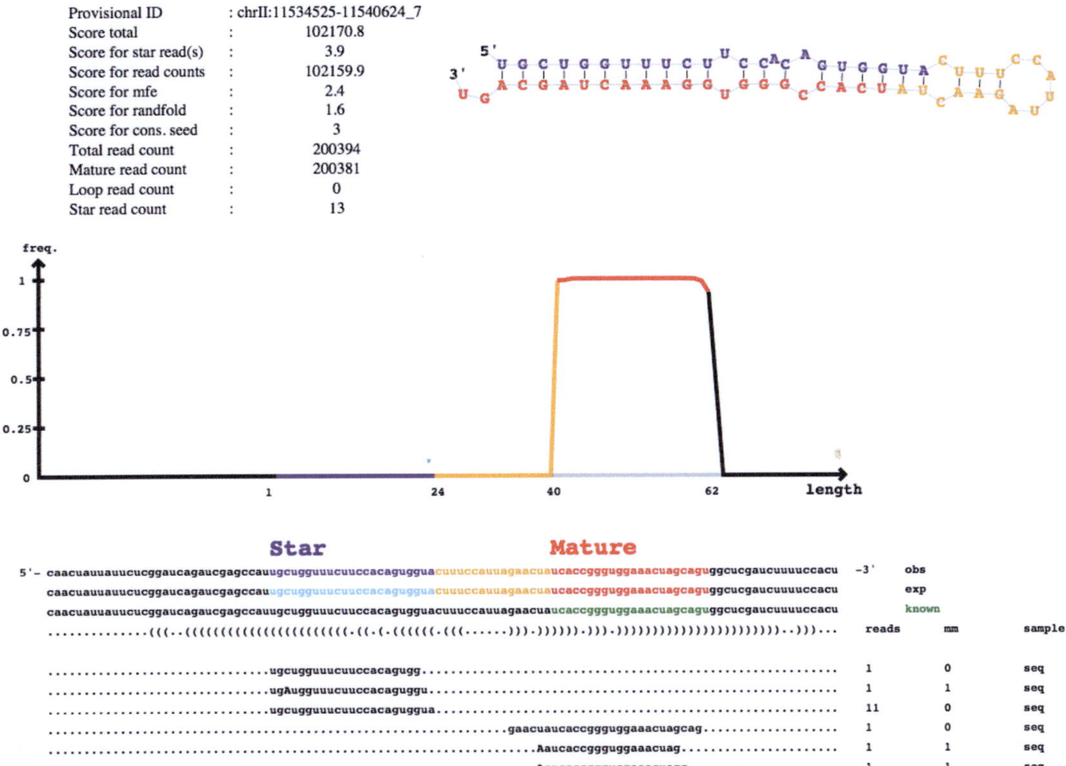

Fig. 2 Identification of novel miRNAs using miRDeep2. Frequency diagram, 2° structure of putative precursor, and identification of potential mature and star sequences from deep sequencing data

(mature, star, and loop regions), homology to other miRNAs, and sequences of predicted mature, star, and precursor hairpins. In addition, there will be links to read pileups, frequency diagrams, and secondary structure diagrams, including predicted mature and star sequences (Fig. 2). The reported miRDeep2 scores and associated information is used to narrow down the top candidate, novel miRNAs that should be further characterized (*see* **Note 10**).

3.3 Validation of miRNA Expression

For validation by qRT-PCR, extract total RNA as described before (Subheading 3.1, **step 4**). To confirm expression changes of known miRNAs during aging, RNA should be obtained from synchronized animals at relevant time-points during adulthood. To validate novel miRNAs, RNA should be obtained from synchronized wild-type N2 animals as well as *alg-1(gk214)* mutants in young adulthood and/or later time points (according to its expression pattern from deep-sequencing) (*see* **Note 11**).

1. Northern analysis of known miRNAs: For confirmation of the expression of known miRNAs, we use ~15–20 µg of total RNA

obtained from animals at different points of adulthood. We design probes using the StarFire Oligonucleotide Labelling Kit (from Integrated DNA Technologies) which are complementary to the mature sequences of miRNAs in question. We use a probe for U6 small nuclear RNA sequence as a normalization control (5′-GCA GGG GCC ATG CTA ATC TTC TCT GTA TT). As an additional control, we utilize a probe for *miR-66* (5′-TCA CAT CCC TAA TCA GTG TCA TG), whose expression remains constant during development [20, 21], during aging or in *daf-2(e1370)* mutants [4] (*see* **Note 12**).

2. Quantitative RT-PCR of novel miRNAs: RNA samples (1–10 μg) are treated with Turbo DNAse according to the manufacturer's protocols (Ambion, Turbo DNAfree kir). The expression of miRNAs is then measured using Taqman small RNA Assays (Applied Biosystems). To validate candidate novel miRNAs, custom Taqman assays are purchased from Applied Biosystems and tested according to the manufacturer's protocols, except that we use a Lightcycler 480 qPCR instrument. We adapted qPCR cycling conditions appropriate for miRNA Taqman detection on LightCycler 480 instruments [22]:Enzyme activation: 95 °C for 10 min; amplification (45 cycles): 95 °C for 15 s (ramp: 4,4 °C/s, analysis mode: quantification), 60 °C for 60 s (ramp: 2,2 °C/s); cooling: 40 °C for 30 s (ramp: 2 °C/s). The detection format was set to "Mono Color Hydrolysis Probe" and the second derivative maximum method was used for absolute quantification. Expression levels are normalized against endogenous control, the small nucleolar RNA (snoRNA), U18 (Taqman). For purpose of validating the expression of these candidate miRNAs, we consider only miRNAs with amplification < 35 cycles and those miRNAs whose expression is reduced in *alg-1(gk214)* mutants (Fig. 3).

3. Quantitative RT-PCR of known miRNAs: For known miR-NAs, in addition to the Taqman method we also use miRScript qRT-PCR (Qiagen). RNA samples (1–10 μg) are treated with Turbo DNase according to the manufacturer's protocols (Ambion, Turbo DNA-free). DNase-free RNA (1 μg) is converted to cDNA as per the manufacturer's protocols (Qiagen), using the "HighFlex" protocol, which allows measurement of the levels of small RNAs and large RNAs simultaneously. PCR cycling conditions are as per the manufacturer's protocols. Typically, we use primers against mRNA genes CDC-42, PMP-3, and Y45F10D.4 for Geometric Means Normalization (*see* **Note 13**).

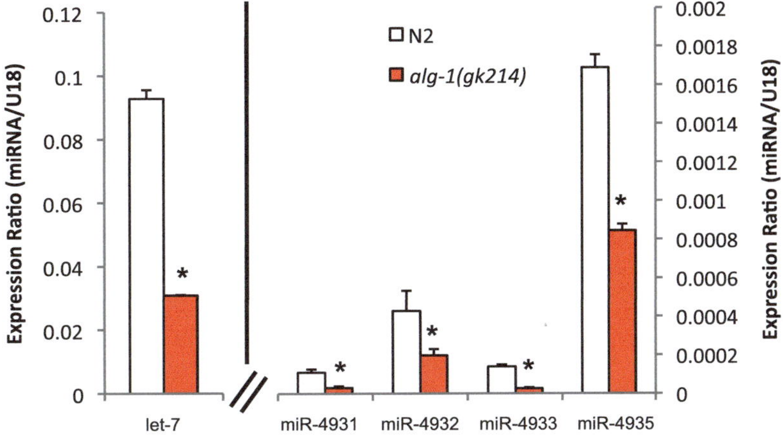

Fig. 3 Validation of expression of novel mi RNAs in aging *C. elegans*. The expression of four candidate miRNAs identified by deep sequencing was confirmed by Taqman qRT-PCR. Consistent with their classification as miRNAs, their expression was significantly reduced in *alg-1*(*gk214*) mutant animals. The expression of known miRNA *let-7* is shown as a positive control (image reproduced from [4] with permission from Elsevier)

4   Notes

1. RNA yields. Total RNA: 8 μg from 25 μl of packed pellet of worms (~300 worms from one small (6 cm) plate). On large plate (16 cm), 2500–3000 worms yielded ~100–150 μl packed worm pellet, which yielded ~40–100 μg of RNA.

2. For maximum yield of eggs, bleach treat a plate enriched for gravid adults. During bleach treatment, vortex tube every ~2 min and observe through microscope. Once gravid adults rupture (body will bend and split), arrest bleach treatment by adding 2 volumes of M9 buffer, spin down, and aspirate supernatant. It is important to then wash bleached worm pellets at least 4–6 times with M9 to remove any residual bleach.

3. Use reagent/conditions that do *not* deplete small RNAs (i.e., use regular TRIzol, not "LS TRIzol"). Make sure to use siliconized, RNase-free tubes throughout to prevent adsorption of RNA to tubing. Glycogen or Glycoblue can be utilized as a carrier to facilitate precipitation and visualization of RNA pellets after precipitation. RNA pellets after precipitations should be air-dried until ethanol is fully evaporated (~5–10 min) but they should not be excessively dried, or the pellet will become difficult to resuspend.

4. Cloning other small RNAs: Piwi-interacting RNAs (piRNAs, i.e., 21U-RNAs) will be also cloned by this procedure. For

cloning of other small RNAs, such as siRNAs, consider alternative protocols [23, 24].

5. Small RNA cloning considerations: To avoid biases in miRNA representation, these are the most important factors to consider during cloning: maintain similar conditions for 3'- and 5'-adapter ligation, use similar concentrations of input RNA for all samples and avoid too many cycles of PCR after RT extensions [25].

6. Additional (optional) parameters in quantifier.pl: Using the -g option to allow mismatches between read and precursor mappings might allow the identification of interesting miRNAs isoforms (such as edited sites). Other possible options to consider are -s star.fa, to compare sequences against a file of star sequences from miRBase. This will allow the determination of mature and star sequences mapping to the precursors. Options -e and -f specify how far upstream (-e, default 2 nucleotides) and downstream (-f, default = 5 nucleotides) of the mature/star sequence the program should consider as a match to the sequencing sequences.

7. As of version 2.0.4 of miRDeep, quantifier.pl normalizes miRNA reads according to total number of miRNAs in each sample. If one suspects that there might be biological reasons for the total numbers of miRNAs to be different in different samples, one might normalize against total number of genome-matching reads. This can be done by recovering the raw miRNA count number from the .csv file generated by quantifier.pl. As an alternative, during RNA preparation one might consider "spiking" the pool with a known amount of one or more known oligonucleotide "calibrator" sequences (that do not match the reference genome) and which can be used as a normalization controls after sequencing [18, 26, 27].

8. Estimation of miRNA abundance: In general, it is not appropriate to compare the abundance of one miRNA versus another within the same sample due to biases inherent to the small RNA cloning procedures, and which depend on the secondary structure and sequence of each miRNA [25]. These biases, however, do not affect the estimation of the relative abundances of each miRNAs between samples [25]. Therefore, with appropriate controls and normalization it is generally possible to determine relative changes in expression of individual miRNAs across different samples.

9. Statistical analysis of differential expression: In order to determine statistical significance of changes in expression of miRNAs read counts determined by miRDeep2, one can export the .csv data into any of a number of tools for differential analysis of deep sequencing data, such as DESeq, DEGseq, edgeR, baySeq, mirZ, and SAMseq [10–15].

10. Analysis and curation of novel miRNA identifications by miRDeep2: The reported miRDeep2 scores and associated information is used to narrow down the top candidate, novel miRNAs that should be further characterized. In particular, we consider characteristics reported by miRDeep2 such as read scores, secondary structure of putative precursor hairpins, and homology with known miRNAs in other species. Manual curation is essential too. Although miRDeep2 attempts to exclude reads that overlap with annotated regions of the genome, it is important to confirm that the latest annotations are consistent with possible miRNA classification. For example, miRNAs should not exist within annotated coding region of an open reading frame (either sense or antisense), and it is unlikely that it would be encoded in $5'$ or $3'$ UTRs of a known gene. Therefore, we manually perform blast analysis of candidate miRNAs against the reference genome to ensure that a candidate miRNA does not overlap with already annotated regions and also to discover possible overlap with annotated small RNAs in other species. Sequences that survive this curation process and exhibit good secondary structures characteristics are then considered for validation by qRT-PCR.

11. Validation of novel miRNA expression: ALG-1 is a miRNA-associated factor and it is known that functional ALG-1 is required for mature miRNA accumulation [28]. Therefore, to confirm that a putative novel miRNA is indeed expressed, we check (a) if it is expressed by qRT-PCR, and (b) if its level is reduced in *alg-1(gk214)* animals. In our experience, we observe a two- to fivefold reduction in bona fide miRNA levels in *alg-1(gk214)* mutants as measured by qRT-PCR.

12. Validation of differential expression of miRNAs obtained by deep sequencing can be accomplished by typical methods of RNA expression analysis, such as Northern analysis or qRT-PCR. However, for miRNAs that are expressed at low levels, especially candidate novel miRNAs, it will be difficult to measure their expression by Northern. Therefore, we typically validate the expression of novel miRNAs using qRT-PCR.

13. Validation of differential expression of known miRNAs: The advantage of quantitative PCR using miScript is that it allows the quantification of small RNAs and large RNAs simultaneously from the same cDNA sample. This permits the use of multiple RNAs as endogenous controls, allowing for better normalization of data. We utilize the genes CDC-42, PMP-3, and Y45F10D.4, and perform geometric means normalization of our qRT-PCR data as recommended [29]. As an additional endogenous control we utilize the small RNA, RNA6B (Qiagen).

Acknowledgement

Some *C. elegans* strains were provided by the CGC, which is funded by NIH Office of Research Infrastructure Programs (P40 OD010440). We thank Dr. Giovanni Stefani and Dr. Masaomi Kato for help with methods. A.d.L. was supported by a National Research Service Award Postdoctoral Fellowship from the National Institutes of Health (NIH; 1F32AG030851). F.J.S. was supported by a Breakthroughs in Gerontology grant from the American Federation for Aging Research, the Ellison Medical Foundation, and the NIH (AG033921).

References

1. Bartel DP (2009) MicroRNAs: target recognition and regulatory functions. Cell 136:215–233

2. Esquela-Kerscher A, Slack FJ (2006) Oncomirs—microRNAs with a role in cancer. Nat Rev Cancer 6:259–269

3. Boehm M, Slack F (2005) A developmental timing microRNA and its target regulate life span in C. elegans. Science 310:1954–1957

4. de Lencastre A et al (2010) MicroRNAs both promote and antagonize longevity in C. elegans. Curr Biol 20:2159–2168

5. Brenner JL, Jasiewicz KL, Fahley AF, Kemp BJ, Abbott AL (2010) Loss of individual microRNAs causes mutant phenotypes in sensitized genetic backgrounds in C. elegans. Curr Biol 20:1321–1325

6. Alvarez-Saavedra E, Horvitz HR (2010) Many families of C. elegans microRNAs are not essential for development or viability. Curr Biol 20:367–373

7. Miska EA et al (2007) Most Caenorhabditis elegans microRNAs are individually not essential for development or viability. PLoS Genet 3, e215

8. Kato M, Chen X, Inukai S, Zhao H, Slack FJ (2011) Age-associated changes in expression of small, noncoding RNAs, including microRNAs, in C. elegans. RNA 17:1804–1820

9. Friedländer MR, Mackowiak SD, Li N, Chen W, Rajewsky N (2012) miRDeep2 accurately identifies known and hundreds of novel microRNA genes in seven animal clades. Nucleic Acids Res 40:37–52

10. Robinson MD, McCarthy DJ, Smyth GK (2010) edgeR: a Bioconductor package for differential expression analysis of digital gene expression data. Bioinformatics 26:139–140

11. Hausser J et al (2009) MirZ: an integrated microRNA expression atlas and target prediction resource. Nucleic Acids Res 37:W266–W272

12. Wang L, Feng Z, Wang X, Wang X, Zhang X (2010) DEGseq: an R package for identifying differentially expressed genes from RNA-seq data. Bioinformatics 26:136–138

13. Anders S, Huber W (2010) Differential expression analysis for sequence count data. Genome Biol 11:R106

14. Li J, Tibshirani R (2013) Finding consistent patterns: a nonparametric approach for identifying differential expression in RNA-Seq data. Stat Methods Med Res 22(5):519–536

15. Hardcastle TJ, Kelly KA (2010) baySeq: empirical Bayesian methods for identifying differential expression in sequence count data. BMC Bioinformatics 11:422

16. Brenner S (1974) The genetics of Caenorhabditis elegans. Genetics 77:71–94

17. Lau NC, Lim LP, Weinstein EG, Bartel DP (2001) An abundant class of tiny RNAs with probable regulatory roles in Caenorhabditis elegans. Science 294:858–862

18. Hafner M et al (2012) Barcoded cDNA library preparation for small RNA profiling by next-generation sequencing. Methods 58:164–170

19. Goecks J, Nekrutenko A, Taylor J, Team G (2010) Galaxy: a comprehensive approach for supporting accessible, reproducible, and transparent computational research in the life sciences. Genome Biol 11:R86

20. Lim LP et al (2003) The microRNAs of Caenorhabditis elegans. Genes Dev 17:991–1008

21. Kato M, de Lencastre A, Pincus Z, Slack FJ (2009) Dynamic expression of small noncoding RNAs, including novel microRNAs and piRNAs/21U-RNAs, during Caenorhabditis elegans development. Genome Biol 10:R54

22. Hofig KP, Feller A, Merz H (2007) New application for the LightCycler 480 system: qPCR-based microRNA-profiling. Biochemica:7–9

23. Pak J, Fire A (2007) Distinct populations of primary and secondary effectors during RNAi in C. elegans. Science 315:241–244

24. Hafner M et al (2008) Identification of microRNAs and other small regulatory RNAs using cDNA library sequencing. Methods 44:3–12

25. Hafner M et al (2011) RNA-ligase-dependent biases in miRNA representation in deep-sequenced small RNA cDNA libraries. RNA 17:1697–1712

26. Fahlgren N et al (2009) Computational and analytical framework for small RNA profiling by high-throughput sequencing. RNA 15:992–1002

27. Farazi TA et al (2011) MicroRNA sequence and expression analysis in breast tumors by deep sequencing. Cancer Res 71:4443–4453

28. Grishok A et al (2001) Genes and mechanisms related to RNA interference regulate expression of the small temporal RNAs that control C. elegans developmental timing. Cell 106:23–34

29. Hoogewijs D, Houthoofd K, Matthijssens F, Vandesompele J, Vanfleteren JR (2008) Selection and validation of a set of reliable reference genes for quantitative sod gene expression analysis in C. elegans. BMC Mol Biol 9:9

Chapter 19

Analysis of DNA Methylation by Pyrosequencing

Colin Delaney*, Sanjay K. Garg*, and Raymond Yung

Abstract

Pyrosequencing is a technique that uses a sequencing-by-synthesis system which is designed to quantify single-nucleotide polymorphisms (SNPs). Artificial C/T SNP creation via bisulfite modification permits measurement of DNA methylation locally and globally in real time. Alteration in DNA methylation has been implicated in aging, as well as aging-related conditions such as cancer, as well as cardiovascular, neurodegenerative, and autoimmune diseases. Considering its ubiquitous presence in divergent clinical pathologies, quantitative analysis of DNA CpG methylation both globally and at individual genes helps to elucidate the regulation of genes involved in pathophysiological conditions. The ability to detect and quantify the methylation pattern of DNA has the potential to serve as an early detection marker and potential drug target for several diseases. Here, we provide a detailed technical protocol for pyrosequencing supplemented by critical information about assay design and nuances of the system that provides a strong foundation for beginners in the field.

Key words Pyrosequencing technique, DNA CpG methylation, Global methylation, Biomarker detection, SNPs, Bisulfide conversation, Assay design

1   Introduction

Epigenetic changes are heritable alterations in DNA that affect gene expression and function by mechanisms other than those from changes in DNA sequence. While each cell in an organism shares the same genetic material, epigenetic instructions define the expression of a gene that is conserved in mitosis. Epigenetic mechanisms regulate many cellular processes including development, differentiation, embryogenesis, X-chromosome inactivation, chromosomal stability, and genomic imprinting [1–4]. A number of epigenetic processes have been described including histone modification, chromatin remodeling, micro RNAs, and DNA methylation. Epigenetic "drift," particularly T cell DNA demethylation, has been shown to contribute to immune dysfunction in aging. DNA methylation involves addition of a methyl group at the 5th carbon of cytosines preceding

---

*These authors made equal contributions to this work.

Albert C. Shaw (ed.), *Immunosenescence: Methods and Protocols*, Methods in Molecular Biology, vol. 1343,
DOI 10.1007/978-1-4939-2963-4_19, © Springer Science+Business Media New York 2015

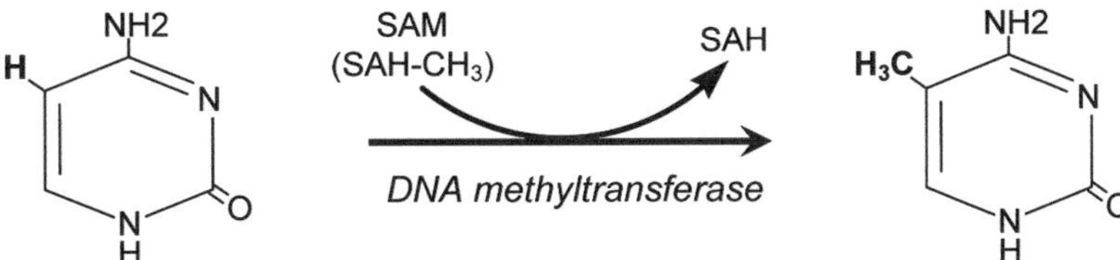

Fig. 1 Methylation of cytosine to 5-methylcytosine. Cytosine preceding guanine (CpG sites) is methylated on carbon 5 (shown in *bold*) in the presence of DNA methyltransferase and SAM. *SAM* S-adenosyl methionine, *SAH* S-adenosyl homocysteine

guanines (CpG dinucleotides), a modification catalyzed by DNA methyltransferases (DNMTs). S-adenosylmethionine (SAM), an intermediate product of methionine metabolism, acts as a methyl donor in the process (Fig. 1). DNA methylation has also been implicated in aging-associated diseases including cancer as well as neurodegenerative and cardiovascular disease and autoimmune syndromes such as lupus and rheumatoid arthritis (RA) [1, 5–7]. Therefore, it may be possible to use DNA methylation as a biomarker for disease risk [1, 8–12]. Among several established methods for measuring DNA methylation including HPLC, methylation-sensitive PCR, bisulfite sequencing, and next-generation sequencing, pyrosequencing offers a robust, versatile platform yielding rapid quantitative results without the onerous time commitment, high costs, and technical difficulty of alternative methods.

1.1 Principle of Pyrosequencing

Pyrosequencing uses a high-throughput platform that can interrogate many CpG sites within an amplicon in real time. The pyrosequencing platform is designed to detect single-nucleotide polymorphisms, or SNPs, which can be artificially created at CpG sites through bisulfite modification. Treating genomic DNA with sodium bisulfite selectively converts cytosine to uracil; however, 5-methylcytosine is protected from deamination and the CG sequence is preserved in downstream reactions (Fig. 2). The technology is distinct from Sanger sequencing, in which labeled dideoxynucleotides are incorporated randomly in the reaction terminating extension of strands representative of each nucleotide position; rather, pyrosequencing uses a sequencing-by-synthesis system in which nucleotides are dispensed one at a time, incorporated into the extending strand and degraded prior to the next nucleotide dispensation (Fig. 3).

1.2 The Pyrosequencing Enzyme Cascade

Pyrosequencing requires a single-stranded PCR amplicon that serves as DNA template, four different enzymes including DNA polymerase, ATP sulfurylase, luciferase, and apyrase, and two different substrates including adenosine 5′ phosphosulfate (APS) and luciferin [13]. First, a sequencing primer is annealed to a single-stranded DNA (ssDNA) template. Upon addition of a single

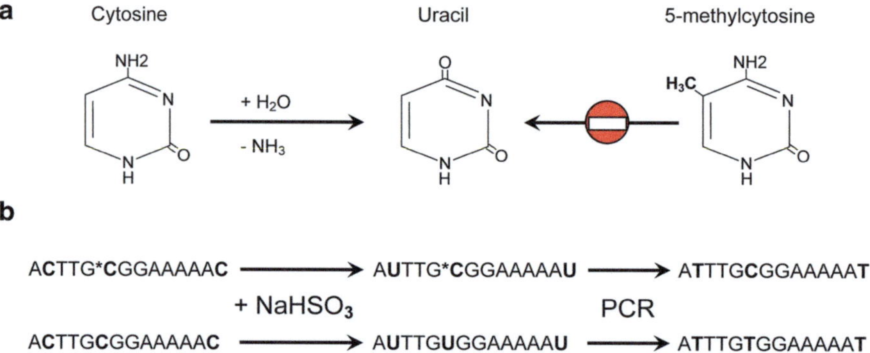

Fig. 2 Deamination of cytosine via sodium bisulfide conversion. (**a**) Deamination of cytosine to uracil is prevented by methylation of the 5-carbon position of cytosine. (**b**) Methylated (*above*) and unmethylated (*below*) CpG-containing DNA undergoes bisulfite conversion. Methylated cytosines are unchanged while unmethylated cytosines are converted to uracil. Following PCR the cytosine is retained while uracil is converted to thymine. *C denotes methylated cytosine. Pyrimidines involved in bisulfite conversion are bolded. *NaHSO3* sodium bisulfite, *PCR* polymerase chain reaction

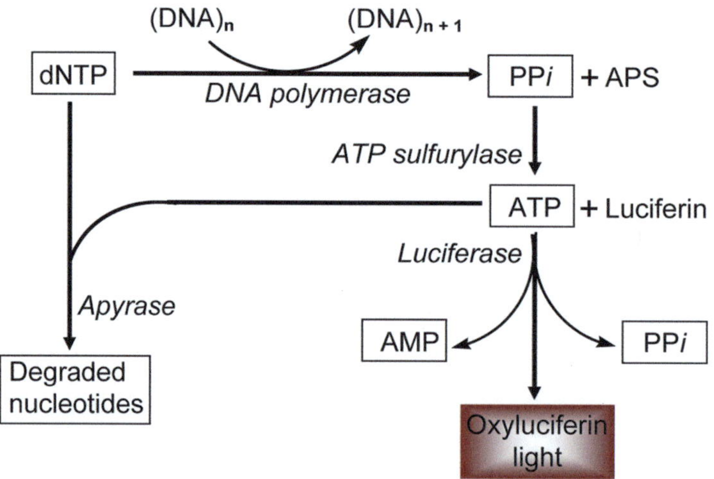

Fig. 3 Enzyme cascade system in pyrosequencing. An ssDNA template is first hybridized with the sequencing primer and mixed with enzymes (written in *italics*) and two substrates (APS and luciferin). After successful incorporation of a nucleotide by DNA polymerase into a growing DNA strands, the released PP*i* reacts with APS in the presence of ATP sulfurylase giving rise to ATP. ATP in the presence of substrate luciferin and enzyme luciferase produces oxyluciferin that generates visible light, which can be detected by inbuilt CCD camera. Any unincorporated nucleotides and ATP are degraded into its building blocks by enzyme apyrase prior to the next nucleotide dispensation. Cascade reactions repeat for every dispensation. *ATP* adenosine triphosphate, *APS* Adenosine 5′ phosphosulfate, *PPi* pyrophosphate

nucleotide, the DNA polymerase incorporates the dNTP into the growing strand, releasing pyrophosphate (PPi). ATP sulfurylase then generates ATP from the PPi and substrate APS, which activates luciferase-mediated conversion of luciferin to the light-emitting oxyluciferin. Light is given off proportionate to the amount of nucleotide added to the elongating strand and recorded by an inbuilt CCD camera. Excess nucleotide is degraded by apyrase, after which the next nucleotide is dispensed. Comparing the peak light emission of incorporation of C or T at a CpG site within the amplicon gives a precise measure of the amount of methylation at that position within the sample.

1.3 Technical Overview of Pyrosequencing

Genomic DNA is bisulfite converted, and then the region of interest is amplified via PCR. Incorporation of a single biotinylated PCR primer allows separation of the two strands of the amplicon to create a ssDNA template for annealing of a pyrosequencing primer and extension of the complementary strand by discrete dispensation of nucleotides. This platform is PCR-based, yields rapid results (i.e., within a single day if starting with PCR), and is highly quantitative. Many different assays can be performed simultaneously (i.e., in a 96-well format, 96 different assays could be performed on one sample, 96 samples could be analyzed with one assay, or anything in between) and the time required is entirely dependent on the number of dispensations needed to cover the region of interest (approximately 5 min + 1 min/dispensation). In addition, pyrosequencing technology can be used to interrogate regulatory elements of specific genes [12, 14–16] or as a means of estimating global methylation [17–19]. However, pyrosequencing assays can be more difficult to design and extensive optimization of these assays is required (*see* Subheading 4). Also, an emerging pitfall of the system is that Bisulfite modification cannot discriminate between 5-methylcytosine and the novel modification 5-hydroxymethylcytosine. Nevertheless, pyrosequencing is a validated means of estimating both global methylation and specific regulatory loci in mammalian samples (*see* **Note 6**).

---

2 Materials

2.1 Consumables

Bisulfite conversion kit (available from multiple suppliers).

PyroPCR kit (Qiagen) or any reliable PCR kit.

96-Well skirted PCR plate, PCR plate stickers.

Agarose.

Ethidium bromide.

Streptavidin Sepharose High Performance beads (GE Healthcare).

PyroMark Gold Q96 Reagent Kit (Qiagen) contains enzymes, substrates, and dNTPs for pyrosequencing reaction.

PyroMark Q96 HS Reagent Dispensing Tip (Qiagen).

PyroMark Q96 HS Nucleotide Tip (Qiagen)—for longer sequencing reads >50 dispensations.

PyroMark Q96 HS Capillary Tip (Qiagen)—for short reads <50 dispensations.

PyroMark Q96 HS Plate (Qiagen).

gDNA of interest.

Control low-methylated gDNA.

Control high-methylated gDNA.

Sss1 methylase (NEB).

5-Azacytidine (Sigma).

PCR primers, one biotinylated and HPLC purified: 100 µM stock in water or TE. Store at –20 °C.

Pyrosequencing primer(s): 0.5 µM in annealing buffer. Store at 4 °C.

2.2 Equipment

PCR machine.

Agarose gel electrophoresis cell, power supply, UV imaging system.

Vacuum Prep work station.

96-Well plate heating block (*not* a PCR machine).

PyroMark MD pyrosequencer or equivalent.

2.3 Buffers

1× TAE: 40 mM Tris–Acetate, 1 mM EDTA, pH 8.

70 % EtOH.

Binding buffer: 10 mM Tris–HCl, 2 M NaCl, 1 mM EDTA, 0.1 % Tween 20, pH 7.6. Store at 4 °C.

Annealing buffer: 20 mM Tris–Acetate, 2 mM $MgAc_2$. Store at 4 °C.

Denaturation buffer: 0.2 N NaOH. Store at RT.

1× wash buffer: 10 mM Tris–acetate pH 7.6. Store at RT.

ddH_2O.

3 Methods

3.1 Generating PCR Amplicon for Pyrosequencing

1. Isolate genomic DNA of interest.

2. Bisulfite modification of DNA of interest: Treating genomic DNA with sodium bisulfite selectively converts cytosine to uracil; however, 5-methylcytosine is protected from deamination and the CG sequence is preserved in downstream reactions (Fig. 2). Many commercial bisulfite modification kits are available for purchase. Follow the manufacturer's instructions. Use 250–1000 ng per conversion reaction and elute with 10–40 µL as appropriate.

3. PCR region of interest (i.e., regulatory element/promoter/enhancer/etc.): Use primers designed specifically to bisulfite-modified DNA. Use 25–100 ng DNA per reaction, 0.1 µM

biotinylated, and 0.2 μM non-biotinylated PCR primers. Designing primers for bisulfite-converted DNA may be more difficult than unmodified DNA because the loss of cytosine increases the degeneracy of the DNA and increases the likelihood of mispriming (*see* **Note 1**).

4. Agarose gel verification of amplicon. Verify that you have a single, strong band and no unincorporated primers. A robust amplicon with no primer dimer is critical for success (*see* **Note 2**).

3.2 Isolation of Biotinylated ssDNA from PCR Amplicon for Pyrosequencing Template

1. Add 14 μL of 0.5 μM pyrosequencing primer in annealing buffer into each appropriate well of a pyrosequencing plate (white, with clear bottoms).

2. Isolate single-stranded pyrosequencing template.

   (a) In a skirted 96-well PCR plate mix together DNA + H_2O to a volume of 40 μL (amplicon DNA usually 5–10 μL per well).

   (b) In a tube combine 40 μL binding buffer and 2 μL streptavidin beads per well (e.g., 10 wells = 400 μL binding buffer + 20 μL beads). For 96-well plate (4 mL + 200 μL beads). Vortex.

   (c) Add 40 μL of the WELL-MIXED binding buffer/bead suspension to each well containing 40 μL of DNA/H_2O in PCR plate.

   (d) Cover plate with plastic PCR sticker to prevent spilling. Shake plate at RT at 1400 rpm for a minimum of 10 min to allow streptavidin beads to bind biotin-labeled strand.

3. While plate is shaking, prepare vacuum prep station (Fig. 4).

   (a) Add ~200 mL of water, 70 % ethanol, denaturation buffer, and 1× wash buffer to the appropriate plastic trays.

   (b) To activate the vacuum, turn on the vacuum pump, and then turn on the switch on the vacuum station.

   (c) Pass water through the filter probe vacuum system to prepare the probes for separation.

   (d) In a 96-well plate, add water in each of the wells that correspond to the same position as your test samples to make sure that the appropriate probes have good suction. A well-functioning probe will clear a full well in about 10 s. If probe fails to suck out water, it is likely blocked by salt buildup and should be replaced. Note the color of the filter tip can be indicative of function. Brighter white tips are usually newer and functional, while duller tips tend to be older and less functional.

4. After vacuum prep station is ready and at least 10 min of shaking has elapsed, stop the shaker. Immediately upon removing the

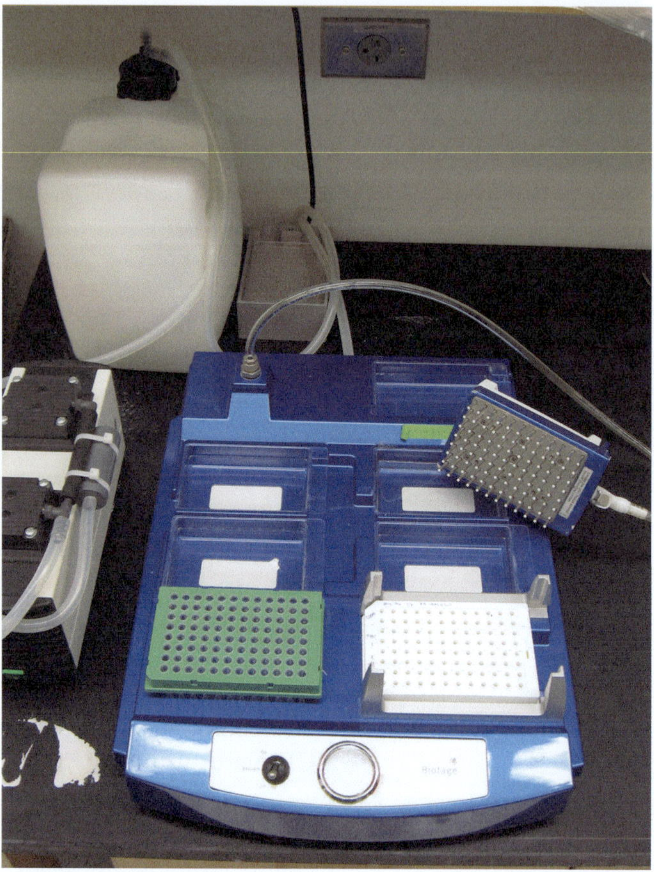

Fig. 4 A representative picture of vacuum prep station showing four different trays, probe connected to vacuum system, and appropriate places for the 96-well plates

plate from the shaker, place the probes into the plate and watch to make sure all fluid is sucked out of the wells. Delay will give beads time to settle out of solution, which will lower your recovery of amplicon.

5. Transfer probes to the tray containing 70 % EtOH. Once fluid is observed passing through the vacuum hose, count to 10 s to wash away residual salts and unlabeled DNA.

6. Transfer probes to the tray containing denaturation buffer and count to 10 as above. Amplicons are denatured and the unlabeled DNA strands are removed from the sample, leaving a ssDNA pyrosequencing template strand.

7. Transfer probes to the tray containing 1× wash buffer and count to 10 to let the fluid drain through. The base in the previous step is neutralized, allowing the pyrosequencing reaction to proceed at proper conditions.

8. Position probes directly above the pyrosequencing plate that has been seated in the appropriate orientation on the vacuum prep station. Do *not* drop probes into the pyrosequencing plate until the vacuum is disengaged lest the annealing primer/buffer be suctioned out of the well. Turn off the vacuum and as soon as pressure gauge has dropped to zero, lower the probes into the pyrosequencing plate. Vigorously agitate the probes to facilitate beads dropping from the filters into the annealing buffer and pyrosequencing primer.

9. Remove the filter probes and place them in the waste water. Shake as above to remove any excess beads/salts, and then pass another 200 mL water through probes to rinse away salts. Store the filter probes dry in an empty 96 tip rack.

3.3 Denaturation and Annealing of Sequencing Primer

1. Place pyrosequencing plate on a heating block pre-heated to 90 °C for 2 min. This eliminates any secondary structure in the single-stranded template that may interfere with primer annealing or enzymatic addition of nucleotides.

2. Remove plate from heat and let cool to RT. (Optional) Turn off heater, but leave pyrosequencing plate on the block for 10 min. This step may facilitate sequencing primer binding by allowing a slower cooldown.

3.4 Preparing the Pyrosequencer

Note that these steps can and should be performed when time permits in the above protocol to eliminate unwanted lag between preparation of the sample and running the pyrosequencing reaction. It is advisable to input the assay into the software prior to strand separation.

1. Create a new assay within a folder in the CpG assay folder by right-clicking the folder and selecting New Assay. Enter the sequence to analyze in the appropriate field and click "Generate Dispensation Order." A theoretical program is displayed (*see* **Note 3**).

2. Turn on machine. It will take about 2 min to warm up and establish communication with the computer. Wait for the info light to begin blinking as an indicator of successful data exchange.

3. Open PyroCpG software.

4. Under the CpG run folder, select the appropriate subfolder (if applicable), right-click, and select "New Run." Name the run.

5. Enter the relevant information (sample ID, assay, notes about experiment, and type of dispensing tips used) into the PyroCpG software for each well you are using for this run. Save often to prevent data loss if software crashes before run commences.

6. Once all wells and assays are entered, select Volume Information from the drop down Tools menu. Note the amount of enzyme, substrate, and nucleotides to add to the appropriate dispensing

tips. Enzyme and substrate always go in black RDTs, while nucleotides in CDTs or NDTs. Tips may be reused several times, so label each tip with its contents (*see* **Note 4**).

7. Add enzyme, substrate, and nucleotides to their respective dispensing tips, and place those tips in the correct slot of the appropriate tip holder. *See* diagram for proper placement.

8. Place tip holder in upper chamber of pyrosequencer manually, with enzyme and substrate tips toward the back of the machine.

9. Using the software, click "Open Process Chamber Lid" either from the shortcut icon or from the Instrument drop-down menu.

10. Cover a new pyrosequencing plate with clear plastic PCR sticker to use to test the dispensation tips. This plate can be reused ad infinitum if consistently maintained.

11. Place plate inside the lower chamber with the notch in the upper left corner. Click "Close Process Chamber Lid" command either from the shortcut icon or from the Instrument drop-down menu.

12. Test the dispensing tips by clicking "Test dispensing tips" icon or from the Instrument drop-down menu. Make sure that your stickered test plate is in position or the dispensations will damage the camera. Each tip will dispense a small volume of fluid, which will be visible on top of the sticker, validating that the tips are functional. Do *not* click "Done" after the dispensation test finishes until the hissing stops or the software may crash!

13. If all six drops are visible on the film, proceed with pyrosequencing. If one or more drops are absent, check to see if there are bubbles in the tips by flicking them gently. Residual salts from repeated use eventually will clog the tips. If tips are blocked, discard and use a new tip. It is recommended to test the dispensation tips twice, once the tips are ready and immediately prior to starting the run, ensuring the tips have not clogged in the interim.

3.5 Run the Pyrosequencing Reaction

1. Once the plate has cooled to RT, open the process chamber door using the software, insert the plate in the correct orientation, and close the process chamber lid using the software.

2. Click "Run." The length of the run is determined only by the number of dispensations in the longest assay selected and is not dependent on the number of wells used.

3.6 Cleanup

1. Immediately after all runs are finished, clean out dispensing tips to prevent salt buildup and tip blockage. RDTs and CDTs can be "milked"; that is, rinse and fill them with water, and then apply pressure to squeeze water in a stream through the tip. NEVER milk NDTs as the bore size of the tip is too small; rather, gently

rinse the tip inside and out with water. Store tips upright in a 5 mL tube rack and avoid contact with the delicate tips, which are easily bent/damaged.

2. Rinse out plastic trays from the vacuum prep station and allow to dry.

3.7 Data Analysis While the pyrosequencer is running, the light trace for each well detected by the camera is presented in real time, generating a pyrogram of peaks, the height of which indicate the stoichiometric incorporation of nucleotides. Each non CpG peak becomes a reference peak that the software uses to calculate the percent methylation of the sample (Fig. 5). However, quantitative analysis cannot be performed until the run is finished.

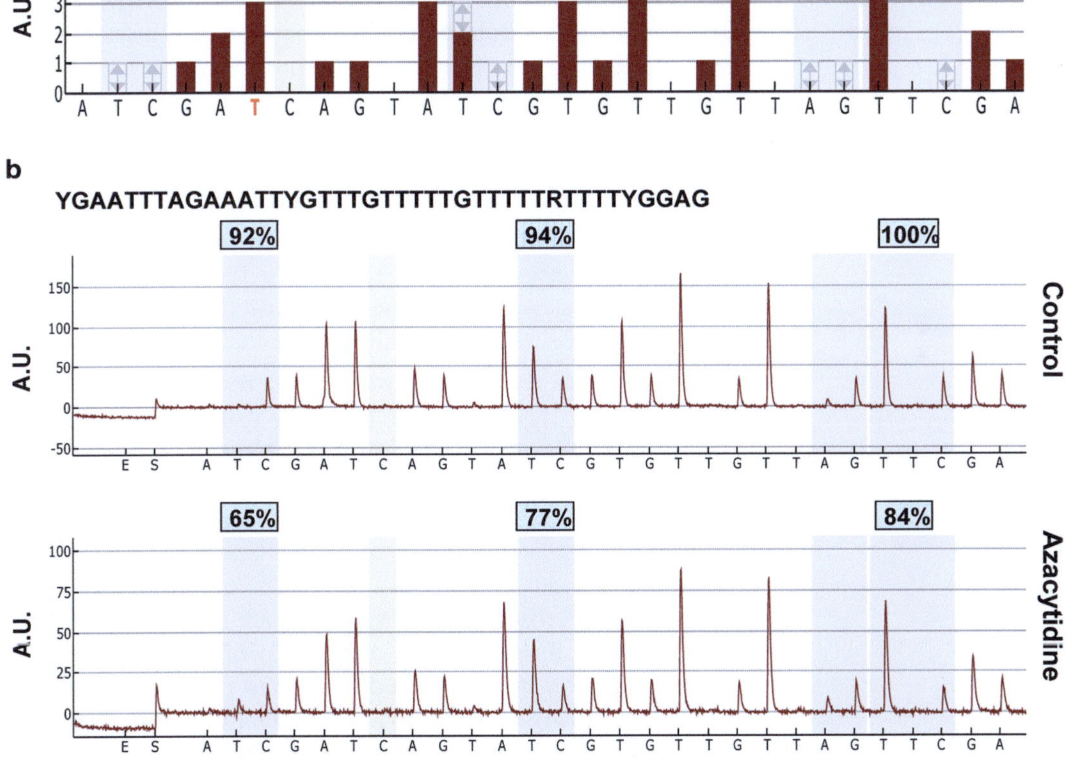

Fig. 5 Representative pyrograms showing hypomethylation of the B1 element following 5-azacytidine treatment. (**a**) Theoretical pyrogram generated by analytical software based on the input sequence to analyze for B1 element pyrosequencing primer 2 (*see* Table 1). (**b**) Pyrograms of DNA isolated from T cells cultured in the absence (*control*) or presence of cytosine analog 5-azacytidine, a known hypomethylating agent. The B1 "sequence to analyze 2" is shown *bolded. Grey shaded* areas indicate CpG sites, *tan shaded bars* indicate bisulfite control dispensations. Percent methylation is indicated above each CpG site

1. Once the run is completed, the 96-well plate map is displayed. Click wells of interest to see the pyrogram.

2. Click "Analyze all" found in the lower right corner of the display. The software will measure the percent methylation at each CpG site and perform quality control analysis of each run. Quality control consists of using the non-CpG dispensations as reference peaks and measuring how well they conform to the theoretical pyrogram generated from the original sequence to analyze input into the assay file. Tolerances are typically set by the manufacturer. CpG sites that pass quality control are indicated in blue, sites that are questionable due to deviation from expected peak heights are yellow, and sites that fail are marked red. It is common to observe different indicated results within the same run and even within the same well at different CpG sites.

   To facilitate data analysis, right click on the pyrogram and select "Show Histogram," which underlays the theoretical pyrogram beneath the real result. Also, "Show Reference Peaks" allows elimination of problematic peaks from contributing to quality control analysis; for example, a long run of nucleotide (>5) may not reach the theoretical peak height due to limitations of detection.

3. Once the run is analyzed, export the raw data to a .txt file by selecting Reports → Analysis Results → Save. The exported file may be opened in spreadsheet format (semicolon delimited) for further analysis, and includes percent methylation of each CpG site, whether that site received a Pass/Check/Fail and any applicable warnings, the mean methylation across the entire sequence to analyze and various statistics.

4. To ensure that the assay is not biased toward methylated or unmethylated DNA, validate the assay using a standard curve of DNA with known methylation (*see* **Note 5**).

4 Notes

1. *Assay design*: Pyrosequencing assays require three steps—bisulfite conversion of unmethylated cytosine to uracil, PCR to generate an amplicon biotin-labeled on one of the two strands, and a pyrosequencing reaction to analyze the nucleotide content of the amplified fragment. Following amplification, the PCR product is purified and denatured, at which time the unlabeled strand is removed to allow the pyrosequencing primer to anneal efficiently to the single-strand template. Typically, assays require at least three primers, a forward and reverse PCR primer as well as a pyrosequencing primer. One and only one of the PCR primers must be biotinylated so that the

single-stranded template can be isolated prior to the pyrosequencing reaction, and the pyrosequencing primer must be complementary to the biotin-labeled strand (i.e., if reverse PCR primer is labeled, the pyrosequencing primer would be oriented in the "forward" direction, and vice versa). Alternatively, it is more economical and feasible to perform a three-primer PCR incorporating a universal biotinylated primer [20]. Also, to interrogate distant CpG sites on the amplicon (greater than ~60 dispensations), multiple pyrosequencing primers may be raised against a single amplicon. There are several software options available to assist in designing pyrosequencing assays as well as companies willing to design and validate custom assays.

2. *Successful PCR conditions*: In order to efficiently capture the biotinylated strand from the amplicon, all biotinylated primer must be incorporated into the PCR product. Unincorporated biotinylated primer will compete with the amplicon during the ssDNA isolation step prior to the pyrosequencing reaction and interfere with the quantification of C/T ratios during the reaction. Therefore, it is common to increase cycles in the PCR step to 45 or greater and use lower concentration of labeled primer to unlabeled primer (e.g., 0.1 µM biotin-primer vs. 0.2 µM unlabeled primer). Increasing the cycles also increases the risk of amplification of unwanted DNA from the environment and care should be taken to minimize exposure to sources of contamination.

3. Understanding and creating proper pyrosequencing assay files: In many ways "pyrosequencing" is an unfortunate term because it leads to confusion in scientists familiar with Sanger sequencing. In contrast to Sanger method, pyrosequencing uses sequencing by synthesis of an already known DNA sequence that contains a SNP at a known position. A proper pyrosequencing run requires entering this "sequence to analyze" into the operating software and indicating in that sequence where the CpG sites are. For CpG methylation detection, inputting the bisulfite converted sequence is necessary. Typically, indicating the cytosines of CpG sites with either a "Y" (for pyrimidine) or "C/T" is understood by the software. For example, a possible bisulfite-converted sequence to analyze could be ATTTGYGGAAAAAT, derived from the gDNA sequence ACTTGCGGAAAAAC (Fig. 2). Note that if a biotinylated forward primer is used, the pyrosequencing primer is in the reverse orientation and the reverse complement sequence must be input (e.g., in the case of the above sequence, the appropriate sequence to analyze would be ATTTTTCCRCAAAT, where the "R" stands for purine or "A/G"). From the sequence to analyze, the software generates a "dispensation order" that takes

into account the order of nucleotides in the sequence to analyze, the length of runs of a single nucleotide, and controls to verify successful bisulfite conversion and integrity of nucleotides. For example, the sequence to analyze ATTTGYGGAAAAAT may generate a dispensation order GATCGCTGAAT. The first G is a negative control, followed by A producing a single-base peak, the run of 3 T's can be measured with a single dispensation of T nucleotide, the first C is a negative control that verifies complete bisulfite conversion, the G is a single-nucleotide peak, the C followed by T is quantifying the CpG site of interest, the next G produces a double-nucleotide peak, and the two A dispensations ensure that the long run of A nucleotide is completely filled in. Incomplete synthesis interferes with downstream nucleotide incorporation, making data analysis difficult or impossible.

Because nucleotide droplets are being added sequentially, as the number of dispensations increases the volume of the reaction increases accordingly. This volume effect dilutes the enzyme and substrate reagents, lowering the signal to noise ratio over time. It follows that there is a finite amount of dispensations per run that will produce usable data. Often data generated after 90–100 dispensations is not usable. It is advisable to use multiple sequencing primers in separate wells to cover a large amplicon rather than attempt to analyze a large region with one reaction.

4. *Dispensing tip selection*: Enzymes and substrates are always dispensed from Reagent Dispensing Tips (RDTs). However, there are different options for dispensing nucleotides, capillary dispensing tips (CDTs) and nucleotide dispensing tips (NDTs). CDTs are easier to maintain and as such may be better for beginners; however, they dispense a larger volume droplet and as such are not suited for longer dispensations >50. NDTs are ideal for longer runs and may produce cleaner results because they dispense smaller droplets, yet they are easier to clog and are harder to clean and maintain.

5. *Bias testing of pyrosequencing assays*: Once an assay is initially optimized to produce a robust amplicon and a clean pyrogram, it is important to validate that the efficiency of the PCR reaction is not altered by differing cytosine content at the CpG sites contained within the region amplified. Differences in efficiencies may skew results, potentially masking or overestimating differences between treatment groups. To check for PCR bias, perform the pyrosequencing assay with amplicons generated from DNA with known methylation content. Start with DNA from low methylated sources—whole genome amplified or cloned plasmid DNA. Treat that DNA with Sss1 methylase enzymes. Alternatively, low-methyl DNA and high-methyl

Table 1
Primers and reaction conditions for the analyses of LINE1 (human) and B1 (mouse) elements

Line 1 (Human)
PCR primer (F): TTTTGAGTTAGGTGTGTGGGATATA   Pyrosequencing primer (F):
PCR primer (R): biotin-AAAATCAAAAAATTCCCTTTC   AGTTAGGTGTGGGATATAGT
Reaction conditions: 95 °C for 5 min; (95 °C 30 s, 50 °C 30 s, 72 °C 30 s)×45 cycles; 72 °C for 5 min
Sequence to analyze: TTYGTGGTGYGTYGTTTTTTAAGTYGGTTTGAAAAGYGTA

B1 element (Mouse)
PCR primer (F): TGGTGGTGGTGGTTGAGAT   Pyrosequencing primer 1 (F):
                                                                                                     TGGTGGTGGTTGAGAT
PCR primer (R):   Pyrosequencing primer 1 (R):
   biotin-AATAACACACACCTTTAATCCCAA   TTTGTAGATTAGGTTGGTTT
Reaction conditions: 95 °C for 15 min; (95 °C 30 s, 63 °C 30 s, 72 °C 30 s)×45 cycles; 72 °C for
   10 min
Sequence to analyze 1: AGYGTTTTTTTGTGTAGTTTTGGTTATTTTGGAATTTATTTTGTAGA
   TTAGGTTGGTTTYGAATTT
Sequence to analyze 2: YGAATTTAGAAATTYGTTTGTTTTTGTTTTTRTTTTYGGAG

DNA are available commercially. Mix these two DNA samples in known ratios to create a standard curve. If the results diverge from linearity, the assay may be biased and must be re-optimized.

6. *Application: global methylation measurement:* Global methylation analysis using pyrosequencing technology utilizes the ubiquity of specific repetitive elements randomly inserted throughout mammalian genomes. Often these elements number in the thousands. In humans, LINE1 and Alu elements have been shown to be useful in measuring changes in global methylation due to cancer, aging, and environmental stressors [17, 21–24]. In mice, the B1 element as well as the intracisternal alpha particle (IAP) can detect changes in methylation in cancer and/or cells treated with hypomethylating agents like the cytosine analog 5-azacytidine [18, 19]. *See* Table 1 for the primer sets and conditions reported to amplify these elements as an estimate of global methylation.

5   Conclusion

Pyrosequencing provides a rapid, high-throughput means of detecting methylation levels at individual loci or estimating global methylation changes. Commercially available bisulfite conversion kits and straightforward PCR amplification step make this technology accessible at reasonable cost while avoiding onerous technical challenges of next-generation sequencing or the delay and labor inherent in cloning fragments for Sanger sequencing. The pyrosequencing platform has been demonstrated to be a versatile means of quantifying DNA methylation globally and at regulatory elements of methylation sensitive genes addition to its broader uses in SNP analysis, association studies, and mutation screening. Thus, pyrosequencing can help elucidate pathogenic dysregulation of gene expression in methylation sensitive genes and advance the pace of biomedical science. Recent advances have focused on high-throughput whole-genome methylation analyses. However, the sensitivity of these assays has not been compared with pyrosequencing.

Acknowledgement

This work was supported by National Institutes of Health National Institute on Aging (AG020628, AG028268), National Institute of Environmental Health Science (P30 ES017885), University of Michigan (Claude D. Pepper Older American Independence Center, Nathan Shock Center for the Basic Biology of Aging, Rheumatic Disease Clinical Center, Caner Center Microarray Core, Michigan Diabetes and Research Training Center Animal Phenotyping Core), Geriatrics Research, Education and Clinical Care Center (GRECC), and the VA Ann Arbor Healthcare System. The content is solely the responsibility of the authors and does not necessarily represent the official views of the National Institutes of Health.

References

1. Portela A, Esteller M (2010) Epigenetic modifications and human disease. Nat Biotechnol 28:1057–1068

2. Eden A, Gaudet F, Waghmare A et al (2003) Chromosomal instability and tumors promoted by DNA hypomethylation. Science 300:455

3. Vera E, Canela A, Fraga MF et al (2008) Epigenetic regulation of telomeres in human cancer. Oncogene 27:6817–6833

4. Jaenisch R, Bird A (2003) Epigenetic regulation of gene expression: how the genome integrates intrinsic and environmental signals. Nat Genet 33 Suppl:245–254

5. Ballestar E, Esteller M, Richardson BC (2006) The epigenetic face of systemic lupus erythematosus. J Immunol 176:7143–7147

6. Brooks WH, Le Dantec C, Pers JO et al (2010) Epigenetics and autoimmunity. J Autoimmun 34:J207–J219

7. Kim M, Long TI, Arakawa K et al (2010) DNA methylation as a biomarker for cardiovascular disease risk. PLoS One 5, e9692

8. Lund G, Andersson L, Lauria M et al (2004) DNA methylation polymorphisms precede any histological sign of atherosclerosis in mice lacking apolipoprotein E. J Biol Chem 279: 29147–29154

9. Jones PA, Baylin SB (2007) The epigenomics of cancer. Cell 128:683–692

10. Warnecke PM, Bestor TH (2000) Cytosine methylation and human cancer. Curr Opin Oncol 12:68–73

11. Urdinguio RG, Sanchez-Mut JV, Esteller M (2009) Epigenetic mechanisms in neurological diseases: genes, syndromes, and therapies. Lancet Neurol 8:1056–1072

12. Strickland FM, Hewagama A, Lu Q et al (2012) Environmental exposure, estrogen and two X chromosomes are required for disease development in an epigenetic model of lupus. J Autoimmun 38:J135–J143

13. Ronaghi M, Uhlen M, Nyren P (1998) A sequencing method based on real-time pyrophosphate. Science 281:363–365

14. Polansky JK, Kretschmer K, Freyer J et al (2008) DNA methylation controls Foxp3 gene expression. Eur J Immunol 38:1654–1663

15. Floess S, Freyer J, Siewert C et al (2007) Epigenetic control of the foxp3 locus in regulatory T cells. PLoS Biol 5, e38

16. Schoenborn JR, Dorschner MO, Sekimata M et al (2007) Comprehensive epigenetic profiling identifies multiple distal regulatory elements directing transcription of the gene encoding interferon-gamma. Nat Immunol 8:732–742

17. Yang AS, Estecio MR, Doshi K et al (2004) A simple method for estimating global DNA methylation using bisulfite PCR of repetitive DNA elements. Nucleic Acids Res 32, e38

18. Jeong KS, Lee S (2005) Estimating the total mouse DNA methylation according to the B1 repetitive elements. Biochem Biophys Res Commun 335:1211–1216

19. Delaney C, Hoeltzel M, Garg SK et al (2012) Maternal micronutrient supplementation suppresses T cell chemokine receptor expression and function in f1 mice. J Nutr 142:1329–1335

20. Royo JL, Pascual MH, Salinas A et al (2006) Pyrosequencing protocol requiring a unique biotinylated primer. Clin Chem Lab Med 44:435–441

21. Yang AS, Doshi KD, Choi SW et al (2006) DNA methylation changes after 5-aza-2′-deoxycytidine therapy in patients with leukemia. Cancer Res 66:5495–5503

22. Bollati V, Baccarelli A, Hou L et al (2007) Changes in DNA methylation patterns in subjects exposed to low-dose benzene. Cancer Res 67:876–880

23. Bollati V, Schwartz J, Wright R et al (2009) Decline in genomic DNA methylation through aging in a cohort of elderly subjects. Mech Ageing Dev 130:234–239

24. Baccarelli A, Wright RO, Bollati V et al (2009) Rapid DNA methylation changes after exposure to traffic particles. Am J Respir Crit Care Med 179:572–578

Immunosenescence

Albert C. Shaw

Albert C. Shaw (ed.), *Immunosenecence: Methods and Protocols*, Methods in Molecular Biology, vol. 1343,
DOI 10.1007/978-1-4939-2963-4, © Springer Science+Business Media New York 2015

DOI 10.1007/978-1-4939-2963-4_20

The spelling of the book title was incorrect. The correct book title should read:
Immunosenescence

Albert C. Shaw
Section of Infectious Diseases
Department of Internal Medicine
Yale School of Medicine
New Haven, CT, USA
e-mail: albert.shaw@yale.edu

The online version of the original book can be found at
http://dx.doi.org/10.1007/978-1-4939-2963-4

INDEX

Albert C. Shaw (ed.), *Immunosenescence: Methods and Protocols*, Methods in Molecular Biology, vol. 1343,
DOI 10.1007/978-1-4939-2963-4, © Springer Science+Business Media New York 2015

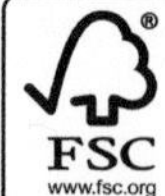